Important
Advances
in Oncology
1992

Edited by

Vincent T. DeVita, Jr., M.D.

Attending Physician and Member
Program of Molecular Pharmacology and
    Therapeutics
Memorial Sloan-Kettering Cancer Center
Benno C. Schmidt Chair in Clinical
    Oncology
Professor of Medicine
Cornell University Medical College
New York, New York

Samuel Hellman, M.D.

Dean and Vice President
Division of the Biological Sciences
Pritzker School of Medicine
University of Chicago
Chicago, Illinois

*Steven A. Rosenberg, M.D., Ph.D.

Chief of Surgery
National Cancer Institute
Professor of Surgery
Uniformed Services University of the Health
    Sciences School of Medicine
Bethesda, Maryland

*This book was co-edited by Dr. Rosenberg in his
private capacity. No official support or endorsement
by the National Institutes of Health is intended or
should be inferred.

With 22 Additional Contributors

Important Advances in Oncology 1992

J. B. Lippincott Company

Philadelphia

New York

London

Hagerstown

Sponsoring Editor: Eileen Wolfberg
Production Supervisor: Robert D. Bartleson
Production: Editorial Services of New England, Inc.
Compositor: Compset, Inc.
Printer/Binder: Arcata Graphics Halliday

6 5 4 3 2 1

LIC 85-64211

ISSN 0883-5896

ISBN 0-397-51157-4

The authors and publisher have exerted every effort to
ensure that drug selection and dosage set forth in
this text are in accord with current recommendations
and practice at the time of publication. However, in
view of ongoing research, changes in government
regulations, and the constant flow of information
relating to drug therapy and drug reactions, the reader
is urged to check the package insert for each drug for
any change in indications and dosage and for added
warnings and precautions. This is particularly
important when the recommended agent is a new or
infrequently employed drug.

Contributors

Thomas C. Chalmers, M.D.
Associate Director
Technology Assessment Group
Harvard School of Public Health
Adjunct Professor of Health
Policy and Management
Harvard School of Public Health
Boston, Massachusetts
Distinguished Physician of the Boston Veterans
    Administration Medical Center
Jamaica Plains, Massachusetts
Dean and President Emeritus
Mt. Sinai Medical Center
New York, New York

Peter D'Arpa, Ph.D.
Postdoctoral Fellow
Department of Biological Chemistry
Johns Hopkins University School of Medicine
Baltimore, Maryland

Vincent T. DeVita, Jr., M.D.
Attending Physician and Member
Program of Molecular Pharmacology and
    Therapeutics
Memorial Sloan-Kettering Cancer Center
Benno C. Schmidt Chair in Clinical Oncology
Professor of Medicine
Cornell University Medical College
New York, New York

Olivera J. Finn, Ph.D.
Associate Professor
Department of Molecular Genetics and
    Biochemistry
University of Pittsburgh School of Medicine
Immunology Program Leader
Pittsburgh, Pennsylvania

Emil Frei III, M.D.
Richard and Susan Smith Professor of Medicine
Harvard Medical School
Physician-in-Chief Emeritus
Chief, Division of Cancer Pharmacology
Dana-Farber Cancer Institute
Boston, Massachusetts

v

Michael L. Grossbard, M.D.
Clinical Fellow in Medicine
Harvard Medical School
Fellow in Medical Oncology
Dana-Farber Cancer Institute
Boston, Massachusetts

Terence S. Herman, M.D.
Associate Professor of Radiation Therapy
Chief, Section of Radiation Therapy
Harvard Medical School
Associate Professor of Radiation Therapy
Chief, Section of Radiation Therapy
Dana-Farber Cancer Institute
Boston, Massachusetts

Waun Ki Hong, M.D.
Professor of Medicine
Chief, Section of Head, Neck and Thoracic
   Medical Oncology
University of Texas
M.D. Anderson Cancer Center
Houston, Texas

Nancy E. Kemeny, M.D.
Associate Attending Physician
Memorial Sloan-Kettering Cancer Center
Associate Professor of Medicine
Cornell University
New York, New York

Joseph M. Khoury, M.D.
Assistant Professor of Urology
Georgetown University Medical Center
Washington, DC

Marc W. Kirschner, Ph.D.
Professor of Biochemistry and Biophysics
School of Medicine
University of California, San Francisco
San Francisco, California

Joseph Lau, M.D.
Assistant Professor of Medicine
Tufts University School of Medicine
Staff Physician
Department of Veteran's Affairs Medical Center
Boston, Massachusetts

Scott M. Lippman, M.D., F.A.C.P.
Assistant Professor of Medicine
Department of Medical Oncology
University of Texas
M.D. Anderson Cancer Center
Houston, Texas

Leroy F. Liu, Ph.D.
Professor, Department of Biological Chemistry
Johns Hopkins University
School of Medicine
Baltimore, Maryland

Dan L. Longo, M.D.
Biological Response Modifiers Program
Division of Cancer Treatment
Frederick Cancer Research and Development
   Center
National Cancer Institute
Frederick, Maryland

Karin B. Michels, M.S.
Department of Epidemiology
Harvard School of Public Health
Harvard University
Boston, Massachusetts

Lee M. Nadler, M.D.
Associate Professor of Medicine
Harvard Medical School
Associate Physician in Medical Technology
Dana-Farber Cancer Institute
Boston, Massachusetts

Jeffrey A. Norton, M.D.
Head, Surgical Metabolism Section
Surgery Branch
National Cancer Institute
National Institutes of Health
Bethesda, Maryland

Michael J. O'Connell, M.D.
Professor
Blanche R. and Richard J. Erlanger Professor of
   Medical Research
Mayo Medical School
Consultant in Medical Oncology
Mayo Clinic
Rochester, Minnesota

Edward H. Oldfield, M.D.
Chief, Surgical Neurology Branch
National Institute of Neurological Disorders and
  Stroke
National Institutes of Health
Bethesda, Maryland

Steven A. Rosenberg, M.D., Ph.D.
Chief of Surgery
National Cancer Institute
Professor of Surgery
Uniformed Services University of Health
  Sciences School of Medicine
Bethesda, Maryland

Thomas H. Shawker, M.D.
Professor of Radiology
Georgetown University School of Medicine
Washington, DC
Chief, Diagnostic Ultrasound
Department of Radiology, Clinical Center
National Institutes of Health
Bethesda, Maryland

Beverly A. Teicher, Ph.D.
Associate Professor of Pathology and Radiation
  Therapy
Harvard Medical School
Associate Professor of Pathology and Radiation
  Therapy
Dana-Farber Cancer Institute
Boston, Massachusetts

James E. Till, Ph.D.
Professor
Institute of Medical Science
University of Toronto
Senior Scientist
Division of Epidemiology and Statistics
Ontario Cancer Institute
Princess Margaret Hospital
Toronto, Ontario, Canada

George D. Webster, M.B., F.R.C.S.
Associate Professor of Urology
Duke University Medical Center
Durham, North Carolina

Preface

Our goal for *Important Advances in Oncology* has been to highlight exciting new areas both in the laboratory and the clinic, even at the risk that what appears to be an advance in one year may turn out not to be an advance in another. Nevertheless, as we look back, it is pleasing to see that the series of texts, now in its eighth year, has tracked what have been substantial advances in cancer research. In fact, certain themes have emerged and have carried over from edition to edition, not out of habit but out of the force of discovery in those fields. For example, the discovery of oncogenes was followed by the description of their function. This edition now explores their influence on the control of the cell cycle as it relates to uncontrolled growth (which is, after all, the essence of cancer itself). Mechanisms of drug resistance, the development of biologics as therapeutics, and the advances in the adjuvant therapy of cancer have also appeared in different garb from edition to edition. This year biologic therapy has advanced to gene therapy and we have focused on a different form of multidrug resistance related to topoisomerase–drug interactions.

The addition of the Controversy section in 1989 grew quite naturally out of the difficulty in drawing the distinction between an obvious important advance and a controversial area. When the editors cannot agree, we let the authors "argue" with each other. In this regard, we have been assisted from time to time by opportune suggestions from readers, which we hope will continue.

VINCENT T. DeVITA, JR., M.D.
SAMUEL HELLMAN, M.D.
STEVEN A. ROSENBERG, M.D., PH.D.

Contents

Part One

Basic Science

Marc W. Kirschner

The Biochemical Nature of the Cell Cycle

1

Transitions in the Cell Cycle and Maturation Promoting Factor ■

The cell cycle can be thought of as being made up of distinct phases which were defined first by morphological and later by biochemical criteria. The concept of phases came from the realization that nuclear division (mitosis) and nuclear replication (DNA synthesis) happened at different times. The cell cycle defined by these primarily nuclear events could then be divided into S-phase, when DNA synthesis occurs, and M-phase, when mitosis occurs. In general cells pause between these events, at stages G1, the gap between M and S, and G2, the gap between S and M (see Fig. 1-1). Differentiated cells often arrest, sometimes permanently, in a state following mitosis but before DNA replication, called G0. Although primacy was given to nuclear events in defining the cell cycle, that cycle could also be defined by the replication of other discrete elements in the cytoplasm, such as the centrosome, or by biochemical requirements to proceed through the cell cycle, such as that part of G1 before the restriction point (a common point of cell cycle arrest due to nutritional or growth factor deprivation) and the part of G1 after the restriction point (Pardee, 1989; Zetterburg and Larson, 1985). Lurking beneath these

morphological events were the expected biochemical regulatory events of the cell cycle. Considerable attention has been devoted to looking for the cyclic appearance of enzymatic activities or translation products that might serve to regulate the various events of the cell cycle. Despite active investigations, the descriptive approach in mammalian cells has been generally disappointing.

Although the direct approach of cataloguing changes in protein synthesis in somatic cells failed to identify important regulators of the mitotic cycle, functional approaches in systems very different from somatic mammalian cells did eventually make the critical contributions to our understanding. Twenty years ago Yoshio Masui and Dennis Smith showed that frog oocytes could be induced to enter meiosis by microinjection of cytoplasm from unfertilized frog eggs that were naturally arrested at meiotic metaphase (see Fig. 1-2) (Masui and Markert, 1971; Smith and Ecker, 1970). Over the years it was demonstrated that cytoplasm from virtually any eukaryotic cell that was in metaphase of either meiosis or mitosis could upon microinjection induce frog oocytes to enter meiosis (Nelkin, *et al,* 1980; Weintraub, *et al,* 1982). The activity in the mitotic cytoplasm was called the maturation-promoting factor (MPF), because the process of meiosis in oocytes was called maturation. Although cumbersome, the frog

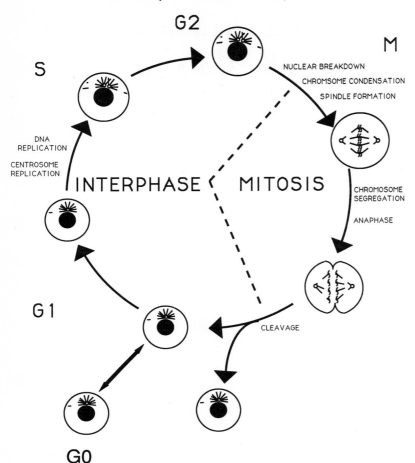

The Eukaryotic Cell Cycle

G2

S

M

NUCLEAR BREAKDOWN
CHROMSOME CONDENSATION
SPINDLE FORMATION

DNA
REPLICATION

CENTROSOME
REPLICATION

INTERPHASE / MITOSIS

CHROMOSOME
SEGREGATION

ANAPHASE

G1

CLEAVAGE

G0

FIG. 1–1 Diagram of a typical somatic cell cycle.

occyte assay allowed the quantitative assay of MPF in the frog cell cycle. MPF activity appeared during prophase and declined at the metaphase-anaphase transition (Gerhart, *et al,* 1984). Injection of MPF activity could cause the cleaving eggs arrested at mitotic interphase to enter mitosis and exit mitosis (Miake-Lye, *et al,* 1983; Newport and Kirschner, 1984). Thus MPF activity was a true oscillating activity that correlated with the morphological events of the mitotic cell cycle. It not only oscillated but possessed the capacity to induce mitotic events in frog eggs. Many of the experimental efforts over the past five years have focused on identifying the composition of MPF, finding out what causes it to oscillate in the cell cycle, and determining how it can control all the disparate reactions of the cell cycle.

The identification of the chemical nature of

MPF came only in part from its biochemical characterization. Paralleling the characterization of the role of MPF in the frog egg was an equally intense attempt to characterize genetically the cell cycle of simple eukaryotic organisms. Normal baker's yeast, *Saccharomyces cerevisiae,* undergoes growth by budding. The size of the bud can be rather simply correlated with the stage of the nuclear cycle. Starting in the early 1970s Lee Hartwell attempted to collect temperature-sensitive mutations in budding yeast that show a uniform point of arrest in the cell cycle, and hence an easily recognizable uniform morphology (see Fig. 1-3) (Hartwell, 1978). Ordinary conditional lethal mutations will eventually arrest anywhere in the cell cycle, but mutations that are inhibited from carrying out specific cell cycle events, such as chromatid separation, would arrest and die at a

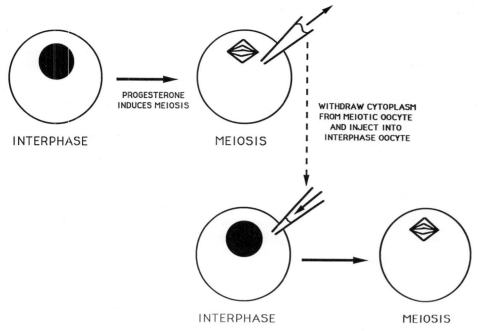

FIG. 1–2 Assay for maturation-promoting factor (MPF). The natural progesterone induced pathway can be circumvented by injection of cytoplasm from oocytes or other cells in either meiotic or mitotic M-phase.

specific point in the cell cycle. As we shall see, it is not at all obvious that specific defects in passing through the mitotic cycle would result in a uniform phenotype of arrest. That this arrest happens is the result of elaborate feedback controls that serve as checks on the successful completion of cell cycle events and halt the process until these events are complete. Specific mutations in cell division cycle or cdc genes could be temporally ordered to give an elaborate pathway with much more experimental detail than the simple morphological cycle. The branching of these pathways indicated that some steps were dependent on the preceding steps while others could proceed through a number of individual steps independently of the other branch. It was expected that important regulatory genes occurred among all the cell cycle genes, although the first few recognized were general housekeeping cell cycle genes such as DNA ligase, or thymidylate synthetase (Pringle and Hartwell, 1981). The general regulatory features that emerged from such studies were that cell cycle control looked like intermediary metabolism with the product of one reaction acting as the substrate of the next. Although this impression was well supported, it was already built into the mode of

isolation, that is, the search for genes that arrested at only a single terminal morphology.

The discovery of the most important of the regulatory genes occurred not directly from budding yeast but from parallel genetic studies in a distantly related yeast, *Schizosaccharomyces pombe*. This yeast has a cell cycle that is more typical of mammalian cells, which increase steadily in mass and then divide by binary fission. A set of cdc genes was identified by Paul Nurse and his colleagues in the United Kingdom (Nurse and Fantes, 1981). One of these genes was particularly interesting since alleles from it could either cause conditional cell cycle arrest or premature entry into mitosis, suggesting that this gene, called cdc2, was not only required for mitosis but was limiting for entry into mitosis. In an outstanding example of conserved function over a billion years of evolution, Nurse's group showed that a human gene carried on a yeast plasmid could complement a temperature-sensitive mutation of the cdc gene (Lee and Nurse, 1987). This led to the identification of the conserved cdc2 genes from many eukaryotic species including the budding yeast, where it had previously been identified.

Obvious parallels existed between the role of

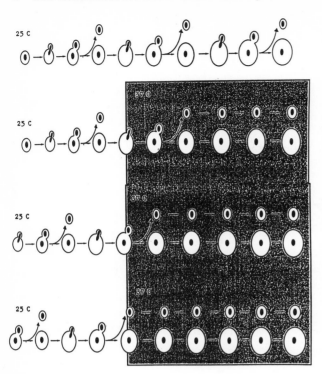

FIG. 1–3 Scheme for identification of temperature-sensitive cell division cycle mutants. No matter what stage the yeast is at the time of the temperature shift, the cells arrest at a specific point, indicated by a uniform morphology.

the cdc2 gene in mitosis in fission yeast and MPF in frogs. Both proteins were required for the entry into mitosis. Both were rate limiting. Both seemed by different criteria to be protein kinases. The actual identification of cdc2 as a component of MPF came by several different molecular experiments, the most direct being the purification of MPF by Lohka and Maller and the demonstration that the principal protein component was a 34kD protein that reacted with antibodies against bona fide cdc2 and its homologs and displayed kinase activity against histone H1 (Lohka, *et al*, 1988).

Cyclin—the Other Subunit of MPF ■

Although the discovery of a ubiquitous kinase, cdc2, was a major step in understanding the control of the cell cycle, it in itself offered little information on how the periodicity of cell divisions was achieved or how all the events of cell division

could be coordinately controlled. The mystery deepened when it was found that the abundance of the cdc2 protein did not change in the cell cycle of yeast or of frog eggs. The regular alternation of M-phase and S-phase, and the regular periodicity of the cell divisions in early embryos implied that some other protein acted on cdc2 to promote its kinase activity. Earlier experiments on MPF suggested that under one set of circumstances (in the first meiotic division in the oocyte) MPF could be activated without protein synthesis, while in all mitotic divisions (as well as the second meiotic division) new protein synthesis was required (Gerhart, *et al*, 1984). These characteristics of MPF activation, which include both translational control of some new component and posttranslational control, are important features of the regulation of MPF activity control in most cells.

The nature of the protein synthesis requirement for MPF activation came from serendipitous experiments on protein synthesis in sea urchin eggs. Tim Hunt and a group of students in the Physiology course at the Marine Biological Laboratory at Woods Hole studied the pattern of proteins labeled during a continuous incorporation of ^{35}S-methionine in sea urchin eggs (Evans, *et al*, 1983). As expected, they found that almost all labeled proteins increased in abundance during the first few cell cycles. One protein, however, showed the curious property of disappearing at each mitosis and accumulating steadily during each interphase; they named it, appropriately, cyclin (see Fig. 1-4). Pulse labeling experiments demonstrated that the rate of synthesis of this protein was constant throughout the cell cycle including mitosis, so that the abrupt disappearance at mitosis was due to its rapid degradation. Although only the weakest circumstantial evidence tied cyclin to the regulation of MPF activity, it was plausible that a simple oscillator be built, whereby cyclin could accumulate during interphase, activating cdc2, which in turn would cause the degradation of cyclin; the absent cyclin would lead to the inactivation of cdc2, allowing the cyclin to accumulate again.

The test of this model came from biochemical experiments in cell extracts (Murray and Kirschner, 1989a; Murray, *et al*, 1989). Concentrated extracts from frog eggs had been prepared that allowed mitotic events, such as chromosome condensation, in response to MPF (Lohka and Maller, 1985; Miake-Lye and Kirschner, 1985). Even more optimized extracts were then prepared that allowed protein synthesis, the accumulation of

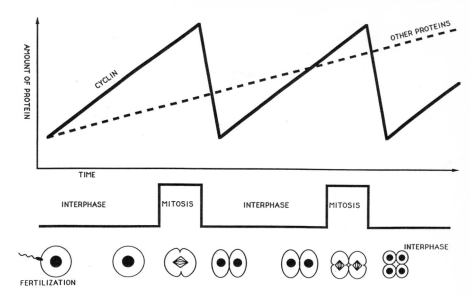

FIG. 1–4 Cell cycle behavior of cyclin protein abundance. Cyclin oscillates in abundance due to its degradation at mitosis. Other proteins accumulate monotonically.

MPF, the mitotic events consequent to MPF induction and the degradation of cyclin and the inactivation of MPF, followed by DNA replication in the next interphase. If protein synthesis were blocked, nuclei could exit mitosis; DNA replication took place but there was no entry into the next mitosis (Kirschner, *et al*, 1985). To test whether cyclin synthesis was required for activation of MPF, Minshull and Hunt found that by destroying cyclin mRNAS specifically with oligonucleotides complementary to the cyclin coding sequence, they blocked the entry into mitosis (Minshull, *et al*, 1989). An even more striking test of cyclin function was the demonstration that cyclin was the only protein whose synthesis was required to enter mitosis (Murray and Kirschner, 1989a). When all the endogenous mRNAs were destroyed by ribonuclease treatment, no appreciable protein synthesis took place and cells remained in G2. If cyclin mRNA—originally from distantly related species like sea urchin—were added, the cell cycle resumed (see Fig. 1-5). As cyclin was the only protein synthesized it was easy to follow its accumulation and degradation. The amount of cyclin mRNA and hence the rate of cyclin synthesis within limits determined the length of the cell cycle. The basic model was fulfilled. It was later shown that cyclin makes a tight noncovalent complex with cdc2 and sometimes another smaller protein, first identified in yeast, called suc1. This complex appears to constitute the active form of MPF (see Fig. 1-6) (Draetta, *et al*, 1989; Solomon, *et al*, 1990).

Posttranslational Activation of MPF ■

From the point of view of clinical medicine we would hope that knowledge of the cell cycle would help us develop means to control it and also help us understand the failures in cell cycle control that occur in pathological processes. In the simple description of the cell cycle in the frog egg, little can be controlled, and in fact the cell cycle will persist even without the nucleus or components of the cytoskeleton (Hara, *et al*, 1980). In continuously growing cells, such as yeast, the synthesis of the cdc2 protein is not regulated and the regulation of the kinase activity falls to cyclin and possibly other molecules (Nurse, 1990). In mammalian cells that are in a nondividing state (called G0), such as freshly isolated T-lymphocytes, the levels of cdc2 protein and its mRNA are very low and upon stimulation with phytohemagglutinin both rise, but as a rather late event after the immediate early genes and the oncogenes c-myb and c-myc (Furukawa, *et al*, 1990). Therefore, in proliferating cells we may expect that many of the controls will be posttranslational, while in quiescent cells there may be complex transcriptional requirements.

In oocyte maturation the first meiotic division can be initiated without protein synthesis if a small amount of MPF is injected into the oocyte (Gerhart, *et al*, 1984). Thus the frog oocyte is arrested in G2 after cyclin synthesis has already occurred; activation of MPF is a posttranslational event (Minshull, *et al*, 1990). In mitotic divisions studied

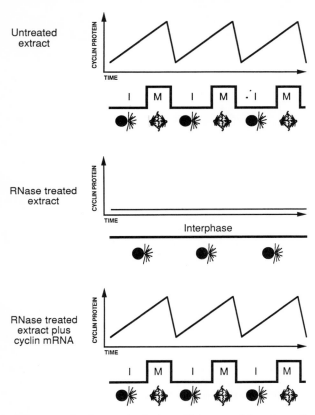

FIG. 1–5 Cyclin synthesis is sufficient to drive the cell cycle. In untreated extracts cyclin oscillates in abundance; cells enter and leave mitosis. Treatment with RNase causes arrest in interphase due to inhibition of protein synthesis. Addition of a mRNA encoding cyclin to the RNase treated extract is sufficient to cause resumption of the cell cycle, even though under these conditions cyclin is the only protein synthesized anew.

in vitro a pause occurs between the production of cyclin and the activation of the kinase activity. This can be most easily seen when purified cyclin protein is added as a bolus (Solomon, *et al,* 1990). Instead of immediate activation of the kinase activity, a lag phase is followed by a rapid activation to maximum level. The lag phase in the frog egg is probably very short in the frog egg cell cycle, but where it is longer it corresponds to the G2 phase of the cell cycle. In both of these cases there must be some limiting reaction that delays activity.

Recent experiments have shown that the lag phase is caused by inhibitory phosphorylations of the cdc2 protein on both threonine and tyrosine (Dunphy and Newport, 1989; Gould and Nurse, 1989; Solomon, *et al,* 1990). These phosphoryla-

tions are generated by kinase activities that are present in the cell but that in turn seem to be regulated by the activity of the cdc kinase. Before cyclin synthesis, which in the frog egg is immediately after mitosis, but in other cells may be any time in G1 or even S-phase, cdc2 is found unphosphorylated and inactive. The binding of cyclin causes cdc2 to become a substrate for kinase activities that generate three phosphorylations on the cdc2 molecule: one phosphorylation is on a threonine residue distant from the ATP binding site and confers activity on the kinase (Krek and Nigg, 1991; Solomon, *et al,* 1990); the other two phosphorylations are on a tyrosine and threonine that are at the ATP binding site of the kinase (Gould and Nurse, 1989). The effect of all three phosphorylations is to modify the kinase in such a way that it is potentially active but in fact inhibited from activity by the inactivating phosphorylations. There are two reasons to hold the kinase in an inactive form. In rapidly proliferating cells, such as frog eggs, it is necessary to accumulate a sufficient pool of MPF in order to enter mitosis with a full complement of kinase activity, rather than generate small quantities of kinase during the first moments of cyclin synthesis. This is understandable given the large number of substrates upon which MPF must act, each of which may have its own rate of phosphorylation or its own threshold of phosphorylation to undergo a mitotic transition. The other reason is that the dephosphorylation of the inactivating sites (the tyrosine and threonine at the ATP binding site) is an important checkpoint in the cell, sensitive to DNA damage and the completion of DNA replication (Broek, *et al,* 1991; Enoch and Nurse, 1990; Lundgren, *et al,* 1991a).

As shown in Figure 1-7, several sets of reactions govern the posttranslational activation and inactivation of cdc2 when complexed to cyclin. The activating phosphorylation is not an autoactivation reaction, mediated by cdc2 itself; although that might have been an attractive autocatalytic scheme for generating an explosive increase in cdc2 activity at mitosis; it is controlled by an unknown kinase. The activating phosphorylation of threonine is essential. Mutants that change the threonine to alanine are unable to enter mitosis, while those that change it to serine are capable of entering mitosis (T. Lee, unpublished). The level of this phosphorylation determines the length of G2 or the level of cyclin required to enter M, and is controlled by a balance of phosphatase activity and kinase activity (Solomon, *et al,* 1990). The phosphatase has been recently purified and shown

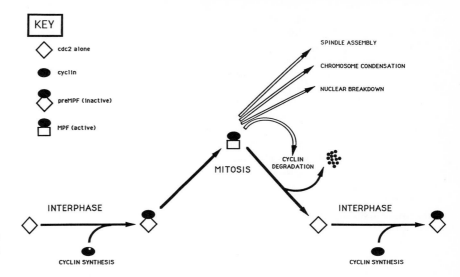

FIG. 1–6 Generation of active MPF activity by the combination of cyclin and cdc2.

to inhibit MPF activity. It is a member of the phosphatase 2a family, inhibitable by okadaic acid (Lee, *et al,* 1991).

The inactivating phosphorylation, particularly the tyrosine phosphorylation, has been studied intensively, since it seems to be the locus of action of a feedback control circuit that monitors the completion of DNA replication or DNA damage (Enoch and Nurse, 1990; Lundgren, *et al,* 1991a). It is known from genetic studies in yeast that a kinase called wee-1 lies on a pathway that leads to tyrosine phosphorylation (Russell and Nurse, 1987). There were two cogent reasons for thinking that wee-1 was not in fact the tyrosine ki-

nase. Deletion of that gene still left appreciable tyrosine phosphorylation. The sequence of wee-1 showed homology to serine/threonine kinases but not tyrosine kinases. The answer to the first objection came in the discovery of a second related gene, called mik-1; together these genes account for the total level of tyrosine phosphorylation (Lundgren, *et al,* 1991b). Deletion of both genes causes what has been called "mitotic catastrophe," the premature entry into mitosis before DNA replication can be completed. The second objection has been partially answered by the finding that wee-1 expressed in bacteria and subsequently purified will phosphorylate both serine

FIG. 1–7 During posttranslational activation of MPF several phosphorylation reactions are shown that distribute MPF among several inactive species and one active species.

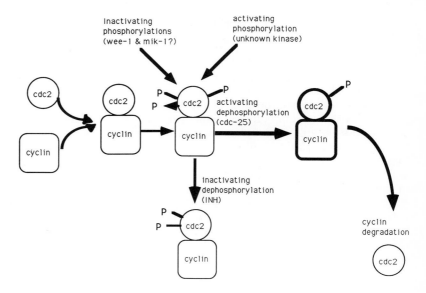

and tyrosine residues on proteins (Featherstone and Russell, 1991). To date, the direct phosphorylation of cdc2 has not been demonstrated. Relatives of wee-1 have now been found in vertebrate organisms and it is highly conserved (Booher, unpublished).

The dephosphorylation reaction is controlled by an enzyme called cdc25, which also seems to be present in all eukaryotes. In humans it is principally expressed in G2 and may be the rate limiting step in entry into M-phase (Sadhu, *et al*, 1990). Although initial evidence suggested that it too was not the enzyme directly acting on cdc2, more recent data suggest that it is the phosphatase (Gautier, unpublished). It is clear that although cyclin is necessary to drive the cell cycle, other enzymatic activities, such as cdc25 or the activating kinase could be rate limiting under some set of conditions. Recently in *Drosophila* embryos it has been shown that the cell cycle in the early embryonic tissues is regulated in a distinctive pattern. This pattern is controlled by the transcription of cdc25 (O'Farrell, *et al*, 1989). Thus although cyclin synthesis still occurs and is required, it accumulates to the required level before cdc25 accumulates and hence it is the cdc25 that is required for entry into M.

The kinetics for the entry into mitosis is controlled by both a positive and negative feedback loop that causes a rapid activation of MPF after cyclin has reached a threshold level. As shown in Figure 1-7, cyclin accumulation leads to a buildup of the inactivated complex of cdc2 and cyclin. This complex is in equilibrium with a small amount of the activated form, whose level is controlled in part by the phosphatase. The activated kinase is part of two nonlinear feedback loops that inhibit the pathway that leads to tyrosine phosphorylation and activates the pathway that leads to tyrosine dephosphorylation. The exact details of this activation and inactivation are not understood. When the level of activated kinase reaches levels high enough to activate the tyrosine dephosphorylation pathway and inactivate the tyrosine phosphorylation pathway, there will be an explosive increase in MPF activity and the cell will be propelled into M. The complicated kinetics of this pathway act like an escapement on a watch, which allows the continuous buildup of potential activity while holding the mechanisms in a suppressed stable state that is capable of releasing that activity in a rapid transition to a new stable state.

Cyclin Destruction and the Escape from Mitosis ■

The feedback loops that cause an autocatalytic entry into mitosis create a stable metaphase state. The high level of MPF activity phosphorylates a number of proteins that cause the vast biochemical changes that characterize mitosis. This process has been studied in some detail for the breakdown of the nuclear envelope, which is made up of a set of intermediate filament proteins, called nuclear lamins (Aebi, *et al*, 1986; McKeon, *et al*, 1986). These proteins assemble into a durable filamentous system that underlies the inner nuclear membrane. Phosphorylation of the lamins leads to disassembly of this lamina (Gerace and Blobel, 1980). MPF phosphorylates directly two sites on the lamin proteins; two other sites are hyper-phosphorylated by pathways that must be indirectly activated by MPF (see Fig. 1-8) (Peter, *et al*, 1990; Ward and Kirschner, 1990). Presumably all other mitotic targets, including the chromatin, the endoplasmic reticulum, and the actin and tubulin cytoskeleton, are also direct or indirect targets of the kinase activity of MPF.

How does the cell exit mitosis? The autocatalytic feedback loops ensure a stable metaphase state. Yet this stable state also includes the seeds of its own destruction. One of the activities induced by MPF is cyclin destruction. Experiments with mutant cyclins, that are defective in their ability to be degraded but are normal in their ability to induce MPF activity, have shown that the destruction of cyclin is necessary for the cell to exit mitosis (Ghiara, *et al*, 1991; Glotzer, *et al*, 1991; Murray, *et al*, 1989). Cyclin degradation is the ratchet of the clock. It is an irreversible step that causes exit from metaphase and entry into the next cell cycle.

Recently some information has been obtained about the biochemical mechanism of cyclin destruction. The destruction mechanism must be very selective. Cyclin is a very stable protein during interphase and is rapidly degraded at the metaphase-anaphase transition. No general increase in cellular protein lability occurs at this transition, so it seems unlikely that a general protease is activated. Recently it has been shown that cyclin contains a recognition sequence for M-phase specific degradation. This recognition domain can be transferred to exogenous proteins to render them degradable in an M-phase specific manner. The

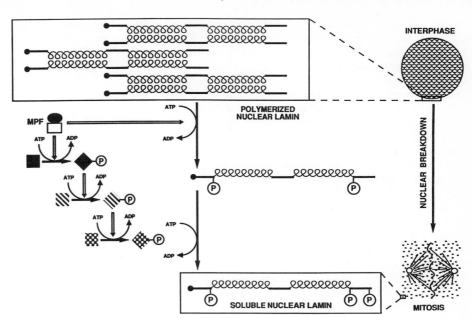

FIG. 1–8 MPF dependent phosphorylation and depolymerization of nuclear lamins during mitosis.

degradation of cyclin is accompanied by the covalent modification of the protein by ubiquitin, a modification that had been known for a long time to occur during the degradation of abnormal or denatured proteins in cells (Ciechanover, *et al,* 1990). Mutations that block cyclin ubiquitination block degradation. Therefore, MPF must somehow cause the cyclin molecule to be recognized by the ubiquitin modification system (Glotzer, *et al,* 1991). Once modified, cyclin is presumably degraded by constitutively present proteases.

Cyclins, cdc2, and the G1/S Transition ■

Most somatic cells arrest in G1 before DNA synthesis with a diploid content of DNA. Arrest at the G2/M transition is unusual for proliferating mammalian cells but is not unusual for eggs or cells with DNA damage. From experiments in yeast it was known that the same kinase, cdc2, was required in both the M-phase and in the G1 phase (Nurse, 1990). Hence, arguably the most important cell cycle gene should give two points of arrest and would not have been a true cell cycle gene by Hartweel's original criteria. The features of the G1/S transition have only recently been under-

stood in budding yeast, though it is likely that they are universal features of all eukaryotic cells. The mechanism of the G1/S transition in budding yeast bears a striking homology to the well-studied G2/M transition in other cells. Both transitions require the same catalytic subunit of cdc2 and both require as an auxiliary factor proteins that are members of the cyclin family. These proteins share similarity of sequence over a 200 amino acid domain, called the cyclin box, but in general show little homology outside this domain. In budding yeast three genes exist for cyclin-like molecules that are required to enter S phase (Wittenberg, *et al,* 1990). These genes play no role in the G2/M transition.

The G1 cyclins in yeast are involved in the nutritional arrest in G1 and are involved in a hormonal pathway, called the mating factor pathway, that causes the cell cycle to stop at G1 to allow the haploid yeast to fuse and later to undergo meiosis. The mating factor pathway regulates the level or activity of the G1 cyclin proteins. It is likely that this regulation is on the level of both transcription and protein stability (Chang and Herskiwoitz, 1990). Thus entry into S is formally analogous to entry into M. In both cases a threshold of cyclin activity is required to advance to the next phase. What is surprising in G1 is the existence of three different cyclic molecules and three different pathways for regulating them. Activation of only one of the cyclins is sufficient to enter S; hence cell cycle arrest requires the negative regulation of all three. It is likely that the role of cdc2 in G1/S transition is somewhat different from its role in the G2/M transition. No evidence exists for large-scale changes in protein phosphorylation in G1 as there is in M. Hence the function of cdc2 at G1 might be to initiate a small number of critical phosphorylations that lead to other biochemical changes, such as changes in gene expression.

The total number of known species of cyclin molecules continues to grow. Hunt and Ruderman originally identified two different cyclin molecules in mitosis (Minshull, *et al*, 1990; Swenson, *et al*, 1986). In eggs and oocytes the A cyclin accumulates before the B and is degraded more rapidly. Recently other cyclin-like molecules have been discovered that act at mitosis. In mammalian somatic cells the A cyclin appears sometime during S, while the B cyclin is tightly coupled to the G2/M transition (Pines and Hunter, 1989). It is not known why there are multiple cyclins. One possibility is that multiple cyclins bring the cell cycle under different forms of regulation. However, as long as the cyclins are redundant, as measured by *in vitro* assays, these pathways can only act to stimulate cell cycle transitions, not to inhibit them. Another possibility is that the cyclins generate different specificities of the kinase activity of cdc2. To date, different target specificities of cdc2 have not been demonstrated. A third possibility is that cyclins could act to target the cyclin–cdc2 complex to different regions of the cell. There are good data that cdc2 is localized in the nucleus and in centrosomes, and it is possible that this is mediated by different cyclins (Alfa, *et al*, 1990; Bailly, *et al*, 1989). In addition to a family of cyclin proteins, there is also a family of kinases related to cdc2, whose function is not understood (Paris, *et al*, 1991).

Mammalian cells depleted in growth factors and then re-fed reenter the cell cycle asynchronously after a long lag (Zetterberg, 1990). This lengthy reentry into the cell cycle has suggested to many people that the depleted cells are in a different cell cycle state called G0. Early responses to growth factors involve several changes in transcription that are thought to be a response to the tyrosine kinase activity of the growth factor receptors. It is not known how this causes entry into the cell cycle but it seems very likely that an early response to the initial transcriptional activation is the increased rate of synthesis of the G1-specific cyclins. The linkage between the G0 proliferative

transition and the fundamental cdc2–cyclin cell cycle mechanism will be an area of considerable interest in the next few years.

Feedback Controls and Cancer Therapy ■

Although in some circumstances, such as early embryos, the cell cycle can proceed from one stage to the other without any feedback control, in most cells there are mechanisms for checking on whether the cell has completed the biochemical steps dictated by the cell cycle machinery. For instance it has been known for a long time that inhibition of DNA synthesis prevents cells from entering mitosis, and inhibition of mitosis prevents cells from entering DNA synthesis. There are two possible explanations as to why cells fail to progress in the cell cycle if specific events are blocked. It could be that the event itself, for example, completion of DNA replication, is required for generating a regulatory signal that would cause the cell cycle to move forward. Alternatively, the failure to complete an event could send a negative signal that would feedback on the intrinsic cell cycle machinery.

It is now thought that there are no positive signals required that would be generated by the completion of DNA replication and that would signal the cell cycle to proceed. In the frog egg the progression through the cell cycle can occur independently of the initiation or completion of mitosis or DNA replication (Murray and Kirschner, 1989b). In somatic mammalian cells treatment with caffeine can cause cells that are arrested in the middle of S-phase to progress into mitosis (Schlegel and Pardee, 1986). In yeast, interfering with the events that lead to tyrosine phosphorylation on cdc2 (either by inactivating the phosphorylation site or by interfering with the kinases) causes premature entry into mitosis and cell death without completion of DNA replication (Enoch and Nurse, 1990; Lundgren, *et al*, 1991a). All of these experiments argue that the act of completing DNA synthesis itself is not required to induce progression of the cell cycle, since many circumstances exist where the MPF cycle can proceed without it. In some cells, however, failure to complete DNA replication sends a negative signal to cause cell cycle arrest.

The control points that are negatively controlled

are the transitions involving either the activation or the inactivation of MPF (Hartwell and Weinert, 1989; Murray and Kirschner, 1989b). It is likely that similar transitions involving the activation and inactivation of cdc2 in the G1/S transition will also come under controls, but these have not been studied. In the G2/M transition the activation of MPF depends on the synthesis of cyclin, phosphorylation at the activating phosphorylation site of cdc2, and the removal of the phosphates on the inactivating phosphorylation sites. Of these, only the removal of the inactivating phosphorylation on tyrosine is known by genetic studies to respond to the failure to complete DNA replication (Gould and Nurse, 1989).

It has been known for many years that DNA damage causes arrest in G2 of the cell cycle. Studies in budding yeast have shown that there is a system of genes involved in assessing DNA damage and in inducing cell cycle arrest to allow time for repair. One such gene, RAD9, has been studied by Hartwell and his colleagues (Weinert and Hartwell, 1988; Weinert and Hartwell, 1990). It is not an essential gene under normal growth conditions but it has an exceptionally high rate of lethality if DNA is damaged with X-rays. Unlike other radiation-sensitive mutations, however, it is not defective in repair. Instead, the lesion is an unusual one, since cells fail to show the usual arrest in G2 after irradiation and proceed with their damaged DNA into mitosis where the chromosomes are torn apart during division. If an artificial arrest is imposed on that mutant by adding the drug nocodazole, which disrupts mitosis, lethality is suppressed, demonstrating that the function of this gene can be replaced by imposing an artificial period between S-phase and mitosis.

In most cells events that block spindle formation impose a block on the metaphase-anaphase transition. For example, colchicine will cause a long-term metaphase arrest, with condensed chromosomes and high MPF activity. Whatever system monitors the successful assembly of the mitotic spindle must be exquisitely sensitive. Nicklas has done experiments in which the microsurgical removal of a single chromosome at metaphase will delay the onset of anaphase (Nicklas and Kubai, 1985). Recently Murray and his colleagues have looked for another set of genes that monitor the successful assembly of the mitotic spindle. The screen for mutants (called MAD mutants for "mitotic arrest deficiency") in this pathway was similar to those for RAD9; they looked for mutations that were sensitive to sublethal concentrations of nocodazole (Li and Murray). Most of these mutations would be expected to be caused by partially defective mitotic spindles, which fall apart at low doses of nocodazole. To find feedback mutations, therefore, a second criterion was used, which demanded that these mutations should not pause at M-phase. Their lethality was due to their leaving mitosis and entering the next cell cycle with damaged DNA or with an incomplete set of chromosomes. Li and Murray further showed that these mutations could be suppressed by inhibiting DNA replication and thus allowing more time for spindle assembly.

Although both the RAD9 and MAD mutations are nonessential, except when the cell is stressed, both show increased frequencies of chromosome loss, suggesting that both pathways are involved in ensuring faithful chromosome replication and segregation. How these mutations feed into the cell cycle machinery is unclear. They act on the MPF transition but on opposite sides of the pathway. Perhaps the RAD9 gene acts indirectly to inhibit the phosphatase activity of cdc25 or to activate the kinase activity of wee-1. Perhaps the MAD mutations act to inhibit cyclin degradation.

Cancer is associated with a high degree of chromosome aberrations and chromosome loss. It is possible that cancer cells show these failures in genetic transmission because they are defective in the feedback circuitry that monitors DNA damage or that monitors spindle defects. Recently Schimke and his colleagues have shown that rodent cells show only transient arrest with nocodazole before they reenter the next cell cycle (Kung, et al, 1990). Cells that show such transient arrest also show high levels of DNA amplification and chromosome abnormalities. Interestingly, human cells were less susceptible to these apparent defects in the MAD-type feedback circuits, suggesting that they have a more stringent feedback control.

Although these feedback circuits seem to be special mechanisms for refined monitoring of basically functional processes, from the point of view of somatic mutation they may be very important. Recent work has shown that cancer may require multiple genetic changes. If a failure in the feedback circuits increases the frequency of mutation even fivefold (a value that comes from looking at the rate of chromosome loss) and malignancy requires five steps, then the chance of generating a malignant phenotype will increase 3000-fold. Feedback circuit genes may even be recessive oncogenes. When the wild type gene is lost, an increased rate of spontaneous mutation and an increased sensitivity to environmental mutagens would occur. Feedback controls are shown in Figure 1-9.

The Cell Cycle and Cancer Therapy ▪

Many cancer therapies may exploit as their therapeutic advantage the deficiencies in cancer cells to monitor and repair DNA damage or to monitor defects in spindle formation. We may imagine that cancer cells are defective in such mechanisms because they quickly accumulate chromosomal rearrangements and amplified DNA and are often aneuploid. Many chemotherapeutic drugs such as 5-flurouracil and methotrexate lead to defects in deoxyribonucleotide pools, and these in turn may lead to DNA damage (Hirota, *et al,* 1989). Other agents, such as X-irradiation or gamma irradiation, also cause DNA damage. Although it has been suggested that cancer cells may have defects in DNA repair, the major defect may lie in the ability of these cells either to sense damaged DNA or to cause the cell cycle machinery to arrest. Current knowledge would suggest that this arrest point is the dephosphorylation of cdc2 on its inhibitory tyrosine and threonine sites. Tumor cells failing to stop would enter a lethal mitosis. Antimicrotubule agents, such as vincristine and taxol, might also have differential effects on tumor cells if these cells have an impaired ability to stop the cell cycle due to a difficulty in assembling the mitotic spin-

dle. Precocious mitosis before the establishment of the metaphase plate would cause cell death. Such models of therapeutic efficiency are more convincing than suggesting that these agents have differential effects on rapidly dividing cells, because often cancer cells are not the most rapidly dividing cells.

Does the new knowledge of the cell cycle now suggest new therapies? The therapeutic index is limited by two factors—general toxicity of drugs and, in the case of therapies directed to dividing cells, collateral killing of non-tumor cells, for example in the bone marrow. If drugs could be developed that would further compromise the feedback controls, these drugs—used in combination with drugs or radiation causing DNA damage or mitotic spindle defects—would allow killing at lower doses and would not be expected to increase the killing of non-tumor cells. It is possible that the failures of the feedback circuits in tumor cells are very specific. Directing drugs at further crippling these pathways could greatly increase the effectiveness of conventional agents. It will be particularly interesting to know if tumors that are resistant to common chemotherapeutic agents have more intact feedback mechanisms.

With regard to the core cell cycle reactions, no attempt has yet been made to design drugs or therapies directed at them. Whether these methods would be particularly effective would depend on whether tumor cells have elaborated specific pathways for stimulating the cell cycle. The availability of *in vitro* assays for these new classes of reactions could facilitate the testing of drugs di-

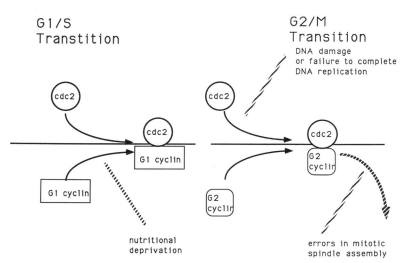

FIG. 1–9 Feedback controls on the core cell cycle reactions.

rected against cyclin, cdc2, and other novel proteins that are involved in the newly discovered phosphorylation and degradation pathways. One of the great surprises of the recent era in cell cycle research is the biochemical uniqueness of the regulatory components. Agents directed against the cell cycle machinery would be expected to have little effect on cell functions independent of cell division.

Acknowledgments. I wish to thank in particular Andrew Murray for his many helpful discussions about feedback control in the cell cycle, for his considerable contributions to the work, and for his construction of several of the figures used in this review. I wish also to thank the members of my laboratory who have participated in this adventure. I thank the National Institute of General Medical Sciences for generous support, even before this work became fashionable.

References ■

Aebi U, Cohn J, Buhle L, and Gerace L. The nuclear lamina is a meshwork of intermediate-type filaments. Nature 1986;323:560–564.

Alfa CE, Ducommun B, Beach D, and Hyams JS. Distinct nuclear and spindle pole body population of cyclin-cdc2 in fission yeast. Nature 1990;347:680–682.

Bailly E, Doree M, Nurse P, and Bornens M. p34cdc2 is located in both nucleus and cytoplasm; part is centrosomally associated at G2/M and enters vesicles at anaphase. EMBO J 1989;8:3985–3995.

Broek D, Bartlett R, Crawford K, and Nurse P. Involvement of p34cdc2 in establishing the dependency of S phase on mitosis. Nature 1991;349:388–393.

Chang F, and Herskiwoitz I. Identification of a gene necessary for cell cycle arrest by a negative growth factor of yeast-far1 is an inhibitor of a G1 cyclin cln2. Cell 1990;63:999–1011.

Ciechanover A, Gonen H, Elias S, and Mayer A. Degradation of proteins by the ubiquitin-mediated proteolytic pathway. New Biol 1990;2:227–234.

Draetta G, Luca F, Westendorf J, Brizuela L, Ruderman J, and Beach D. Cdc2 protein kinase is complexed with both cyclin A and B: evidence for proteolytic inactivation of MPF. Cell 1989;56:829–838.

Dunphy WG, and Newport JW. Fission yeast p13 blocks mitotic activation and tyrosine phosphorylation of the Xenopus cdc2 protein kinase. Cell 1989;58:181–191.

Enoch T, and Nurse P. Mutation of fission yeast cell cycle control genes abolishes dependence of mitosis on DNA replication. Cell 1990;60:665–673.

Evans T, Rosenthal ET, Youngblom J, Distel D, and Hunt T. Cyclin: a protein specified by maternal mRNA in sea urchin eggs that is destroyed at each cleavage division. Cell 1983;33:389–396.

Featherstone C, and Russell P. Fission yeast p107wee1 mitotic inhibitor is a tyrosine serine kinase. Nature 1991;349:808–811.

Furukawa Y, Piwnica-Worms H, Ernst TJ, Kanakura Y, and Griffin JD. cdc2 gene expression at the G1 to S transition in human T lymphocytes. Science 1990;250:805–808.

Gerace L, and Blobel G. The nuclear envelope lamina is reversibly depolymerized during mitosis. Cell 1980;19:277–287.

Gerhart J, Wu M, and Kirschner MW. Cell cycle dynamics of an M-phase specific cytoplasmic factor in Xenopus laevis oocytes and eggs. J Cell Biol 1984;98:1247–1255.

Ghiara JB, Richardson HE, Sugimoto K, Henze M, and Reed SI. A cyclin-B homolog in S. Cerevisiae-chronic activation of the cdc28 protein kinase by cyclin prevents exit from mitosis. Cell 1991;65:163–174.

Glotzer M, Murray AW, and Kirschner MW. Cyclin is degraded by the ubiquitin pathway. Nature 1991;349:132–138.

Gould KL, and Nurse P. Tyrosine phosphorylation of the fission yeast cdc2+ protein kinase regulates entry into mitosis. Nature 1989;342:39–45.

Hara K, Tydeman P, and Kirschner MW. A cytoplasmic clock with the same period as the division cycle in Xenopus eggs. Proc Natl Acad Sci USA 1980;77:462–466.

Hartwell LH. Cell division from a genetic perspective. J Cell Biol 1978;77:627–637.

Hartwell LH, and Weinert TA. Checkpoints: Controls that ensure the order of cell cycle events. Science 1989;246:629–634.

Hirota Y, Yoshioka A, Tanaka S, Watanabe K, Otani T, Minowada J, Matsuda A, Ueda T, and Wataya Y. Imbalance of deoxyribonucleoside triphosphates, DNA double-strand breaks, and cell death caused by 2-chlorodeoxyadenosine in mouse FM3A cells. Cancer Res 1989;49:915–919.

Kirschner M, Newport J, and Gerhart J. The timing of early developmental events in Xenopus. TIGS 1985;1:41–47.

Krek W, and Nigg EA. Differential phosphorylation of vertebrate p34cdc2 kinase at the G1/S and G2/M transition of the cell cycle-identification of major phosphorylation sites. EMBO J 1991;10:216–305.

Kung AL, Sherwood SW, and Schimke RT. Cell line-specific differences in the control of cell cycle progression in the absence of mitosis. Proc Natl Acad Sci USA 1990;87:9553–9557.

Lee MG, and Nurse P. Complementation used to clone a human homologue of the fission yeast cell cycle control gene cdc2. Nature 1987;327:31–35.

Lee TH, Solomon MJ, Mumby MC, and Kirschner MW. INH, a negative regulator of MPF, is a form of a protein phosphatase 2A. Cell 1991;64:415–423.

Li R, and Murray AW. Feedback control of mitosis in budding yeast. Cell 1992;66:519–531.

Lohka MJ, Hayes MK, and Maller JL. Purification of maturation-promoting factor, an intracellular regulator of early mitotic events. Proc Natl Acad Sci USA 1988;85:3009–3013.

Lohka MJ, and Maller JL. Induction of nuclear-envelope breakdown, chromosome condensation, and spindle formation in cell-free extracts. J Cell Biol 1985;101:518–523.

Lundgren K, Walworth N, Booher R, Kirschner MW, and Beach D. Mik-1 and wee-1 cooperate in the inhibitory tyrosine phosphorylation of cdc2. Cell 1991a;64:1111–1122.

Masui Y, and Markert C. Cytoplasmic control of nuclear behavior during meiotic maturation of frog oocytes. J Exp Zool 1971;177:129–146.

McKeon F, Kirschner M, and Caput D. Homologies in both primary and secondary structure between nuclear envelope and intermediate filament proteins. Nature 1986; 319:463–468.

Miake-Lye R, and Kirschner MW. Induction of early mitotic events in a cell-free system. Cell 1985;41:165–175.

Miake-Lye R, Newport J, and Kirschner MW. Maturation promoting factor induces nuclear envelope breakdown in cycloheximide-arrested embryos of Xenopus laevis. J Cell Biol 1983;97:81–91.

Minshull J, Blow JJ, and Hunt T. Translation of endogenous B-type cyclin mRNA is necessary for extracts of activated *Xenopus* eggs to enter mitosis. Cell 1989;56:947–956.

Minshull J, Golsteyn R, Hill C, and Hunt T. The A- and B-type cyclin associated cdc2 kinases in Xenopus turn on and off at different times in the cell cycle. EMBO J 1990;9:2865–2875.

Murray AW, and Kirschner MW. Cyclin synthesis drives the early embryonic cell cycle. Nature 1989a;339:275–280.

Murray AW, and Kirschner MW. Dominoes and clocks: two views of the cell cycle. Science 1989b;246:614–621.

Murray AW, Solomon MJ, and Kirschner MW. The role of cyclin synthesis and degradation in the control of maturation promoting factor activity. Nature 1989;339:280–286.

Nelkin B, Nichols C, and Vogelstein B. Protein factors from mitotic CHO cells induce meiotic maturation in Xenopus laevis oocytes. FEBS Letters 1980;109:233–238.

Newport JW, and Kirschner MW. Regulation of the cell cycle during early Xenopus development. Cell 1984;37: 731–742.

Nicklas RB, and Kubai DF. Microtubules, chromosome movement, and reorientation after chromosomes are detached from the spindle by micromanipulation. Chromosoma 1985;92:313–324.

Nurse P. Universal control mechanism regulating onset of M-phase. Nature 1990;344:503–508.

Nurse P, and Fantes PA. Cell cycle controls in fission yeast: a genetic analysis. In: Glover SW and Hopwood DA, eds. Genetics as a tool in microbiology. Society for General Microbiology Symposium 31. Cambridge: Cambridge University Press, 1981:85–98.

O'Farrell PH, Edgar BA, Lakich D, and Lehner C. Directing cell division during development. Science 1989;246:635–640.

Pardee AB. G1 events and regulation of cell proliferation. Science 1989;246:603–608.

Paris J, Le GR, Couturier A, Le GK, Omilli F, Camonis J, MacNeill S, and Philippe M. Cloning by differential screening of a Xenopus cDNA coding for a protein highly homologous to cdc2. Proc Natl Acad Sci USA 1991; 88:1039–43.

Peter M, Nakagawa J, Doree M, Labbe JC, and Nigg EA. In vitro disassembly of the nuclear lamina and M phase-specific phosphorylation of lamins by cdc2 kinase. Cell 1990;61:591–602.

Pines J, and Hunter T. Isolation of human cyclin cDNA: Evidence for cyclin mRNA and protein regulation in the cell cycle and for interaction with p34[cdc2]. Cell 1989;58:833–846.

Pringle JR, and Hartwell LH. The *Saccharomyces cerevisiae* cell cycle. In: Strathern JN, Jones EW, and Broach JR, eds. The molecular biology of the yeast *Saccharomyces*— Life cycle and inheritance. Cold Spring Harbor, New York: Cold Spring Harbor Laboratory Press, 1981:97–142.

Russell P, and Nurse P. Negative regulation of mitosis by wee1[+], a gene encoding a protein kinase homolog. Cell 1987;49:559–567.

Sadhu K, Reed SI, Richardson H, and Russell P. Human homolog of fission yeast cdc25 mitotic inducer is predominantly expressed in G2. Proc Natl Acad Sci USA 1990;87:5139–43.

Schlegel R, and Pardee AB. Caffeine-induced uncoupling of mitosis from the completion of DNA replication in mammalian cells. Science 1986;232:1264–1266.

Smith LD, and Ecker RE. Regulatory processes in the maturation and early cleavage of amphibian eggs. Curr Topics in Dev Biol 1970;5:1–38.

Solomon MJ, Glotzer M, Lee T, Philippe M, and Kirschner MW. Cyclin Activation of p34[cdc2]. Cell 1990;63:1013–1024.

Swenson KI, Farrell KM, and Ruderman JV. The clam embryo protein cyclin A induces entry into M phase and the resumption of meiosis in Xenopus oocytes. Cell 1986; 47:861–870.

Ward GE, and Kirschner MW. Identification of cell cycle-regulated phosphorylation sites on nuclear lamin C. Cell 1990;61:561–577.

Weinert TA, and Hartwell LH. The RAD9 gene controls the cell cycle response to DNA damage in *Saccharomyces cerevisiae*. Science 1988;241:317–322.

Weinert TA, and Hartwell LH. Characterization of RAD9 of *Saccharomyces cerevisiae* and evidence that its function acts posttranslationally in cell cycle arrest after DNA damage. Mol Cell Biol 1990;10:6554–6564.

Weintraub H, Buscaglia M, Ferrez M, Weiller S, Boulet A, Fabre F, and Baulieu E-E. Mise en evidence d'une activitie "MPF" chez *Saccharomyces cerevisiae*. Paris: CR Acad Sci 1982;295:787–790.

Wittenberg C, Sugimoto K, and Reed SI. G1-specific cyclins of *S. cerevisiae:* cell cycle periodicity, regulation by mating pheromone, and association with the p34[cdc2] kinase. Cell 1990;62:225–237.

Zetterberg A. Control of mammalian cell proliferation. Curr Opin Cell Biol 1990;2:296–300.

Zetterburg A, and Larson O. Kinetic analysis of regulatory events in G1 leading to proliferation or quiescence of Swiss 3T3 cells. Proc Natl Acad Sci USA 1985;82:5365–5369.

Steven A. Rosenberg

Gene Therapy of Cancer

2

Gene therapy can be defined as a therapeutic technique in which a functioning gene is inserted into the cells of a patient to correct an inborn genetic error or to provide a new function to the cell. Increased understanding of gene regulation in eukaryotic cells and the development of improved techniques for inserting and expressing foreign genes into mammalian cells have opened new possibilities for cancer therapy based on these gene transfer techniques. In May 1989 the first successful transfer of foreign genes into a human was performed in a patient with advanced melanoma.[1] This trial using a bacterial "marker" gene led to the first gene therapy approaches with advanced cancer, which began in January 1991. This paper will review the current status of gene therapy and its potential future applications in the treatment of patients with cancer.

The Introduction of Foreign Genes into Mammalian Cells ■

A variety of techniques are available for the introduction of DNA into eukaryotic cells including coprecipitation with calcium phosphate, the use of polycations or lipids complexed with DNA, encapsulation of DNA in lipid vesicles or erythrocyte ghosts, or the exposure of cells to rapid pulses of high voltage electric current (electroporation).[2] DNA has also been introduced into cells by direct microinjection or by the use of high velocity tungsten microprojectiles. These techniques are capable of integrating multiple copies of DNA into the genome although the efficiency of the integration varies widely with the technique, type of gene, and cell type. The efficiency of most of these physical transfection techniques is less than one in ten thousand and can be lower than one in a million.

Recently, techniques have been developed utilizing viral vectors to introduce DNA into mammalian cells.[2-12] These techniques have the potential for infecting all cells exposed to the virus. In developing techniques for the use of viral vectors, it was necessary to develop vectors that stably incorporated into the target cell without damaging it. Early work used transforming DNA viruses such as papovaviruses, simian virus 40, polyoma virus, or adenoviruses. More recently, murine and avian retroviruses have been used for DNA transduction and have proved both practical and safe. These retroviral vectors can infect multiple cell types, although cell replication is necessary for integration into the genome utilizing this approach.

Retroviruses are viruses in which the viral genes are encoded in RNA rather than DNA. Following infection of the cell, the viral RNA is converted to DNA by the action of reverse transcriptase. The DNA then enters the nucleus and integrates randomly into the genome. This integrated provirus is indistinguishable from other cellular genes and replicates along with the cell during mitosis. The integration of the provirus into the cell genome and the subsequent formation of progeny virus may have no effect on the viability of the infected cell.

Because practical applications of gene therapy involve introduction of the foreign gene by the retrovirus without actual replication of new retroviral particles in the host, special techniques have been developed that use packaging cell lines.[2–12] Retroviral vectors can be produced with the deletion of the viral protein coding sequences and introduction of the exogenous gene. These modified retroviruses retain the encapsidation sequences required for production of RNA transcripts into virions as well as the necessary sequences for integration and expression of the vector in the host cell genome.

To obtain these replication defective vector preparations, special "packaging cell lines" were produced that contain the helper virus genome but lack the encapsidation or psi sequence. Thus the packaging cell line cannot produce active virions that contain viral RNA. Introduction of the retroviral vector provides the necessary encapsidation sequence that, in conjunction with the viral coding sequences in the packaging cell line, produces virions containing the vector RNA. The most popular packaging cell lines have been derived from NIH 3T3 cells.[2–12] The possibility exists, however, that replication competent virus may be produced by recombination of the vector encapsidation sequences with the viral coding sequences present in the packaging cell line. Several workers have engineered modifications of the packaging cell lines and the retroviral vectors to minimize the possibility of helper virus generation including deletions of specific sequences in the 5′ and 3′ LTR, thereby requiring at least two recombinations to produce replication competent virus. The particular retroviral vector that we have used, designated LNL6,[7] which is derived from the N2 vector,[6] was also engineered to contain a stop codon at the site of the gag start codon, thereby further reducing the possibility that any competent virus would be produced.

The development of improved retroviral vectors for introduction of genes into eukaryotic cells is an active area of current investigation. The need exists for the consistent production of high titer virus capable of efficient transduction into a broad array of target cell lines. The need for cell replication and DNA synthesis required for provirus integration limits the usefulness of these retroviruses to the introduction of DNA into rapidly dividing cells. Although integration of the retroviral genome is often stable, in some cases there is substantial instability of the inserted genes, and loss of inserted genetic material with cell replication can occur. The random integration of the retrovirally derived DNA into the cell genome can lead to insertional mutagenesis through disruption of essential cellular genes or through activation of otherwise quiescent cellular genes. A major area of current interest involves the development of retroviral vectors with appropriate internal promoters that can express multiple genes in the same retroviral construct. In those retroviral vectors in which one gene is promoted by the retroviral LTR and another from internal promoters the interactions between these promoters can lead to marked inhibition of expression of one of the inserted genes.

Despite these problems, retroviral vectors represent the most efficient means of stably integrating DNA into large numbers of target cells, by coincubation of either the packaging cell line or the retroviral vector preparation with the target cell. Future developments, however, are aimed at the development of retroviral vectors that can be introduced systemically into an intact animal and be targeted specifically for selected cells. Although techniques for accomplishing this goal are not currently feasible, this area is being actively investigated.

Viruses other than the murine and avian retroviruses are being explored for possible use as expression vectors.[13] Human adeno-associated viruses can be achieved in high concentrations and appear to be nonpathogenic; however, difficulties in producing these preparations in the absence of contaminating helper viruses and concern about the long-term consequences of integration of these adenoviruses into cells have limited their usefulness. Vaccinia viruses, herpes viruses, bovine and papilloma viruses, and others are also being explored for their usefulness in gene transduction into human cells.

Gene Therapy of Cancer Using Gene Modified Tumor-Infiltrating Lymphocytes (TIL) ■

Studies of Murine TIL in Cancer Treatment ■

Tumor-infiltrating lymphocytes (TIL) are lymphocytes that infiltrate into growing tumors and can be grown by culturing single cell suspensions obtained from tumors in interleukin-2 (IL-2).[14–21] TIL cultures can be readily established from most murine and human tumors. To prepare TIL a single cell suspension is made from a freshly resected tumor, generally by enzymatic digestion and is incubated in a complete medium containing IL-2. Although lymphocytes comprise just a minor subpopulation of the enzymatic digest, some lymphocytes contain IL-2 receptors, presumably because of their interaction with antigens on the tumor cell surface. These lymphocytes begin to grow under the influence of IL-2 in the culture medium. Although tumor cells also grow, the lymphocytes outgrow the tumor cultures; when these lymphocytes have either specific lytic activity or lymphokine activated killer activity, tumor cells are destroyed. Thus by two to three weeks after initiating the culture, pure populations of lymphocytes without contaminating tumor cells can be obtained.

Extensive studies of murine TIL have been conducted both *in vitro* and *in vivo*. *In vitro,* murine TIL are CD8+ and often have specific cytolytic function directed against the tumor from which they were derived.[22] Recently, we have found that TIL can specifically secrete cytokines when cocultured with their specific tumor.[23,24] Extensive *in vivo* studies have demonstrated the effective therapeutic impact of the administration of TIL into mice with established cancer.[14,15,23,25] A summary of the immunotherapeutic effects of TIL plus IL-2 in mice is shown in Table 2-1.

The administration of TIL plus IL-2 is from 50 to 100 times more effective than LAK cells and IL-2 in treating established three day lung micrometastases.[14,15] Although TIL can be specifically lytic, it appears that specific secretion of cytokines such as gamma interferon and tumor necrosis factor are the best correlates of the *in vivo* antitumor effectiveness of TIL.[23] Although most specifically lytic TIL are therapeutically effective *in vivo,* nonlytic TIL that specifically secrete

Table 2–1

Immunotherapy of Murine Tumors with Tumor Infiltrating Lymphocytes (TIL) and IL-2

1. The administration of TIL plus IL-2 is 50–100 times more effective than LAK cells plus IL-2 in reducing established (day 3) lung micrometastases.
2. The administration of TIL plus IL-2 plus cyclophosphamide is effective in treating mice with advanced lung (day 14) or liver (day 8) metastases. All three agents are required for effective treatment.
3. The phenotype of TIL effective *in vivo* is CD3+, CD4−, CD8+.
4. TIL raised from tumors that express Class I antigens only after transfection with genes coding for Class I can mediate the regression of micrometastases from the parental tumor after treatment of the mouse with gamma-interferon.
5. Local tumor irradiation synergizes with TIL and IL-2 administration in mediating the regression of established metastases. Local irradiation can substitute for cyclophosphamide.
6. TIL with improved antitumor activity *in vivo* can be generated from tumor suspensions by using immunomagnetic beads to isolate lymphocytes followed by incubation of lymphocytes in low dose IL-2.
7. In mice cured of lung micrometastases by administration of TIL, live TIL can be identified *in vivo* three months after injection.
8. The specific secretion of gamma interferon by TIL when cultured with tumor is the best *in vitro* correlate of the *in vivo* antitumor effectiveness of TIL. Nonlytic TIL that specifically secrete gamma-interferon can effectively treat established lung micrometastases.

gamma interferon can also effectively eliminate established lung micrometastases.

These studies of transplantable mouse tumors led us to the study and application of TIL derived from human cancers.

In Vitro and *in Vivo* Studies of Human TIL ■

We have successfully grown TIL from approximately 80% of over 300 human cancers of varying histologies, including melanoma, renal cell cancer, colon cancer, breast cancer, bladder cancer, and others. Many groups have successfully grown human TIL from tumors.[16–21] The *in vitro* characteristics of human TIL as determined from our studies are shown in Table 2-2. From approximately a third of patients with melanoma, TIL can be derived that have specific cytolytic activity for fresh cancer cells and not normal cells from the same patient, including lymphocytes, fibroblasts, or

Table 2–2
In Vitro Studies of Human Tumor Infiltrating Lymphocytes (TIL)

1. TIL can be grown in IL-2 from approximately 80% of human cancers of a variety of histologic types including melanoma, renal cell cancer, colon cancer, breast cancer, ovarian cancer, and others.
2. TIL with specific cytolytic activity for fresh cancer cells can be grown from approximately one-third of patients with melanoma.
3. TIL are mainly CD3+ and can be either CD8+, CD4+, or mixtures of both. Smaller numbers of CD56+ TIL can also be present.
4. Specific lysis of TIL can be inhibited by antibodies to CD3 or to MHC class I molecules.
5. Growth of TIL from melanoma patients in IL-2 plus IL-4 results in increased *in vitro* lytic specificity for autologous melanoma.
6. Incubation of cultured tumors in gamma-interferon increases their susceptibility to lysis by TIL.
7. TIL with lytic specificity for autologous tumor have not been obtained from patients with colorectal cancer, breast cancer, or sarcomas and only rarely from patients with renal cell cancer.
8. Direct positive panning techniques using antibody coated flasks can be used to separate and grow highly purified subpopulations of CD4+ and CD8+ TIL.
9. Repeated immunoselection using TIL with specific lysis can be used to identify tumor lines resistant to lysis by autologous TIL. These immunoselected tumors can be used to identify multiple tumor antigens on a single tumor.
10. Shared tumor antigens on allogeneic melanomas that are recognized in an MHC-restricted fashion can be identified by testing lysis of specific TIL on panels of HLA typed melanoma cultures. HLA-A2 is a common restriction element in the recognition of melanoma antigens.
11. MHC-restricted recognition of shared melanoma antigens on allogeneic melanomas was demonstrated by using HLA-A2 restricted specific TIL to lyse allogeneic melanomas transfected with the gene for HLA-A2.
12. Nonlytic TIL with specific immune recognition of human tumor antigens can be recognized by the specific release of cytokines (such as GM-colony stimulating factor, tumor necrosis factor, and gamma-interferon) following incubation with autologous tumor. Specific reactivity has been identified in patients with melanoma and breast cancer.
13. *In vitro* lysis of autologous tumor by TIL exhibits mild but significant correlation with clinical response.

EBV transformed B cells.[16,17,21] It is difficult, however, to generate specifically cytolytic TIL from tumors other than melanoma, and we have been unsuccessful in finding TIL with specific lysis in patients with colon cancer and breast cancer. Rare cultures from patients with renal cancer can exhibit specific cytolytic activity.[26] TIL derived from human tumors are mainly CD3+ and can be CD8+ or CD4+ or mixtures of both. Some cultures contain CD56+ non-MHC restricted killer cells. The specific lysis of autologous tumor by TIL is MHC restricted. Specific lysis of TIL can be inhibited by antibodies to either CD3 or MHC class I molecules.[21] When specific TIL are tested against a panel of HLA-typed allogeneic melanomas, cross reactivity of lysis can be seen that follows a pattern of specific HLA specificities.[27] HLA-A2 appears to be a common restriction element for the recognition of melanoma antigens on allogeneic melanomas. Recently, we have transfected the gene for HLA-A2 into allogeneic non-HLA-A2 melanomas and have shown that HLA-A2 restricted TIL can lyse allogeneic melanomas expressing the transfected HLA-A2 gene in six of six patients (Kawakami, *et al,* submitted for publication).

The recognition of specific antigens by TIL has led to studies attempting to define the nature of these antigens. By repeated immunoselection using TIL with specific lysis we have isolated tumor lines resistant to lysis by autologous TIL.[28] These immunoselected tumors have been used to identify multiple tumor antigens present on a single tumor.

In seeking other assays for detecting tumor specific antigens we have determined that specific cytokine release by TIL cocultured with the autologous human tumor is also an indicator of specific immune recognition of tumor antigens.[24] The specific secretion of cytokines such as GM colony stimulating factor, tumor necrosis factor, and gamma interferon following incubation with autologous tumor have shown patterns similar to that seen with the use of lytic TIL. Using this cytokine release assay specific reactivity has been identified in TIL from patients with breast cancer and melanoma. We are currently exploring the use of this assay to identify tumor specific antigens present in other tumors.

In pilot trials, the treatment of patients with advanced melanoma using TIL plus IL-2 has resulted in objective responses in 38% of 50 patients.[29] This is approximately twice the level of response seen with IL-2 alone or LAK cells plus IL-2 (see Table 2-3). Interestingly, prior nonresponsiveness to therapy with IL-2 based regimens does not compromise the ability to respond to TIL plus IL-2 therapy. We are currently actively searching for *in vitro* correlates of TIL that will predict *in vivo* antitumor effectiveness. *In vitro* lysis of autologous tumor by TIL has a weak but significant correlation with clinical response, and we are currently testing whether specific cytokine

Table 2–3
TIL Treatment of Patients with Melanoma*

	No Response (NR)	Objective Response (PR + CR)	PR + CR All	Percent
No previous IL-2				
IL-2 + CY†	17	11	11/28	39
IL-2 (No CY)	7	4	4/11	36
Previous IL-2				
IL-2 + CY**	3	3	3/6	50
IL-2 (No CY)	4	1	1/5	20

*Excludes patients with brain metastases at start of treatment (all NR)
**Excludes two patients who received IL-2 at 30,000/kg; both were NR
†cyclophosphamide

release bears a correlation to clinical response as well.[30]

Studies have been conducted *in vivo* in patients with metastatic melanoma treated with TIL labeled with Indium-111 to test whether or not administered TIL localized to tumor deposits.[31,32] Clear tumor localization of TIL was seen on 13 of 18 nuclear scan series. Similarly, paired biopsies of tumor and normal skin showed a substantial concentration of Indium-111 TIL in tumor compared to normal skin. It thus appears that TIL can concentrate in tumor deposits. Approximately 0.015% of the injectate accumulates per gram of tumor. The accumulation of TIL in tumor has played an important role in our development of gene therapies utilizing TIL transduced with cytokine genes.

Gene Transfer into Humans Using TIL ■

Our attempts to follow the *in vivo* distribution and survival of human TIL following systemic administration to humans were limited by the problems associated with using radioactive Indium-111 as a label for the cells. Indium-111 has a half-life of 2.8 days, and the combination of the natural decay of the isotope and the spontaneous release of Indium-111 from the cell limited the time we could use these cells for study to one to two weeks. Further, the autoirradiation of the TIL by the Indium-111 led to potential damage of the TIL that could alter their function. We thus required a different method for studying the fate of TIL following *in vivo* injection. Information was needed about how

long infused TIL persisted *in vivo,* where they were located in the body, and whether the *in vivo* accumulation of TIL at the tumor site, draining lymph nodes, or in the circulation correlated with clinical antitumor effect. The opportunity to reisolate administered TIL from the tumor site would also provide us with information about the functional characteristics of TIL that traffic to tumor sites and whether or not any of these properties correlated with *in vivo* antitumor effects.

The introduction of new genes into TIL provided a possibility for genetically marking the cell to answer many of these questions. An introduced gene has many potential advantages as a cell marker that no other exogenous label can provide. The label becomes part of the permanent genome of the cell and will not leach away from the original cell as would a radioactive label. The label is not diluted as the cells proliferate, and every daughter cell is labeled. The label is lost as soon as the cell dies and will not become sequestered or reutilized in other cells. Further, the vital function of the cells is not changed by the marker label. In fact, a new functional property such as the use of a selectable marker gene might be introduced into the cell that would permit the specific recovery of the marked cells. Finally, depending on the gene inserted, very sensitive detection methods are available such as the polymerase chain reaction, which would enable the identification of as few as one marked cell in one million unmarked cells.

We thus proposed a clinical protocol to use retroviral mediated gene transfer to introduce the gene coding for neomycin phosphotransferase, a bacterial protein capable of rendering the cell resistant to G418, a neomycin analog otherwise lethal to all eukaryotic cells.[1] Because gene transfer studies had never been approved in humans, the potential risks and benefits of this proposed technology were carefully analyzed by a variety of review groups including the Clinical Research Committees of the National Cancer Institute, the National Heart, Lung and Blood Institute, the NIH Biosafety Committee, the Gene Therapy Subcommittee of the Recombinant DNA Advisory Committee (RAC), the full RAC, and the Food and Drug Administration. Final approval was also required from the Director of the NIH, who gave his approval to proceed in January 1989. A variety of factors were considered by these review groups. We had to demonstrate that we could insert and express the marker gene in human TIL, that the marked TIL were not significantly altered, that the marked cells could be detected in animal models, and that there was low risk to the patient and no risk to the public in using this new technology.

In our initial studies, TIL obtained from cancer patients were grown in culture and transduced with the retroviral vector N2, from the PA317 packaging cell line.[6] The N2 was a derivative of the Moloney murine leukemia virus in which the gag, pol, and env genes were removed or truncated and the bacterial Neo[R] gene inserted. To further decrease the development of replication-competent virus, the LNL6 vector was derived from the N2 vector.[7] This vector contained a stop codon at the site of the gag start codon. In addition, substitution of the 5′ Moloney leukemia virus sequences with those of the Moloney sarcoma virus sequences minimized the homology between the vector and helper virus genome, which also decreased the potential frequency of recombination. The PA317/LNL6–C8 cell line was used to produce the transduction vector used in our clinical studies and has provided high titer retroviral vector without helper virus contamination.

To produce LNL6 virions for use in transducing human TIL, cryopreserved vials of the PA317/LNL6–C8 cell line were thawed and grown in culture.[1] When the cell cultures approached confluence they were harvested, pooled, and filtered before titering on NIH 3T3 cells. Supernatants were frozen at −70°C until immediately before use. In our studies viral titers ranged from 2×10^5 to 2×10^6 G418 resistant colony forming units/ml. A variety of tests were performed on the retroviral supernatant, including sterility tests for aerobic and anaerobic bacteria and mycoplasma, MAP tests, tests for lymphocytic choriomeningitis virus, and an S+L− assay for ecotropic, xenotropic, and amphotropic viruses after 3T3 amplification. General safety tests in mice and guinea pigs were also performed in accordance with FDA requirements.

The TIL cell transductions were performed when TIL cultures reached from 1 to 10×10^8 cells.[1] An aliquot of the cells were exposed to the LNL6 supernatant at a multiplicity of infection between one and three in the presence of 5 mg/ml of protamine. The cells were incubated for two hours, washed, and then placed in culture; the transduction procedure was repeated one day later. The recovery rate of TIL after the transductions varied from 70 to 100%.

A variety of preclinical studies preceded the clinical administration of gene transduced TIL into humans.[33,34] These studies were conducted with both the N2 and the LNL6 vectors.

The gene coding for neomycin phosphotransferase could be readily introduced into human TIL using these vectors.[1,33,34] An example of the growth of the nontransduced and transduced TIL in IL-2 is shown in Figures 2-1 and 2-2. Examples of the ability of the transduced cells to resist exposure to the neomycin analogue G418 are also shown in these figures. Only the transduced and not the nontransduced cells could grow in G418 concentrations of 0.4 mg or higher.

The presence of proviral sequences in transduced TIL populations was demonstrated on Southern blots by hybridization of Sac 1 digested DNA with P32 labeled Neo[R] probes (see Fig. 3). A single copy of the expected 3.2 kilobase Neo[R] hybridizing fragment was present without rearrangement or deletion in the transduced TIL populations but was not detectable in nontransduced cells. The integration and expression of the transduced TIL appeared stable during extended cell cultures even in the absence of G418. Restriction digest with Sca I which did not cut within the provirus revealed multiple clones of transduced TILs containing proviral DNA integrated into different sites of the chromosome. NPT activity could also be demonstrated in the transduced cells.

Extensive tests were performed on the transduced and nontransduced populations to test whether the transduction procedure altered the phenotypic and functional characteristics of the TIL.[1,33] Because the antigenic specificity of the TIL was dependent on the presence of T-cell receptors, we used human genomic and cDNA probes specific for beta and gamma T-cell receptors to study the pattern of gene rearrangement in the TIL.[33] As illustrated in Figure 2-4, T-cell receptor

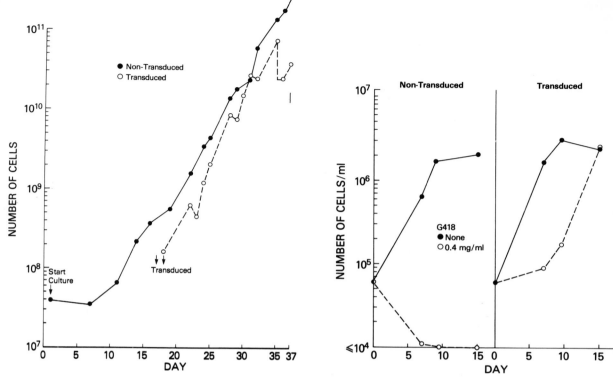

FIG. 2–1 Growth of non-transduced and transduced human TIL in culture. When TIL reach approximately 3×10^8 cells an aliquot is transduced and the transduced and nontransduced cells are grown in parallel. (left) Growth rates for the two populations appear to be similar. (right) The effect of 0.4 mg/ml of G418 on nontransduced and transduced TIL. The nontransduced TIL die in the presence of G418. The transduced TIL show a short lag after exposure to G418 and then begin to grow at a rate equivalent to that of the nontransduced cells. This figure is from previously published material.[33]

beta gene rearrangements appeared similar in the nontransduced and transduced selected populations. Similarly the study of Northern blots for cytokine mRNA expression also revealed similar patterns between the transduced and the nontransduced TIL; both TIL expressed mRNA for TNF alpha, TNF beta, but not for IL-6, GMCSF, IL-1 beta, or gamma-interferon.[33] Similarly, studies of the phenotype and cytotoxicity of transduced and nontransduced cells appeared to reveal substantial similarity unaffected by cell transduction. The phenotype and cytotoxicity of TIL actually administered to humans as part of our clinical trial is shown in Table 2-4.[1] It thus appeared from these studies that the gene for Neo[R] could be inserted and expressed in human TIL and that the marked TIL were not significantly altered.

Prior to initiating clinical trials, studies were performed to see if marked cells could be detected in animal models.[34] Despite extensive efforts we have been unable to introduce genes into short-term murine lymphocyte cultures by any available technique. Extensive efforts have been made using retroviral vectors, calcium phosphate precipitation, and electroporation to stably insert genes into short-term murine cultures, but have met with no success. It has, however, been possible to insert genes into selected long-term mouse lymphocyte lines, and thus these long-term cultures were used to test the detection and recovery of marked cells in animal models. Culver and his associates inserted the Neo[R] gene into long-term cultures of sperm whale myoglobin specific murine T helper cells (clone 14.1), which were maintained by repeated cycles of stimulation *in vitro* with myoglobin in the presence of antigen presenting cells.[34] These murine T helper cells were transduced with the N2 vector as well as the retroviral SAX vector

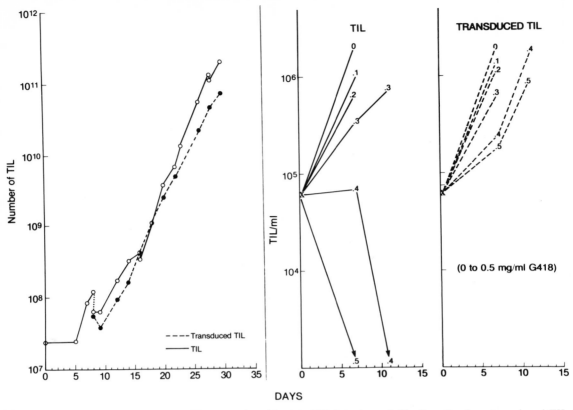

FIG. 2–2 Growth of transduced and nontransduced human TIL in culture (left). Growth of nontransduced TIL in varying concentration of G418 (middle). Note that at concentrations of 0.4 and 0.5 mg/ml G418 nontransduced TIL die. (right) Growth of transduced TIL in varying concentrations of G418. Note that transduced TIL grow successfully in G418 concentrations as high as 0.5 mg/ml. This figure is from previously published material.[1]

which expressed both Neo[R] and human adenosine deaminase genes. Following selection of these cells in G418, they were injected into nude mice to test the persistence of the cells *in vivo*. In these studies G418 resistant cells were readily recovered from the spleens of recipient animals several months after injection. These cells could be grown *in vitro* and shown to express neomycin phosphotransferase activity. Thus animal models suggested that marked cells could survive and could be recovered in animal models although it should be emphasized that these studies were not performed with murine TIL.

Safety considerations were paramount in our preclinical evaluation of the use of retroviral vectors for transduction of human cells.[1,35] Sterility tests and tests for replication-competent virus capable of detecting one viral particle/ml of solution were performed on the viral supernatants as well as on the gene modified cells after expansion in culture. In no case did we ever find evidence of replication-competent viruses in cells administered to patients.

Following presentation of much of this information to the appropriate regulatory committees, permission was received to treat up to 10 patients having advanced melanoma and life expectancies of 90 days or less. In these trials patients received an aliquot of gene modified cells along with nonmodified cells as part of their standard TIL treatment for advanced melanoma.[1] The clinical protocol was similar to that we have previously described but was modified to exclude cyclophosphamide from the treatment.[29] In brief, tumor deposits were resected and TIL grown in culture by techniques similar to those previously described.[29] After approximately two to three weeks of growth an aliquot of cells was removed for retroviral transduction and grown in parallel with the parent culture. A maximum of 2 to 3 × 10[11] cells were

Detection of Vector DNA (N2) in Infected Human TIL

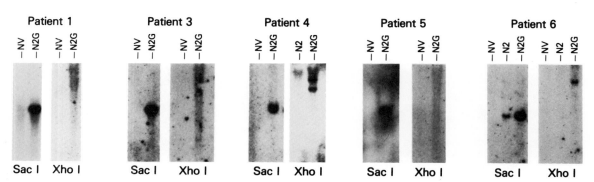

FIG. 2–3 Detection and integration of vector DNA in human TIL transduced with the NeoR gene. The Sac1 digested DNA shows the expected 3.2 kilobase NeoR hybridizing fragment in the transduced cells but not in the nontransduced ones. The Sac1 digested DNA revealed multiple clones of transduced TIL containing proviral DNA integrated into different sites of the host chromosome. This figure is from previously published material.[33]

FIG. 2–4 T-cell receptor beta gene rearrangements in nontransduced and transduced TIL. Similar patterns of gene rearrangements were seen in the transduced and nontransduced populations. This figure is from previously published material.[33]

TCR-β Gene Rearrangement and Expression in N2-Transduced Human TIL

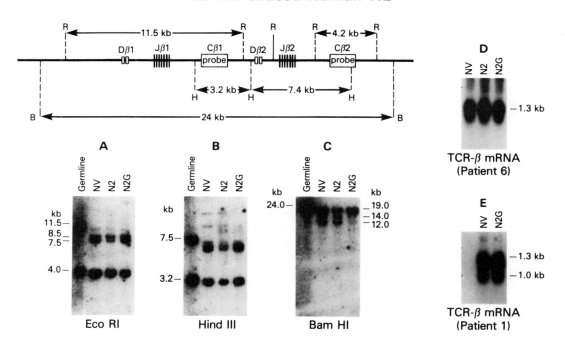

Table 2–4
Phenotype and Cytotoxicity of Infused Cells

| Patient | Cells Tranduced | Phenotype† | | | | | | | | | | | Cytotoxicity versus | | |
| | | CD3 | CD4 | CD8 | CD11 | CD14 | CD16 | CD20 | CD25 | DR | CD56 | CD57 | K562 | Daudi | Autologous Tumor |
						(% positive cells)							(% lysis at 80:1)*		
1	No	95	7	85	7	0	0	4	26	95	14	8	28	28	−5
	Yes	97	4	85	0	0	1	3	22	87	11	0	3	−2	1
2	No	98	5	95	1	5	4	5	5	92	24	0	20	2	13
	Yes	99	0	96	1	0	1	5	6	94	45	0	5	−5	16
3 A	No	95	2	85	36	0	1	1	1	79	17	17	41	30	6
	Yes	89	3	87	3	0	1	0	12	83	N.D.**	6	17	18	14
B	No	97	9	87	10	0	0	3	1	80	5	13	17	17	7
	Yes	83	16	68	0	0	1	0	9	74	2	5	4	5	10
4	No	95	15	55	2	5	2	0	15	80	9	3	1	1	4
	Yes	96	7	94	14	0	2	6	38	96	9	1	3	22	20
5	No	91	14	83	0	1	1	0	30	91	7	5	14	21	51
	Yes	96	20	74	2	0	0	1	21	89	2	6	10	13	40

*80:1 effector target ratio.

**Not done.

†CD3 is expressed on mature T-cells, CD4 and CD8 represent major T-cell subsets; CD16 is the FcR III present on null cells. CD11 (C3bi receptor) is present on some T-cells and null cells as is CD56 (NKHI). CD57 (Leu 7) is expressed primarily on null cells. CD14 is present on monocytes; CD16 and 20 on B cells. CD25 is one chain of the IL-2 receptor (Tac) and DR is a Class II MHC molecule present on B cells, macrophages, and activated T-cells. This table is from previously published material.[1]

infused. After the completion of infusions, patients received 720,000 IU/kg of IL-2 intravenously every eight hours for up to five days, although doses were omitted depending on the patient's tolerance for the drug. The side effects of the administration of IL-2 and the cell infusions were treated with acetaminophen, indomethacin, ranitidine, and meperidine as described previously.[29] After one to three weeks for recovery, the patients returned to the hospital for a planned second cycle of therapy with TIL and IL-2. Transduced TIL were given either on the first or second cycle but not both.

The Director of the NIH gave approval to begin this human gene transfer study on January 19, 1989. The first patient received an infusion of gene modified cells on May 22, 1989. To the present we have treated ten patients with advanced melanoma, using Neo[R] gene modified cells. The results in the first five patients have been published previously.[1] The characteristics of these patients are presented in Table 2-5. They vary in age from 26 to 52; all had extensive melanoma with multiple lesions, including lesions in brain, lung, liver, subcutaneous tissue, adrenal gland, and other sites. Characteristics of the infused gene transduced and nontransduced TIL administered to the first five patients are presented in Table 2-6.

Lymphocytes grew to a maximum of 63,400-fold over a 65-day period. Estimates of the percent of transduced cells by semiquantitative polymerase chain reaction analysis revealed that 1–11% of the cells were transduced. Semiquantitative Southern blot analysis estimated that 4–18% of cells were transduced. Studies of these cell surface determinants as well as cytotoxicity of the transduced cells are shown in Table 2-4. In each patient, evidence for the insertion of the NeoR gene was demonstrated using Southern blots. Expression of the neomycin phosphotransferase was also detected in all of the transduced cell populations and none of the nontransduced cells. We further demonstrated the expression of the NeoR gene by successfully culturing TIL from four of the five initial patients in the neomycin analogue G418.

A primary goal of our studies was the detection of these gene marked cells in blood and tumor samples. Samples of peripheral blood and tumor were taken from all patients before and at varying times after the infusion. Because of the pattern of tumor spread, multiple tumor biopsies could not be obtained from all patients. Polymerase chain reaction analyses were performed in a blinded fashion by at least two investigators, and the results on all positive samples were confirmed in a second independent assay. The results of these as-

Table 2–5
Patient Characteristics

Patient	Age/Sex	Primary Site	Prior Treatment	Tumor Harvest							Sites of Evaluable Disease
				Site	Size (cm)	Total No. of Cells Obtained ($\times 10^{-7}$)	Number of Cells to Start Culture* ($\times 10^{-7}$)	% Lymphocytes	% Tumor Cells		
1	52/M	Neck	Wide local excision	Lymph node	$4 \times 4 \times 2$	33	12	15	85		Lung, liver, spleen
2	46/F	Finger	Amputation finger Lymph node dissection	Lymph node	$5 \times 5 \times 3$	157	50	70	30		Lymph nodes, intramuscular
3	42/M	Back	Wide local excision Lymph node dissection Melanoma "vaccine" Interleukin-2/ Alpha-Interferon	Lymph node Subcutaneous Subcutaneous	$6 \times 5 \times 4$ $2 \times 2 \times 2$ $2 \times 2 \times 2$	205	120	31	69		Lung, subcutaneous
4	41/M	Chest	Wide local excision Lymph node dissection Interleukin-2/ Alpha-Interferon	Subcutaneous Subcutaneous	$2 \times 1 \times 1$ $5 \times 4 \times 4$	41	4	39	61		Lung, liver, lymph nodes, subcutaneous, brain
5	26/F	Arm	Wide local excision	Subcutaneous (6)	$2 \times 2 \times 2$ to $5 \times 4 \times 2$	71	15	16	84		Lung, lymph nodes, subcutaneous

*Denotes the number of cells used to start the cultures that were ultimately administered to the patient.

This table is from previously published material.[1]

Table 2–6
Characteristics of Infused Cells

Patient	Cells Transduced	Day of Transduction	Number of Cells Transduced ($\times 10^{-8}$)	Multiplicity of infection‡	Total Days of Growth	Fold Expansion*	Doubling Time** (days)	Number of Cells Infused ($\times 10^{-10}$)	Estimate of Cells Transduced (%)	Cycle Administered	Number of IL-2 doses to patient
1	No	—	—	—	36 and 37	63,400	2.5	22.8	—	1	7
	Yes	13	1.8	2.3	60	16,100	7.5	7.1	1	2	
2	No	—	—	—	65	209	3.5	0.2	—	1	15
	Yes	19	2.5	1.3	65	5,030	3.5	13.2	11	1	
3 A†	No	—	—	—	35	874	2.8	10.8	—	1	13
	Yes	12	1.8	1.6	48	35,100	2.5	14.5	1	2	
B	No	—	—	—	35	324	2.3	3.5	—	1	
	Yes	12	1.4	1.6	48	21,400	3.5	5.5	1	2	
4	No	—	—	—	36	8,470	2.0	26.0	—	1	10
	Yes	16	1.8	1.7	36	9,480	2.0	3.3	4	1	
5	No	—	—	—	30	18,900	2.0	15.0	—	1	7
	Yes	8	0.6	1.6	30	5,250	2.3	6.2	10	1	

*Calculated fold expansion of cells administered. Not all cultured cells were given; some cells were diverted for experimental studies or lost to contamination. Nontransduced cells shown here are those in conjunction with the transduced cells administered to the patient.

**Varied during culture growth; doubling time at time of final cell infusion is presented here.

†Two separate cultures transduced and expanded separately. Culture A was started in AIM-V medium; culture B was started in RPMI 1640 plus 10% human serum.

‡Ratio of number of virions to number of TIL during the transduction procedure.

This table is from previously published material.[1]

says on the first five patients is presented in Figure 2-5. Circulating peripheral blood mononuclear cells containing the NeoR gene were consistently present in the first 19–22 days after cell infusion. Cells were detected in the peripheral blood on day 51 in one patient and on day 60 in another patient. One of the patients underwent resection of a lesion 64 days after the infusion of gene modified cells. TIL in this specimen contained the NeoR gene and were reinfused on day 94. In this patient gene modified cells were detected in the circulation on day 121 and day 189 following the initial infusion.

An attempt was made to estimate the number of gene modified cells in the circulation using semi-quantitative PCR analysis.[1] In patient 1 the incidence of transduced TIL in peripheral blood was approximately 1:5000 mononuclear cells on day 1, 1:8000 on day 2 and 1:16,000 on day 4 after cell infusion. Another patient had one transduced cell in 300 on day 3, 1:1500 on day 6, 1:3000 on day 14, and 1:10,000 on day 19. TIL grown from the tumor in one of the patients grew successfully in G418, indicating that the Neo^R gene was not only present but was expressed in these cells. Multiple specimens taken at autopsy performed on three patients who received gene modified cells about

six months earlier revealed no PCR positive cells with the exception of one specimen in a single renal cortex biopsy that was thought to be a false positive; the opposite renal cortex was negative.

Two of the initial five patients had an objective regression of cancer; they included one patient who had complete regression of multiple lung lesions, subcutaneous deposits, and oral mucosal deposits that has persisted for over two years. The antitumor effects were due to the TIL/IL-2 treatment and not to any direct function of the modified gene.

All of the safety studies in the patients have been negative. All viral supernatants used for gene transduction and all infused TIL were sterile for bacteria, fungi, and mycoplasma and negative on $S + L -$ assays for ecotropic, xenotropic, and amphotropic infectious viruses as well as on NIH 3T3 amplification tests. Polymerase chain reaction analysis for the presence of the amphotropic helper virus 4070A envelope genes and reverse transcriptase assays of all TIL were negative. All infused TIL stopped growing shortly after IL-2 was withdrawn from the culture medium. Western Blot assays of the patient's serum to antibodies to 4070A viral P30 gag protein and $S + L -$ assays for

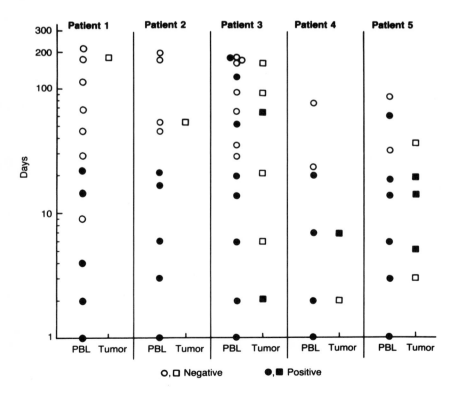

FIG. 2–5 Results of polymerase chain reaction assays on peripheral blood mononuclear cells and tumor biopsy of five patients receiving NeoR gene modified TIL. Circulating gene modified cells were consistently seen in the circulation for approximately 21 days after infusion. NeoR gene modified TIL were found in tumor biopsies up to 64 days after TIL infusion. This figure is from previously published material.[1]

virus performed at various times up to 180 days after cell infusion were negative.[1]

These studies demonstrated that it was possible to utilize retroviral mediated gene transfer to introduce foreign genes into cells which could be readministered safely to humans.[1] These studies also showed that at least small numbers of lymphocytes could persist for long periods both in the circulation and at tissue sites and suggested that TIL might be suitable vehicles for the introduction of other genes that might improve the therapeutic efficacy of these cells or might be suitable for the introduction of genes to correct inherited genetic defects such as severe combined immunodeficiency disease based on adenosine deaminase deficiency.

Gene Therapy of Cancer Using TIL Transduced with the Gene for Tumor Necrosis Factor (TNF) ∎

Our initial studies utilizing TIL transduced with the gene for NeoR provided the basis for attempts of the gene therapy of cancer utilizing TIL transduced with genes that would increase their therapeutic efficacy. The first gene selected for these studies was the gene coding for production and secretion of the cytokine tumor necrosis factor (TNF).

A variety of considerations led to the hypothesis that TIL secreting large amounts of TNF would increase the therapeutic efficacy of the TIL. Extensive animal research in the Surgery Branch, NCI, and in many other groups demonstrated that the injection of recombinant TNF could mediate the necrosis and regression of a variety of established experimental murine cancers.[36-38] The combined administration of TNF and IL-2 mediated far greater antitumor effects against subcutaneous and liver tumors than either cytokine alone.[39] The exact mechanisms of the antitumor effects of TNF are not clearly understood although it appears that TNF has a significant effect on the vascular supply of tumors.[38] Membrane bound TNF may be involved in direct tumor lysis as well.[40] These animal experiments led to extensive tests of recombinant human TNF administered to humans with advanced cancer.[41-45] In the Surgery Branch, NCI, we treated 38 patients with advanced cancer, using escalating doses of recombinant TNF administered in conjunction with IL-2.[41] No antitumor effects of TNF administration were seen in these studies nor were antitumor responses seen following either bolus or continuous infusion administration of TNF in multiple other studies as well.[42-45]

The reason for the discrepancy between the effectiveness of TNF in mice and humans is not fully understood although an important factor appears to be the substantial differences in tolerance of mice and humans to the administration of TNF. Tumor-bearing mice can tolerate from 400 to 500 ug/kg of TNF, and these doses are required to mediate tumor regression; the administration of less TNF is far less effective.[38] In contrast, the maximum dose of TNF tolerated by humans is approximately 8 mg/kg/day.[41] Thus when injected intravenously, only 2% of the TNF dose required to mediate antitumor effects in the mouse can be administered to a person. Because of the unique effectiveness of TNF in the treatment of a variety of murine malignancies we sought means to selectively increase the local concentration of TNF at the tumor site. Because TIL were shown to accumulate at tumor deposits, we hypothesized that TIL producing large amounts of TNF might generate very high TNF concentrations in the local tumor microenvironment and thus achieve concentrations capable of mediating antitumor effects.

Although it would be ideal to test this hypothesis directly using gene transduced murine TIL, it has thus far not been possible to perform gene transduction of murine TIL. We and many other groups have expended substantial effort attempting to introduce genes into short-term murine cytolytic T-lymphocytes or TIL by a variety of techniques including retroviral gene transduction, DNA calcium phosphate precipitation, electroporation, and liposome mediated transfection. These techniques have all been unsuccessful in introducing genes into short-term murine TIL although we have been able to introduce the TNF gene into some long-term noncytotoxic murine T-cell lines. It has thus been essential to utilize indirect evidence to support the hypothesis that human TIL transduced with a TNF gene will mediate antitumor effects.

Using Indium-111 labeled TIL our measurements in humans showed that about 0.015% of the injected cells can traffic to each gram of tumor.[31,32] Thus of 3×10^{11} injected TIL approximately 4.5×10^7 will traffic to each gram of tumor. If highly selected TNF transduced TIL can produce up to 2500 mg of TNF/10^6 cells per 24 hours, then the TIL accumulating at the tumor site will produce approximately 112 mg of TNF/kg of tumor. If we estimate that only a small percentage of the tumor is the interstitial fluid volume, then the equivalent TNF concentration in the interstitial fluid should exceed the 400 ug/kg that murine models predict will be necessary to mediate tumor destruction. These concentrations at the tumor site are approximately 100 times the concentration that can be achieved at the tumor in humans by the intravenous injection of TNF.

An indirect estimate of the impact of high local concentrations of TNF at the tumor site may be achieved by introducing the gene for TNF into murine tumors and studying the effects of this TNF secretion on the growth of these tumor cells when injected *in vivo*. These studies using cytokine genes transduced into tumors will be considered in more detail in a subsequent section of this review. In brief, however, we have shown that transduction of tumors with the TNF gene can result in the production of from 10 to 12 ng of TNF/10^6 cells/24 hrs.[46] Nontransduced tumor cells do not produce TNF. When these murine tumors producing TNF are injected into syngeneic mice, they grow to about 5 mm and then often spontaneously regress, leading to the cure of the mice. Nontransduced tumors or tumors transduced with the NeoR gene alone grow and kill the mice. In similar studies we have introduced the TNF gene into human melanoma cells and injected them into nude mice. These tumor cells also will grow and then often regress while nontransduced human tumors will grow and kill the nude mice. Thus local production of TNF by human tumors can also lead to their destruction. In these studies we have not detected TNF in the serum of animals bearing TNF transduced tumors. When transduced tumors have been removed from animals and placed back into culture, assays of culture supernatants have shown that these cells are continuing to make TNF.

Thus these studies have shown that high local concentrations of TNF in the tumor microenvironment can lead to tumor regression and hold promise that TIL accumulating at tumor sites producing large amounts of TNF might indeed lead to tumor regression in humans.

In further support of this hypothesis are studies in which TNF has been injected directly into tumor nodules in humans. Bartsch and associates injected TNF directly into tumors and showed tumor regression in one of three melanoma patients.[47] In this study an additional patient with a squamous cell cancer of the oral pharynx and a patient with malignant histiocytoma also showed significant shrinkage when TNF was injected into the tumor. A double blind, randomized, placebo controlled study of the intralesional injection of recombinant TNF was reported by Kahn and colleagues.[48] In this study, one Kaposi's sarcoma lesion was injected with recombinant TNF and another Kaposi's sarcoma lesion in the same patient was injected with the same volume of sterile saline. As reported by these authors "TNF reduced the cross sectional area of 12 of 13 (92%) of the injected KS lesions and caused a complete disappearance of two lesions. The placebo response rate was 7% with no complete response observed (p<0.01). There was no observed disease progression in any TNF treated lesion." These studies also suggested that achieving high local concentrations of TNF at the tumor site could lead to tumor regression in humans.

Finally, in 25 patients with metastatic renal cell cancer reported by Blay and associates using lymphokine activated killer (LAK) cells and IL-2, a correlation was found between serum levels of TNF at 48 hours after the end of IL-2 infusion and response to this immunotherapy.[49] Studies in the Surgery Branch using TIL in animal models also suggested that those TIL that specifically secreted cytokines, including TNF, were the TIL with the most potent antitumor activities, and this cytokine secretion correlated far better than did direct tumor lysis with the antitumor efficacy of TIL against established metastases.[23] These studies suggested that secretion of TNF by lymphocytes might play a role in the response to immunotherapy and thus increased production of TNF might increase therapeutic effects. For these reasons we have begun clinical trials in humans utilizing the systemic administration of TIL transduced with the gene for TNF.

The TNF retroviral vector used in these studies was generated by inserting the native full length human TNF-cDNA gene containing the native signal peptide sequence into the retroviral vector LXSN developed by Miller and colleagues.[10-12] A schematic representation of the TNF retroviral vector is shown in Figure 2-6. The human TNF gene is promoted by the retroviral LTR and the Neo^R gene by the SV40 early promoter. Both the promoters are placed in the same orientation. To prevent synthesis of viral proteins from the vector, alterations have been made in the basic vector backbone, including insertion of a stop codon in

TNF-Neo^R Retroviral Construct

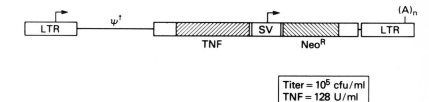

FIG. 2–6 Schematic diagram of the TNF Neo^R retroviral construct. The TNF gene is promoted by the retroviral LTR and the Neo^R gene promoted by the SP40 early promoter.

Titer = 10^5 cfu/ml
TNF = 128 U/ml
(L929)

place of the gag start codon. Similarly, part of the vector has been replaced with the homologous region from the Moloney murine sarcoma virus which is very similar to the Moloney murine leukemia virus but does not make a glycosylated protein. The TNF vector producing cell lines was generated by transfection of the PA317 packaging cell line as discussed earlier in this review.

Although it has been relatively easy to utilize this retroviral vector to transduce both murine and human tumor cells with the genes for TNF and Neo^R, as will be summarized later in this report, it has proven far more difficult to get consistent transduction and expression of the TNF gene in human TIL. Despite multiple attempts to optimize the transduction procedure, transduction efficiencies in the range of 0.1 to 10% have been common. Some patients' TIL appear to be more readily transduced than others, and the reasons underlying this difference are unclear. It has been possible to achieve TNF production by transduced TIL in selected patients in excess of 100 picograms/10^6 cells/24 hours and in selected cells TNF levels in excess of 1000 picograms/10^6 cells/24 hours have been achieved in some patients. TIL producing TNF grow well in culture and retain their growth dependence on IL-2.

Following extensive review, the protocol for the use of these TNF gene modified TIL was approved and treatment of patients with TNF modified TIL begun on January 29, 1991. A schema of the protocol is shown in Table 2-7. In this protocol escalating numbers of TNF transduced TIL are administered to patients in the absence of IL-2 administration. This cautious escalation of the use of TNF transduced TIL was instituted because of the potential toxic side effects that could be induced in patients due to the TNF secretion. Thus far four patients have been entered into this protocol and it is too early to determine whether or not TIL producing TNF will be more effective than unmodified TIL. These studies represent, however, a prototype for the use of TIL potentially modified by other genes for use in the gene therapy of cancer.

Other Potential Modifications of TIL for Use in the Gene Therapy of Cancer ■

In addition to the introduction of the gene for TNF into TIL several other genetic modifications of TIL might improve their therapeutic efficacy. A list of some of these possibilities is shown in Table 2-8.

The increased local secretion of alpha-interferon or gamma-interferon by TIL might have antitumor effects for several reasons. Alpha-interferon has been shown to have a direct antiproliferative effect against some tumor cell types and thus high local concentrations at the tumor site might im-

Table 2–7
Protocol Schema—Revised

TNF-gene Modified TIL
1. Escalate TNF TIL *twice weekly*. No IL-2.
10^8 cells
3×10^8
10^9
3×10^9
10^{10}
3×10^{10}
10^{11}
3×10^{11}
2. Reduce cell dose to *one-tenth* maximum tolerated dose. Escalate as in (1) every *three weeks* with 180,000 IU/kg IL-2.
3. After three patients discuss with the FDA. (Possibly start at a higher cell dose with IL-2.)

Table 2–8
Possible Genetic Modifications
of Tumor-Infiltrating Lymphocytes
to Improve Antitumor Activity

Tumor necrosis factor (interferes with blood supply)
Interferon-alpha or -gamma (upregulated MHC antigens)
Other cytokines such as IL-6, IL-1 alpha, IL-7, RANTES
    (modulates immune response to tumors)
Fc receptor (mediate antibody dependent cellular
    cytotoxicity—ADCC)
Chimeric T-cell receptors (constant region of T-cell
    receptor plus variable region of monoclonal antibody
    alters specificity of T-cell)
IL-2 receptor (increase sensitivity to administered IL-2)

pede tumor growth. In addition, both alpha- and gamma-interferon can upregulate major histocompatibility antigens and other molecules on the cell surface such as tumor antigens or adhesion molecules and thus increase the immunogenicity of these tumor cells. The introduction of other cytokine genes that may be involved in antitumor activity, such as IL-6, IL-1 alpha, IL-7, and RANTES, may also have antitumor effects because of their ability to modulate the immune response at the tumor site.

Modifications of tumor cells that do not affect secretory functions but rather might alter a different functional aspect of the cell might also be useful. TIL do not bear Fc receptors and therefore cannot mediate antibody dependent cellular cytotoxicity. However, because TIL target to tumor sites and have cytolytic capacity, the transduction of TIL with the gene for Fc receptors might induce the ability to mediate antibody-dependent cellular cytotoxicity and thus be a potent therapeutic tool in conjunction with the administration of monoclonal antibodies.

TIL are dependent on IL-2 for their continued survival, and the high doses of IL-2 required to cause TIL proliferation *in vivo* can be associated with substantial toxicity when administered to patients. Transduction of the gene for IL-2 receptors into TIL might increase the sensitivity of TIL to administered IL-2 and thus lessen the need for the high doses of IL-2 currently required.

Recent work by Eshhar and his coworkers has provided an intriguing possibility for extending the use of TIL to tumors for which reactive monoclonal antibodies exist.[50] These workers have made chimeric T-cell receptors by combining the genes coding for the constant region of the T-cell receptor with the variable region of monoclonal antibodies. When these genes are transfected into hybridoma cells, they confer the reactivity of the monoclonal antibody to the hybridoma. These chimeric T-cell receptors can result in triggering lysis or cytokine release from the appropriate hybridoma line. An example of this phenomenon is shown in Table 2-9. We are currently attempting to produce chimeric T-cell receptors by utilizing the constant region of the human T-cell receptor with the variable region of monoclonal antibodies that recognize human gastrointestinal or ovarian tumors. The transduction of these chimeric T-cell receptor genes into TIL may induce the TIL to exhibit the non-MHC-restricted reactivity of the monoclonal antibody.

Table 2–9
Transfecting Chimeric T-Cell Receptor Genes Can Alter
the Specificity of MD.45* Hybridoma Line

Transfected chimeric genes†	Stimulator Cells					
	EL-4	A20**	TNP A20	TNP Mouse Spleen	TNP Human Lymphocyte	TNP KLH
	(IL-2 production, u/ml)					
—	17	0	0	0	0	0
$V_L C_\beta$	50	0	0	1	1	0
$V_H C_\beta$	15	0	23	5	2	6
$V_H C_\beta + V_L C_\alpha$	72	0	108	10	20	150

*MD.45: Murine hybridoma that lyses H-2^b target cells (EL-4)

**A20: B-cell lymphoma from BALB/c mice (H-2^d)

†Variable region from anti-TNP antibody plus constant region of T-cell receptor

This table is adapted from previously published material.[50]

Gene Therapy of Cancer Using Tumor Transduced with Cytokine Genes to Increase Immunogenicity ■

Recent studies have shown that the introduction of genes coding for cytokines into tumor cells can increase the immunogenicity of tumor cells and result in decreased tumor growth.[46,51-58] The potential use of these gene modified tumor cells, either for active immunization against cancer or for the generation of lymphocytes to be used in adoptive immunotherapy, represents an attractive approach to the gene therapy of cancer. The introduction of cytokine genes into tumor cells can also provide a sensitive assay for identifying cytokines with antitumor activity and to elucidate the types of tumor cells susceptible to this type of cytokine gene therapy. A summary of studies of the introduction of cytokine genes into murine tumors is shown in Table 2-10.

Tepper and associates introduced the gene for interleukin-4 (IL-4) into the J558L BALB/c plasmacytoma and the K485 mammary cancer.[51] IL-4 was studied because of its ability to activate MHC-restricted and MHC-unrestricted cytotoxic lymphocytes and macrophages. Tumor cells expressing the IL-4 gene showed reduced tumor growth that was related to the secretion of IL-4. The mixture of nontransfected with transfected tu-

Table 2–10
Introduction of Cytokine Genes into Murine Tumors

Gene inserted	Reference	Tumor	Method	Comments
IL-4	Tepper, et al[51]	J558L BALB/c plasmacytoma K485 mammary cancer	Electroporation or calcium phosphate	Tumor growth reduced or eliminated; related to IL-4 secretion; Nontransfected cells at same site inhibited; Dense macrophage and eosinophil infiltrate
IL-2	Fearon, et al[52]	CT26 BALB/c colon cancer B16 C57BL/6 melanoma	Calcium phosphate	Mediated generation of CTL; activity blocked by anti CD8 and anti MHC Class I antibodies; Tumor growth inhibited; CD8+ cells required *in vivo*
	Gansbacher, et al[53]	CMS-5 BALB/c sarcoma	Retroviral transduction	Tumor growth inhibited; correlated with IL-2 secretion; CTL activity induced; Nontransduced cells at same site inhibited
	Ley, et al[54]	P815 DBA/2 mastocytoma	(not stated)	Growth inhibited
TNF	Asher, et al[46]	MCA-205 C57BL/6 sarcoma	Retroviral transduction	Tumor growth inhibited; correlated with TNF secretion; blocked by anti-TNF antibody Membrane associated TNF detected Nontransduced cells at same site inhibited
	Blankenstein, et al[55]	J558L BALB/c plasmacytoma	Retroviral transduction	Tumor growth inhibited; blocked by anti-TNF antibody and anti-TNF antibody and anti-CR3 antibody Dense macrophage infiltrate (IL-6 transfected tumor showed no growth inhibition)
	Teng, et al[56]	1591 UV induced skin tumor	Lipofection or calcium phosphate	Tumor growth inhibited; Mediated generation of CTL; Increased membrane Class I expression
Gamma-Interferon	Gansbacher, et al[57]	CMS-5 BALB/c sarcoma	Retroviral transduction	Tumor growth inhibited; Mediated generation of CTL; Increased membrane Class I expression
G-CSF	Colombo, et al[58]	C-26 BALB/C colon cancer	Retroviral transduction	Tumor growth inhibited; blocked by anti GCSF antibody; tumor growth inhibited in nude mice

mor cells also resulted in growth inhibition, indicating that the local production of IL-4 could lead to antitumor effects against parental tumor cells at the same site although no effect was seen on tumor cells at distant sites. The rejection of the IL-4 producing tumors was associated with a dense macrophage and eosinophil infiltrate at the tumor site.

Many workers, including Fearon and associates,[52] Gansbacher and colleagues,[53] and Ley and coworkers[54] have introduced the gene for IL-2 into tumor cells, using either calcium phosphate transfection or retroviral mediated gene transduction. These workers used different tumors including colon cancer, melanoma, sarcomas, and mastocytomas, and all showed that introduction and expression of the IL-2 gene could lead to inhibition of growth of the tumor. This activity could be blocked by anti-CD8 or anti-MHC Class I antibodies. Thus CD8+ cells were required *in vivo* to mediate these effects. Fearon and associates hypothesized that the failure of the immune response to the parental tumor was due, in part, to the failure of T-cell help that could be overcome by the local production of cytokines such as IL-2.[52]

Asher and colleagues conducted extensive studies of the retroviral mediated transduction of the TNF gene into mouse sarcomas; these studies are used here as an example of the results obtained by other workers using the TNF gene as well as genes coding for other cytokines.[46] The introduction of TNF genes into a murine sarcoma and subsequent cloning of the tumor cells revealed that different clonal tumor populations had widely varying but stable expression of TNF secretion. An example of the variation of TNF secretion in clonal tumor lines is shown in Figure 2-7. TNF can exist in a secreted or membrane bound form; both types of TNF were found in these tumor cells.

Cells secreting high levels of TNF would grow to a size of several millimeters and then often spontaneously regress. In contrast, cells producing low or no levels of TNF grew progressively and resulted in death of the animals (see Fig. 2-8). The growth inhibition could be inhibited by the administration of anti-TNF antibodies as shown in Figure 2-9. The mechanism of tumor rejection was shown to be related to an immune effect in the host; lymphocyte depletion in the mouse using antibodies to either CD4+ or CD8+ T-cell subpopulations could result in abrogation of tumor inhibition. It thus appeared that both cell subpopulations were necessary to mediate antitumor effects. As was shown by other investigators using other cytokine genes the mixture of cytokine producing cells and noncytokine producing parental cells resulted in the inhibition of the mixture. Studies by Blankenstein and associates[55] and Teng and colleagues,[56] using a BALB/c plasmacytoma and a UV induced skin tumor respectively, have also shown tumor growth inhibition that could be

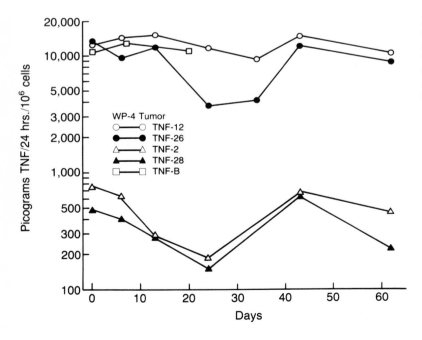

FIG. 2–7 Secretion of TNF by transduced murine tumor cell lines. Note that some clones produced higher levels of TNF compared to other clones and that this production was consistent over 2 months of growth in culture. This figure is from previously published material.[38]

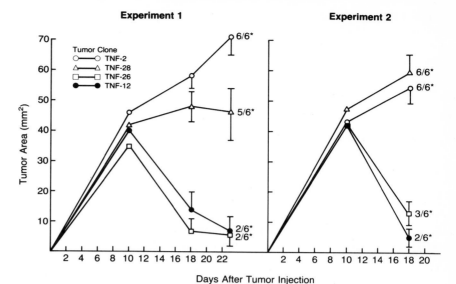

Experiment 1

Experiment 2

Days After Tumor Injection

*Number with tumor/total at day 28

FIG. 2–8 Growth of TNF producing murine tumor clones following injection into mice. High-producing TNF clones grew for about 10 days and then regressed, whereas low-producing clones grew progressively and resulted in death of the mice. This figure is from previously published material.[38]

blocked by anti-TNF antibody and TNF gene modified tumor cells.

Other cytokines are being studied for their potential to reduce tumor growth when introduced into tumor cells. No effect was seen by Blankenstein and associates[55] when introducing the IL-6 gene into tumors. Gansbacher and colleagues[57] saw tumor growth inhibition when introducing the gene for gamma interferon into the CMS-5 BALB/c sarcoma. Interestingly, this growth inhibition was associated with an increased expression

of membrane Class I antigens. Colombo and associates[58] introduced the gene for granulocyte colony stimulating factor (G-CSF) into the C26 BALB/c colon cancer and showed growth inhibition that could be blocked by anti-G-CSF antibody.

No studies have yet demonstrated that active immunization with gene modified tumor cells can reduce the growth of established tumor deposits at distant sites in mice. It is possible, however, that the use of other cytokines or cytokines in combi-

FIG. 2–9 Growth of TNF producing murine tumor clones in mice receiving either anti-TNF antibody or a control anti-TPA antibody. In animals receiving control antibody the tumor grew for approximately 11 days and then regressed. Progressive tumor growth was seen when anti-TNF antibody was administered, indicating that TNF production is involved in the regression of these TNF gene modified tumors. This figure is from previously published material.[38]

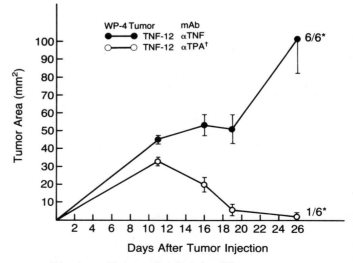

Days After Tumor Injection

*Number with tumor/total at day 28

Table 2–11
Protocol Schema for the Use of Tumor Cells Transduced with the Genes for TNF or IL-2 for the Treatment of Patients with Advanced Cancer

1. Tumor resected as part of standard treatment
2. Tissue culture line established
3. Cytokine gene transduced into culture and cultures selected in G418 (cytokine greater than 100 pg/10^6 cells/ 24 hours)
4. Inject 2×10^8 gene-modified tumor subcutaneously into right thigh and 2×10^7 cells intradermally at two nearby sites.
5. Three weeks later remove draining lymph node and grow in vitro in IL-2
6. Adoptive immunotherapy using these cells plus IL-2

nation may provide a more potent immune stimulus sufficient to reduce growth or cause regression of distant tumors.

Alternatively, gene modified tumor cells could potentially be used to generate immune lymphocytes for use in the adoptive immunotherapy of cancer. Fearon and associates[52] and Gansbacher and colleagues[53] showed that IL-2 modified tumor cells could induce the generation of specific cytotoxic T-lymphocytes that could not be raised to the original parental tumor. Experiments are underway to attempt to use these cytolytic cells for the adoptive therapy of established tumor deposits.

Based on these considerations, a clinical protocol has begun in the surgery branch of the NCI to utilize tumor cells modified by transduction with the gene for IL-2 and TNF for the treatment of patients with advanced cancer. A schema of the protocol is shown in Table 2-11.

Concluding Comments ■

Studies are underway to attempt to use gene transfer technology for the development of new approaches to cancer treatment. Initial studies using TIL modified by transduction with the gene for Neo[R] have shown that retroviral mediated gene transfer can be safely and practically used for the introduction of genes into humans. Attempts are underway to utilize this technology to introduce the genes for tumor necrosis factor into TIL to attempt to improve the therapeutic efficacy of these cells. Other approaches to the gene therapy of cancer involve attempts to modify tumor cells in an attempt to increase their immunogenicity for use in either active immunization against cancer or to raise immune lymphocytes for use in adoptive transfer. Attempts are currently underway to attempt to clone the gene that codes for tumor antigens in both animal and human systems. The identification of these genes could potentially result in their incorporation into viruses for use in active immunization against cancer that may have applications for cancer treatment and prevention.

References ■

1. Rosenberg SA, Aebersold P, Cornetta K, et al. Gene transfer into humans: Immunotherapy of patients with advanced melanoma, using tumor-infiltrating lymphocytes modified by retroviral gene transduction. N Engl J Med 1990;323:570–578.
2. Kriegler, M. Gene transfer and expression. A laboratory manual. New York: Stockton Press, 1990:1–242.
3. Gilboa E, Eglitis MA, Kantoff PW, et al. Transfer and expression of cloned genes using retroviral vectors. BioTechniques 1986;4:504–512.
4. Eglitis MA, Anderson WF. Retroviral vectors for introduction of genes into mammalian cells. BioTechniques 1988;6:608–614.
5. Adam MA, Miller AD. Identification of a signal in a murine retrovirus that is sufficient for packaging of nonretroviral RNA into virions. J Virol 1988;62:3802–3806.
6. Armentano D, Yu SF, Kantoff PW, et al. Effect of internal viral sequences on the utility of retroviral vectors. J Virol 1987;61:1647–1650.
7. Bender MA, Palmer TD, Gelinas RE, et al.: Evidence that the packaging signal of Moloney murine leukemia virus extends into the gag region. J Virol 1987;61:1639–1646.
8. Danos O, Mulligan RC. Safe and efficient generation of recombinant retroviruses with amphotropic and ecotropic host ranges. Proc Natl Acad Sci USA 1988;85:6460–6464.
9. Markowitz D, Goff S, Bank A. Construction and use of a safe and efficient amphotropic packaging cell line. Virol 1989;167:400–406.
10. Miller AD, Buttimore C. Redesign of retrovirus packaging cell lines to avoid recombination leading to helper virus production. Mol Cell Biol 1986;6:2895–2902.
11. Miller AD, Trauber DR, Buttimore C. Factors involved in the production of helper virus-free retrovirus vectors. Somatic Cell Mol Genet 1986;12:175–183.
12. Miller AD, Rosman GJ. Improved retroviral vectors for gene transfer and expression. BioTechniques 1989;7:980–986.
13. Friedmann T. Progress toward human gene therapy. Science 1989;244:1275–1281.
14. Rosenberg SA, Spiess P, Lafreniere R. A new approach to the adoptive immunotherapy of cancer with tumor-infiltrating lymphocytes. Science 1986;223:1318–1321.
15. Spiess PJ, Yang JC, Rosenberg SA. *In vivo* antitumor activity of tumor-infiltrating lymphocytes expanded in recombinant interleukin-2. JNCI 1987;79:1067–1075.
16. Muul LM, Spiess PJ, Director EP, et al. Identification of

specific cytolytic immune responses against autologous tumor in humans bearing malignant melanoma. J Immunol 1986;138:989–995.

17. Itoh K, Tilden AB, Balch CM. Interleukin-2 activation of cytotoxic T-lymphocytes infiltrating into human metastatic melanomas. Cancer Res 1986;46:3011–3017.

18. Kurnick JT, Kradin RL, Blumberg R, et al. Functional characterization of T-lymphocytes propagated from human lung carcinomas. Clin Immunol Immunopathol 1986;38:367–380.

19. Rabinowich H, Cohen R, Bruderman I. Functional analysis of mononuclear cells infiltrating into tumors: lysis of autologous human tumor cells by cultured infiltrating lymphocytes. Cancer Res 1987;47:173–177.

20. Miescher S, Whiteside TL, Moretta L, et al. Clonal and frequency analyses of tumor-infiltrating T-lymphocytes from human solid tumors. J Immunol 1987;138:4004–4011.

21. Topalian SL, Solomon D, Rosenberg SA. Tumor-specific cytolysis by lymphocytes infiltrating human melanomas. J Immunol 1989;142:3714–3725.

22. Barth RJ, Bock SN, Mulé JJ, et al. Unique murine tumor-associated antigens identified by tumor-infiltrating lymphocytes. J Immunol 1990;144:1531–1537.

23. Barth RJ, Mulé JJ, Spiess PJ. Interferon gamma and tumor necrosis factor have a role in tumor regressions mediated by murine CD8+ tumor-infiltrating lymphocytes. J Exp Med 1991;173:647–658.

24. Schwartzentruber DJ, Topalian SL, Mancini M, et al. Specific release of granulocyte-macrophage colony-stimulating factor, tumor necrosis factor-α, and IFN-υ by human tumor-infiltrating lymphocytes after autologous tumor stimulation. J Immunol 1991;146:3674–3681.

25. Yang JC, Perry-Lalley D, Rosenberg SA. An improved method for growing murine TIL with in vivo antitumor activity. J Biol Response Modif 1990;9:149.

26. Belldegrun A, Muul LM, Rosenberg SA. Interleukin-2 expanded tumor-infiltrating lymphocytes in human renal cell cancer: isolation, characterization, and antitumor activity. Cancer Res 1988;48:206–214.

27. Hom SS, Topalian SL, Simoni ST, et al. Common expression of melanoma tumor-associated antigens recognized by human tumor-infiltrating lymphocytes: analysis by HLA restriction. J Immunotherp 1991;10:153–164.

28. Topalian SL, Kasid AL, Rosenberg SA. Immunoselection of a human melanoma resistant to specific lysis by autologous tumor-infiltrating lymphocytes: possible mechanism for immunotherapeutic failures. J Immunol 1990;144:4487–4495.

29. Rosenberg SA, Packard BS, Aebersold PM, et al. Use of tumor-infiltrating lymphocytes and interleukin-2 in the immunotherapy of patients with metastatic melanoma: a preliminary report. N Engl J Med 1988;319:1676–1680.

30. Aebersold P, Hyatt C, Johnson S, et al. Lysis of autologous melanoma cells by tumor-infiltrating lymphocytes is associated with clinical response. J Natl Cancer Inst, in press.

31. Fisher B, Packard BS, Read EJ, et al. Tumor localization of adoptively transferred indium-111 labeled tumor-infiltrating lymphocytes in patients with metastatic melanoma. J Clin Oncol 1989;7:250–261.

32. Griffith KD, Read EJ, Carrasquillo JA, et al. In vivo distribution of adoptively transferred indium-111 labeled tumor-infiltrating lymphocytes and peripheral blood lymphocytes in patients with metastatic melanoma. J Natl Cancer Inst 1989;81:1709–1717.

33. Kasid A, Morecki S, Aebersold P, et al. Human gene transfer: characterization of human tumor-infiltrating lymphocytes as vehicles for retroviral-mediated gene transfer in man. Proc Natl Acad Sci USA 1990;87:473–477.

34. Culver K, Cornetta K, Morgan, R, et al. Lymphocytes as cellular vehicles for gene therapy in mouse and man. Proc Natl Acad Sci USA 1991;88:3155–3159.

35. Cornetta K, Morgan RA, Anderson WF. Safety issues related to retroviral-mediated gene transfer in humans. Human Gene Therapy, in press.

36. Carswell EA, Old LJ, Kassel RC, et al. An endotoxin-induced serum factor that causes necrosis of tumors. Proc Natl Acad Sci USA 1975;72:3666–3670.

37. Wang AM, Creasy AA, Ladner MB, et al. Molecular cloning of the complementary DNA for human tumor necrosis factor. Science 228:149–154.

38. Asher AL, Mulé JJ, Reichert CM, et al. Studies of the antitumor efficacy of systemically administered recombinant tumor necrosis factor against several murine tumors in vivo. J Immunol 1987;138:963–974.

39. McIntosh JE, Mulé JJ, Merino MJ, et al. Synergistic antitumor effects of immunotherapy with recombinant interleukin-2 and recombinant tumor necrosis factor-alpha. Cancer Res 1988;48:4011–4017.

40. Kriegler M, Perez C, DeFay K, et al. A novel form of TNF/cachectin is a cell surface cytotoxic transmembrane protein: ramifications for the complex physiology of TNF. Cell 1988;53:45–53.

41. Rosenberg SA, Lotze MT, Yang JC, et al. Experience with the use of high-dose interleukin-2 in the treatment of 652 cancer patients. Ann Surg 1989;210:474–485.

42. Spriggs DR, Sherman ML, Michie H, et al. Recombinant human tumor necrosis factor administered as a 24-hour intravenous infusion: a phase I and pharmacologic study. J Natl Cancer Inst 1988;80:1039–1044.

43. Sherman ML, Spriggs DR, Arthur KA, et al. Recombinant human tumor necrosis factor administered as a five-day continuous infusion in cancer patients: Phase I toxicity and effects on lipid metabolism. J Clin Oncol 1988;6:344–350.

44. Feinberg B, Kurzrock R, Talpaz M, et al. A phase I trial of intravenously administered recombinant tumor necrosis factor-alpha in cancer patients. J Clin Oncol 1988;6:1328–1334.

45. Moritz T, Niederle N, Baumann J, et al. Phase I study of recombinant human tumor necrosis factor-alpha in advanced malignant disease. Cancer Immunol Immunother 1989;29:144–150.

46. Asher AL, Mulé JJ, Kasid A, et al. Murine tumor cells transduced with the gene for tumor necrosis factor-α: evidence for paracrine immune effects of tumor necrosis factor against tumors. J Immunol 1991;146:3227–3234.

47. Bartsch HH, Pfizemaier K, Schroeder M, et al. Intralesional application of recombinant human TNF factor-alpha induces local tumor regression in patients with advanced malignancies. Europ J Cancer Clin Oncol 1989;25:285–291.

48. Kahn J, Kaplan J, Zeigler P. Phase II trial of intralesional recombinant tumor necrosis factor-alpha (rTNF) for AIDS associated Kaposi's sarcoma (ks). Proc Am Soc Clin Oncol 1989;8:4.

49. Blay JY, Favrot MC, Negrier S, et al. Correlation be-

tween clinical response to interleukin-2 therapy and sustained production of tumor necrosis factor. Cancer Res 1990;50:2371–2374.

50. Gross G, Waks T, Eshhar Z. Expression of immunoglobulin-T-cell receptor chimeric molecules as functional receptors with antibody-type specificity. Proc Natl Acad Sci 1989;86:10024–10028.

51. Tepper RI, Pattengale PK, Leder P. Murine interleukin-4 displays potent antitumor activity *in vivo*. Cell 1989;57:503–5121.

52. Fearon ER, Pardoll DM, Itaya T, et al. Interleukin-2 production by tumor cells bypasses T-helper function in the generation of an antitumor response. Cell 1990;60:397–403.

53. Gansbacher B, Zier K, Daniels B, et al. Interleukin-2 gene transfer into tumor cells abrogates tumorigenicity and induces protective immunity. J Exp Med 1990;172:1217–1224.

54. Ley V, Roth C, Langlade-Demoyen P, et al. A novel approach to the induction of specific cytolytic T-cells *in vivo*. Res Immunol 1990;141:855–863.

55. Blankenstein T, Qin Z, Uberla K, et al. Tumor suppression after tumor cell-targeted tumor necrosis factor-α gene transfer. J Exp Med 1991;173:1047–1052.

56. Teng MN, Park BH, Koeppen HKW, et al. Long-term inhibition of tumor growth by tumor necrosis factor in the absence of cachexia or T-cell immunity. Proc Natl Acad Sci 1991;88:3535–3539.

57. Gansbacher B, Bannerji R, Daniels B, et al. Retroviral vector-mediated υ-interferon gene transfer into tumor cells generates potent and long lasting antitumor immunity. Cancer Res 1990;50:7820–7825.

58. Colombo MP, Gerrari G, Stoppacciaro A, et al. Granulocyte colony-stimulating factor gene transfer suppresses tumorigenicity of a murine adenocarcinoma *in vivo*. J Exp Med 1991;173:889–897.

Beverly A. Teicher

Terence S. Herman

Emil Frei III

Perfluorochemical Emulsions: Oxygen Breathing in Radiation Sensitization and Chemotherapy Modulation

3

Cancer patients are usually anemic, and evidence is accumulating that anemia is an important prognostic factor. Furthermore, increasing hemoglobin levels into the normal range can improve prognosis and treatment outcome.[1] Solid tumor masses are very heterogeneous in oxygenation and contain regions of hypoxia.[1,2] External pressure on capillaries resulting from rapid and uncontrolled cell proliferation within malignant tumors causes blood vessels to constrict or collapse so that red blood cell passage is restricted.[3–9] Furthermore, deficient vascular beds within solid tumors cause areas of severe vascular insufficiency and, often, regions of frank necrosis.[10–13] Thomlinson and Gray[3] described the occurrence of small necrotic volumes in tumors at sites distant from capillaries and were able to calculate, based on the diffusion characteristics of O_2, that hypoxic but still viable cells would be present at distances of about 130 μm from the axis of the capillary blood vessels.[1–3] This pattern of tumor growth has been observed in many animal and some human tumors.

In situ observations of growing tumors have revealed rapidly opening and closing blood vessels.[9] Recently, the therapeutic significance of acute or partial hypoxia, which are consequences of vascular flux, as well as chronic hypoxia have been reviewed.[14,15] As measured by radiobiologic methods[16,17] and by direct pO_2 measurements,[18–20] hypoxia is present in most animal solid tumor models. Several recent studies with oxygen electrodes have reaffirmed the occurrence of significant hypoxic areas within human tumors.[1,21,22] Preclinical studies both *in vitro* and *in vivo* have established that hypoxia protects cells from the cytotoxic actions of radiation and many chemotherapeutic agents and thereby may be a significant factor in therapeutic resistance.[2,23–25] Gatenby and associates[22] have measured the oxygen distribution in nodal metastases of human squamous cell carcinoma and have been able to correlate the oxygen tension in these masses with the response of the tumors to radiation therapy. Twelve of 31 tumors studied had greater than 26% of their volume containing a pO_2 less than 8 mm Hg.[22] Vaupel and coworkers,[20] Groebe and Vaupel,[26] and Kallinowski and colleagues[27] found in human breast cancer xenografts growing in nude rats that, as tumor mass increased, the O_2 consumption rate per unit weight significantly decreased. This decreased O_2 consumption rate of the cancer cells *in vivo* was the result of the increasingly deficient blood supply, with increasing tumor size. Even in small tumors, however, some areas of hypoxia were commonly found.[20,26,27] Kallinowski and coworkers[21] and Vaupel[1] have reported oxygen measurements from human breast carcinoma and human cervix cancer as well as adjacent normal tissue. A relatively high percentage of hypoxic regions was found in many human malignancies. It now appears certain that the vast majority of solid tumors contain hypoxic cells, which frequently constitute 10–20% of the total viable tumor-cell population.[28,29]

Cells grown in culture as spheroids (i.e., small balls of tightly packed cells) show central necrosis and evidence of hypoxia when grown to greater than 0.35 mm in diameter.[30] It is quite probable, therefore, that even in occult metastases, too small to be detected by standard diagnostic techniques, foci of hypoxic cells are present and have therapeutic implications.

Importance of Hypoxic Cells in Cancer Therapy ■

Hypoxia has long been known to protect cells from the cytotoxic effects of radiation. Hypoxic cells surviving large doses of radiation are capable of either reestablishing the tumor *in situ* or producing tumors in other animals after transplantation.[11–13] This effect is most marked after administration of large single fractions of radiation. Fractionated radiotherapy of animal tumors results in a more complex situation, because "reoxygenation" may occur between treatments. During reoxygenation, the tumor cells that were hypoxic at the time of irradiation become better perfused, presumably because of the death of radiosensitive normally oxygenated cells situated between them and tumor capillaries. These previously hypoxic cells then reacquire the radiosensitivity characteristic of aerobic cells. As a consequence, the sensitivity of the tumor to subsequent irradiation is increased. Patterns of reoxygenation in tumors vary widely, however. Some tumors reoxygenate rapidly and extensively but others reoxygenate slowly.[31,32]

The importance of hypoxic cells in limiting the sensitivity of human tumors to conventional, fractionated radiotherapy regimens is still debated extensively. Some clinical data[33] and extrapolations from animal tumors in which reoxygenation occurs quite slowly suggest that hypoxic cells probably limit the curability of certain types of human cancer by fractionated radiotherapy.

The relative antineoplastic selectivity of many chemotherapeutic agents in current clinical use for the treatment of cancer derives from the toxicity of the drugs to cells that are actively traversing the cell cycle. Cycle-active agents are relatively ineffective against quiescent tumor cells that are not actively cycling at the time of treatment and cells in nutritionally deficient environments are typically noncycling. Quiescent cells are present in both animal and human tumors, and the quiescent cells of animal tumors are "clonogenic" (i.e., capable of proliferation). Even for anticancer agents that are capable of readily killing noncycling cells, hypoxic cells may be resistant for the following reasons: (1) These cells may have prolonged cell cycle times or may be blocked in their progression through the G_1 phase. Cells that remain out of mitosis for prolonged periods are better able to repair DNA damage caused by many anticancer drugs.[29,31] (2) Appropriate concentrations of drugs that have physiochemical properties not conducive to diffusion into tumor tissue or that are unstable or metabolized rapidly may not reach chronically hypoxic tumor cells located in regions of severe vascular insufficiency.[3,4,24,25] (3) Some chemotherapeutic agents require the presence of O_2 for maximal cytotoxicity.[24–25]

A variety of strategies have been developed in the laboratory to overcome the problem of hypoxia. These strategies include (1) the use of hypoxic cell selective cytotoxic agents, (2) the use of "oxygen mimics" as radiation and chemosensitizers, (3) the use of hyperbaric oxygen, and (4) the use of perfluorochemical emulsions with oxygen or carbogen (95% oxygen/5% carbon dioxide) breathing.[2,23,25,34–39] Each of four methods for producing an increased therapeutic attack on hypoxic cells is currently undergoing clinical trial.[40–45]

Perfluorochemical Emulsions: Oxygen Carriers ■

Increased delivery of oxygen from the lungs can be a useful way of improving the oxygenation of solid tumor masses by altering the gradient of oxygen as it is absorbed from the vasculature and distributed into the tissue. The use of hyperbaric oxygen in conjunction with radiation therapy was tested in clinical trials in England over about a 12-year period beginning in the mid-1960s.[46,47]

Bush and associates[33] reported that hypoxia influences the local control rate with radiotherapy for patients with advanced carcinoma of the cervix. In this study of 2803 patients a significant difference existed in the local control rates, for all patients analyzed according to hemoglobin levels.

Those patients with hemoglobin concentrations <12g% had a poorer prognosis than those with higher hemoglobin concentrations. The hyperbaric oxygen trials were positive for certain tumor types.[33,47] Much less work has been done with hyperbaric oxygen and chemotherapy.

The use of perfluorochemical emulsions and carbogen or oxygen breathing has been explored extensively with very positive results in preclinical solid tumor models in conjunction with radiation therapy.[38,39,48–59] Some initial clinical trials of the perfluorochemical emulsion, Fluosol-DA, and oxygen breathing with radiation therapy have been carried out and some are still underway.[42–45] The effect of perfluorochemical emulsions and carbogen or oxygen breathing with many chemotherapeutic agents has also been studied in preclinical solid tumor models.[25,35,36,60–72] With many chemotherapeutic agents very positive therapeutic results were also obtained, and several initial clinical trials have been carried out with Fluosol-DA and oxygen breathing with single anticancer drugs.[73–75]

Clark and Gollan[76] demonstrated in 1966 that liquid perfluorochemicals could sustain life when mice were immersed in them for long periods. Then in 1967, Sloviter and Kamimoto[77] reported successful perfusion of rat brains with perfluorochemicals. In 1986, Geyer[78] demonstrated by total blood replacement in rats that perfluorochemicals in an emulsified form can function as oxygen carriers as well as red blood cells. Intravenous infusions of perfluorochemical (PFC) liquids, however, cause the death of animals because these substances are imiscible in aqueous media and thus form emboli. Therefore, these substances must be suspended as fine particles (emulsions) when they are used as artificial blood substitutes.

The size of the particles is important in relation to the retention and behavior of the particles in circulation. The half-life of a fine emulsion in rabbits (with a particle size of 0.1 μm in average diameter) was about 85 hours, whereas that of a coarse emulsion (0.25 μm in average diameter) was about 30 hours. By comparison, the average diameter for red blood cells is 5–10 μm. In emulsions with larger particles, the emulsion particles tend to clump and also form emboli.

Perfluorochemicals are metabolically inert and are transpired through the lungs. After many perfluorocarbons had been screened, perfluorodecalin was found to be the best compound with respect to rate of excretion. It was difficult, however, to form a stable emulsion from perfluorodecalin alone; therefore, other perfluorocarbons

were used in combination with perfluorodecalin.[79,80] Using the mixed perfluorocarbon technique developed by Geyer, the Green Cross Corporation of Japan found that the addition of perfluorotripropylamine significantly increased the stability of the emulsion. The perfluorochemical emulsion selected for clinical testing was named Fluosol-DA.

Composition of Fluosol-DA 20%		
Perfluorodecalin	14.0	w/v%
Perfluorotripropylamine	6.0	w/v%
Pluronic-F68	2.7	w/v%
Yolk phospholipids	0.4	w/v%
Potassium oelate	0.032	w/v%
Glycerol	0.8	w/v%
NaCl	0.6	w/v%
KCl	0.034	w/v%
Glucose	0.180	w/v%
$MgCl_2$	0.020	w/v%
$CaCl_2$	0.028	w/v%
$NaHCO_3$	0.210	w/v%
pH: 7.4-7.6		

The emulsion consists of 20% perfluorochemical, with seven parts of perfluorodecalin and three parts of perfluorotripropylamine, Pluronic-F68, and phospholipids as emulsifier, and glycerol as a cryoprotecting agent. To furnish the preparation with physiological osmolarity and oncotic pressure, Kreb's Ringers bicarbonate solution was included.

The volume of oxygen dissolved in Fluosol-DA changes linearly with oxygen partial pressure, according to Henry's law. The uptake and release of oxygen (and CO_2) are completely reversible, as with hemoglobin, and the rate is very fast, twice as fast as that of hemoglobin. The combined surface area of the particles is 1.82×10^8 cm^2 per liter available for oxygen diffusion. This is about 100 times greater than that of blood, which contains a surface area of 1.86×10^6 cm^2 oxygen-carrying particles per liter.

Perfluorochemicals have limited oxygen-transport capability at ambient pressures. Oxygen content is linear with respect to oxygen tension, as opposed to blood, in which the relation is sigmoid for oxygen. Blood delivers approximately 6 vol% oxygen to tissues at ambient pressures, whereas at these same pressures, Fluosol-DA 20% can deliver only about 2 vol%. If oxygen pressure is increased to 1 atm of inspired gas (FiO$_2$ 1.0), however, the amount of oxygen that can be delivered by Fluosol-DA 20% is about 6.5 vol%. Evidence suggests that a lower oxygen pressure (FiO$_2$ 0.85) can be used if the concentration of perfluorochemicals is increased.

The particle size distribution of the Fluosol-DA emulsion, as determined by centrifugal sedimentation and electron microscopy, is in a narrow range, and 90% or more of the particles are smaller than 0.2 μm in diameter. The particles are coated with a layer of phospholipid and the detergent Pluoronic F-68. The small size allows the emulsion particles to flow through very small capillaries, leading to tissue volumes where red cells cannot reach. The corollary to this is that oxygen can at least enter areas of small capillary microcirculation. The particle size also will influence emulsion stability and viscosity. Biologically, particle size also will affect transit time, distribution, and therefore possibly toxicity.

Fluosol-DA/Oxygen Breathing and Radiation ■

Three times more radiation is required to kill fully anoxic cells than normally oxygenated cells. Radiosensitization, however, occurs at relatively low concentrations of oxygen. A concentration of 0.25% oxygen moves the dose-response curve halfway toward the fully aerated condition, with essentially identical dose-response curves obtained for cells in 2, 20, or 100% oxygen. Therefore, a small amount of oxygen delivered to hypoxic regions of a solid tumor would significantly increase the radiosensitivity of those tumor regions. The potential of perfluorochemical emulsions and carbogen breathing to improve the oxygenation of hypoxic regions in the several murine tumors has been investigated by Song and coworkers using oxygen microelectrodes.[52,53,58,81,82] Measurement of intratumoral pO$_2$ by oxygen microelectrodes demonstrated significant increases in pO$_2$ when Fluosol-DA was injected into the animals and the animals breathed carbogen (95% O$_2$, 5% CO$_2$). Hiraga and colleagues[83] and Klubes and associates[84] found that cerebral vascular flow increased approximately twofold following complete blood-perfluorochemical exchange and 1.5-fold after partial exchange. A similar 1.5-fold increase in flow was measured in intraparenchymal tumors following partial exchange. Thus, it appears that

perfluorochemical emulsions are capable of improving tumor oxygenation both by serving as a carrier for oxygen and by increasing tumor vascular flow.

The perfluorochemical emulsion Fluosol-DA in combination with breathing a 100% or 95% oxygen atmosphere has enhanced the response of several solid rodent tumors to single dose and fractionated radiation treatments.[37–39,48–58,81,82,85–87]

In the application of this methodology to the clinic, questions arise regarding the lowest effective dose and the scheduling of perfluorochemical emulsion in a course of fractionated radiation therapy. We have used the Lewis lung-tumor model to address these questions in an animal tumor system.[49] X-rays were delivered as three Gy fractions twice per day. Fluosol-DA was administered once per day at a dose of 4 mL, 8 mL, or 12 mL per kg of body weight (Fig. 3-1). The dose-modifying factors (DMF) observed at a tumor growth delay time of six days were 1.42 ± 0.16 at 4 mL/kg, 1.85 ±

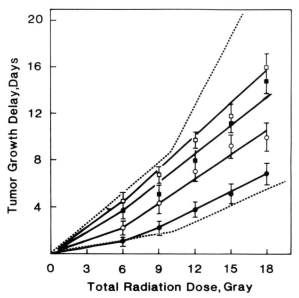

FIG. 3–1 Growth delay of the Lewis lung tumor produced by various doses of Fluosol-DA and fractionated X-ray treatment. Radiation was delivered in 3 Gy fractions twice per day and Fluosol-DA administered once per day. In all groups, carbogen breathing was maintained for 1 hour prior to and during each fraction. (□) 12 mL/kg Fluosol-DA; (■) 8 mL/kg Fluosol-DA; (0) 4 mL/kg Fluosol-DA; (●) no Fluosol-DA; (•••, upper) single dose x-ray treatment and 12 mL/kg Fluosol-DA; (•••, lower) single dose x-ray treatment in the absence of Fluosol-DA. Teicher, Rose[48,49]

0.23 at 8 mL/kg, and 2.17 ± 0.34 at 12 mL/kg. Although the dose modification seen at 12 mL/kg was greater than that seen at 8 mL/kg, this difference was not statistically significant (p < 0.5). Both 12 mL/kg and 8 mL/kg were significantly better than 4 mL/kg (p < 0.0006 and p < 0.0024, respectively). For all treatments, the enhancement in tumor growth delay was highly significant, as compared with results in carbogen-breathing controls (p < 0.0001 with 12 mL/kg and 8 mL/kg and p < 0.005 with 4 mL/kg.

In clinical practice, it is unlikely that perfluorochemical emulsions would be administered daily. In an effort to somewhat mimic a clinical regimen, we administered a single dose of Fluosol-DA (12 mL/kg) on day 1 of the treatment program and delivered radiation in 2, 3, or 4 Gy fractions on days 1 to 5, one fraction per day (Fig. 3-2).[49] The DMF observed in Fluosol-DA treated animals when carbogen breathing was maintained for one hour prior to and during each radiation fraction, was 2.60 ± 0.54, which is not significantly different from the dose modification seen with Fluosol-DA/carbogen and a single dose of x-rays.[49] This indicates that some effect of Fluosol-DA persists over several days or that breathing a high oxygen content atmosphere even after the Fluosol-DA effect is diminished can be of therapeutic benefit. In this protocol, Fluosol-DA and air breathing did not lead to dose modification. Although Fluosol-DA/air breathing, as compared with carbogen in the absence of Fluosol-DA, produced 0.5 to 1.0 additional days of tumor growth delay, this difference was not statistically significant.

As an approach to determining the optimal dose schedule for Fluosol-DA during a course of fractionated radiation therapy, a total dose of 16 mL/kg of Fluosol-DA was administered either as two doses of 8 mL/kg on days 1 and 3 or as four doses of 4 mL/kg on days 1, 2, 3 and 4 of a four-day protocol using the Lewis lung tumor model system (Fig. 3-3). The Lewis lung tumor was grown s.c. in the flanks of C57BL/6J mice. Treatment was initiated when the tumors were 50–100 mm.[3] Radiation was delivered as 4 daily fractions of 2.5, 4.0, or 5.0 Gray. Fluosol-DA was administered i.v. prior to irradiation. Each day carbogen breathing was maintained for 1 hour prior to and during each x-ray treatment. When Fluosol-DA was administered as two doses of 8 mL/kg, the DMF observed was 1.7 ± 0.3. When Fluosol-DA was given as

FIG. 3–2 Growth delay of the Lewis lung tumor produced by a single dose of 12 mL/kg of Fluosol-DA and five daily fractions of x-rays. (0) Fluosol-DA and 1 hour of carbogen breathing prior to and during each x-ray fraction; (▢) Fluosol-DA and air breathing; (●) 1 hour of carbogen breathing prior to and during each x-ray fraction (•••, upper) Fluosol-DA and carbogen breathing with single dose x-ray treatment; (•••, lower) carbogen breathing with single x-ray treatment. Holden, Herman, Teicher[35,36]

FIG. 3–3 Growth delay of the Lewis lung tumor produced by two schedules of Fluosol-DA and four daily fractions of x-rays. (●) Fractionated x-ray treatment with carbogen breathing for 1 hour prior to and during each fraction. (■) Fluosol-DA (0.1 mL; 4 mL/kg) was administered prior to each x-ray treatment with carbogen breathing 1 hour prior to and during each fraction. (0) Fluosol-DA (0.2 mL; 8 mL/kg) was administered on treatment days 1 and 3, carbogen breathing was maintained for 1 hour prior to and during each fraction. Teicher, McIntosh[85]

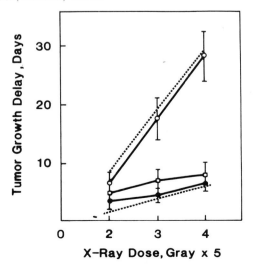

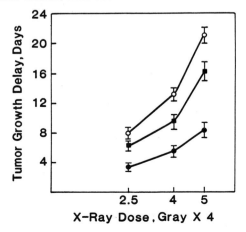

four doses of 4 mL/kg, the DMF was 1.5 ± 0.3 compared to x-ray treatment with carbogen breathing. It appears, therefore, that administering Fluosol-DA at a therapeutic dose less frequently with carbogen breathing with every radiation fraction may produce a better treatment outcome than giving more frequent lower doses.

Fluosol-DA emulsion particles are taken up by the reticuloendothelial system, causing reversible hepatomegaly and splenomegaly. No enhanced radiation toxicity has been seen in sensitive normal tissues in animals treated with Fluosol-DA and oxygen breathing with radiation.[88] An exciting possibility for Fluosol-DA in radiation therapy is to use Fluosol-DA in combination with hyperbaric oxygen, which will significantly increase the amount of oxygen carried by the perfluorochemical.[89]

Fluosol-DA/Oxygen Breathing and Alkylating Agents ■

The level of cellular oxygenation is also an important factor in the action of many antineoplastic agents, several of which have been classified *in vitro*[24] and *in vivo*[25] by their selective cytotoxicity toward oxygenated and hypoxic tumor cells. Fluosol-DA and carbogen breathing have been shown to enhance the antitumor activity and cytocidal activity of each of the antitumor tumor alkylating agents studied here: cis-diamminedichloroplatinum(II) (CDDP) (19-21),[25,36,63,72] carboplatin, cyclophosphamide,[25,36,63,72] N,N′,N″-triethylenethiophosphoramide(thioTEPA),[90] 1,3-bis (2-chloroethyl)-1-nitrosourea(BNCU),[51,66] and L-phenylalanine mustard().[60-63] The Fluosol-DA/oxygen approach is perhaps best adapted to chemotherapy, since chemotherapy can be delivered effectively in every-three-week courses, which may consist of only one or two days of treatment. This would fit in more effectively with Fluosol-DA/oxygen than would, for example, daily radiotherapy.

However, because of the short diffusion distance and metabolic instability of oxygen, it is unlikely that Fluosol-DA and carbogen or oxygen breathing can be 100% efficient in oxygenating tumor masses.[81,82] Using micro-oxygen electrodes, Hasegawa and colleagues[82] and Song[81] showed substantially increased oxygenation of tumors in the presence of Fluosol-DA/carbogen, but some

hypoxic regions remained. These regions of hypoxic cells may remain viable and contribute to tumor regrowth. Use of selective hypoxic cell cytotoxic agents in conjunction with Fluosol-DA plus oxygen breathing is, therefore, a logical combination approach.

It has been well established that the nitroimidazole radiosensitizing agents can also act as selective cytotoxic drugs for hypoxic cells.[91-94] In addition, these compounds, which are said to mimic the effect of oxygen in cells, have been shown to enhance the cytotoxicity of several antitumor alkylating agents including L-PAM, cyclophosphamide, BCNU, and 1-(2-chloroethyl)-3-cyclohexyl-1-nitrosourea *in vitro* and *in vivo*. This phenomenon has been termed chemosensitization.[13,95] The presence of hypoxic cells in solid tumors may account for the preferential effect, since chemosensitization *in vitro* occurs only when cells are exposed to misonidazole under hypoxic conditions, that is, conditions in which reduction of misonidazole through formation of oxygen-mimicking free radical can occur. For these reasons, we examined the ability of the 2-nitroimidazole etanidazole to act as a chemosensitizer of a series of antitumor alkylating agents in conjunction with Fluosol-DA and carbogen breathing.

Tumor cell survival assay in the FSaIIC murine fibrosarcoma demonstrated that when the modulator Fluosol-DA (0.3 mL; 12 mL/kg i.v.) was administered just prior to an alkylating agent plus carbogen breathing for 6 h or the modulator etanidazole (1 g/kg i.p.) was administered just prior to an alkylating agent, the combination treatment produced significantly more tumor cell killing across the dosage range of each alkylating agent tested compared with the alkylating agent alone.[96] Each alkylating agent produced a dose-dependent log-linear tumor cell survival curve. There was a five- to tenfold increase in tumor cell killing when either Fluosol-DA/carbogen or etanidazole was added to treatment with the alkylating agent. For CDDP and thioTEPA, the modulators used in combination increased tumor cell killing by only two- to threefold over that obtained with a single modulator, but for the other alkylating agents, tumor cell killing was increased by ten- to fiftyfold when the combination of modulators was used. Bone marrow granulocyte-macrophage colony-forming unit survival assay showed that the combination of modulators with the alkylating agents result in only small increases in bone marrow toxicity of the alkylating agents except for thioTEPA, and L-PAM, for which the toxicity to the bone

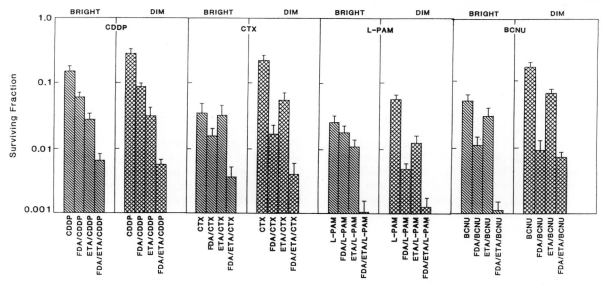

FIG. 3–4   Survival of subpopulations based on Hoechst 33342 fluorescence intensity of FSaIIC cells from FSaIIC tumor treated with a single dose of CDDP (10 mg/kg). CTX (150 mg/kg), L-PAM (10 mg/kg) or BCNU (50 mg/kg) with or without etanidazole (1 g/kg) and/or Fluosol-DA (12 mL/kg) and carbogen breathing (6h). *Points*, means of 3 independent determinations ± SE (*bars*). Reprinted from Teicher, *et al.*[96]

Table 3–1

Growth Delay of the FSaIIC and EMT-6 Tumors by Alkylating Agents With or Without the Combined Modulation of Etanidazole and Fluosol-DA/Carbogen (6h)

	Tumor Growth Delay[b] (days)			
Treatment Groups	Drug Alone[a]	Fluosol-DA/Carbogen[c]	Etanidazole[d]	Etanidazole/ Fluosol-DA/ Carbogen
		FSaIIC fibrosarcoma		
No drug		0.2 ± 0.3	0.3 ± 0.5	2.7 ± 0.5
CDDP (10 mg/kg)	7.7 ± 0.7	12.8 ± 1.3	12.3 ± 1.6	16.1 ± 1.1
Carboplatin (50 mg/kg)	5.2 ± 0.5	16.4 ± 1.7	7.8 ± 1.3	22.1 ± 3.2
Cyclophosphamide (150 mg/kg)	4.2 ± 0.5	13.9 ± 1.5	5.3 ± 0.7	15.11 ± .2
ThioTEPA (10 mg/kg)	3.0 ± 0.4	6.2 ± 1.2	4.2 ± 0.4	87.91 ± .1
BCNU (15 mg/kg)	2.5 ± 0.4	5.5 ± 0.9	4.3 ± 0.7	9.4 ± 1.3
L-PAM (10 mg/kg)	2.9 ± 0.5	9.9 ± 1.7	5.2 ± 0.5	15.2 ± 2.0
		EMT-6 mammary carcinoma		
No drug				3.8 ± 1.1
CDDP (10 mg/kg)	7.5 ± 0.8			32.7 ± 3.2
Carboplatin (50 mg/kg)	4.5 ± 0.5			12.4 ± 1.2
Cyclophosphamide (150 mg/kg)	6.3 ± 0.5			25.2 ± 2.1
ThioTEPA (10 mg/kg)	3.0 ± 0.4			10.7 ± 1.5
BCNU (15 mg/kg)	2.7 ± 0.4			10.5 ± 1.3
L-PAM (10 mg/kg)	3.0 ± 0.4			11.4 ± 1.4

[a]All drugs given i.p.

[b]Tumor growth delay is the difference in days for treated tumors to reach 500 mm³ compared with untreated control tumors. Mean of 14 animals ± SE.

[c]Fluosol-DA dose was 0.3 mL; 12 mL/kg i.v. just prior to alkylating agents. Carbogen breathing began just after Fluosol-DA and continued for 6 h.

[d]Etanidazole dose was 1 g/kg i.p. just prior to alkylating agents.

marrow granulocyte-macrophage colony-forming unit was increased by five- to tenfold compared with the alkylating agents alone.

The Hoechst 33342 dye diffusion defined tumor cell subpopulation assay,[107,116–120] also in the FSaIIC tumor, demonstrated that the combination of modulators increased the toxicity of CDDP, cyclophosphamide, L-PAM, and BCNU by 9- to 55-fold compared with the alkylating agent alone in both the bright (euoxic-enriched) and dim (hypoxic-enriched) cells (Fig. 3-4). For each alkylating agent except BCNU, the increase in tumor cell killing was greater in the dim cells than in the bright cells. Finally, tumor growth delay studies in both the FSaIIC tumor and the EMT-6 murine mammary adenocarcinoma confirmed that the combination of modulators significantly increased the tumor growth delay caused by CDDP, carboplatin, cyclophosphamide, thioTEPA, and BCNU (Table 3-1). The greatest increases (four- to fivefold) were observed for carboplatin and L-PAM in the FSaIIC tumor and CDDP and cyclophosphamide in the EMT-6 tumor. These results suggest that Fluosol-DA/carbogen together with etanidazole may be an effective modulator combination of alkylating agents in the clinic.

Studies Combining Fluosol-DA/Oxygen Breathing with Chemotherapy and Radiation ■

With most solid tumors, however, it is unlikely that Fluosol-DA and carbogen breathing will be 100% efficient in oxygenating the entire tumor mass. It is likely that pockets of viable hypoxic cells will remain and prevent tumor cure. This residual hypoxic cell component of solid tumors must be considered in the design of curative therapeutic regimens.

The addition of treatment with a perfluorochemical emulsion combined with breathing a high oxygen atmosphere has been shown to improve the response of several animal tumor systems to treatment with BCNU[51,97,98] as well as to other cancer chemotherapeutic agents.[35,36,60–72] We have examined the use of Fluosol-DA, and carbogen breathing with single dose radiation treatment, BCNU, and combined drug and radiation treatment in intracranially implanted 9L gliosarcoma.[51] The median enhancement in life span produced by Fluosol-DA and carbogen breathing in addition to

radiation was two days at 10 Gy and six days at 20 Gy compared to radiation treatment alone (Fig. 3-5). In the group receiving 20 Gy with Fluosol-DA and carbogen breathing, 2 of 20 lived 120 days. Treatment with a single intraperitoneal injection of BCNU (10 mg/kg) on day 7 post tumor cell implantation produced an increase in life span of 2 days compared to untreated control animals. The combination of drug treatment with Fluosol-DA and carbogen breathing produced an increase in life span of 26 days, which was significantly different from BCNU treatment with air breathing ($p < 0.001$) (Fig. 3-6). Finally, when BCNU and Fluosol-DA and carbogen were combined with radiation treatment (20 Gy), an increase in life span of nearly 85 days compared to untreated controls was produced, with 47% (9 of 19) surviving 120 days (Fig. 3-7).[51] These results suggest that this combination might be effective in the treatment of malignant brain tumors.

The effects of the combination of Fluosol-DA and carbogen on the response of BA1112 rat rhabdomyosarcomas to continuous low-dose rate irradiation were examined.[99] Tumors were irradiated locally in unretrained, unanesthetized rats at a dose rate of 0.98Gy/hr, using a specially designed [241]Am irradiator system. Cell survival was measured using a colony formation assay. Slightly less radiosensitization was observed with continuous low-dose-rate irradiation than in previous experiments using acute high-dose-rate irradiation. The diminished sensitization with Fluosol-DA/carbogen during continuous low-dose-rate irradiation probably reflects the intrinsically lower oxygen enhancement ratio (OER) of low-dose/low-dose-rate irradiation, reoxygenation of the tumors during the prolonged treatment times used for continuous low-dose-rate irradiation, and the decrease in the levels of circulating perfluorochemicals during the 30-hour irradiations. More importantly, the significant level of radiosensitization observed in the experiments with continuous low-dose-rate irradiation suggests that hypoxic cells persist in BA112 tumors during continuous low-dose-rate irradiations and that the response of these tumors to continuous low-dose-rate irradiation can be improved by adjunctive treatments which oxygenate these radioresistant hypoxic cells.[99]

The antitumor efficacy of adding the nitroimidazole radiosensitizing drugs misonidazole and etanidazole or hyperthermia (43°C for 30 min) to Fluosol-DA/carbogen (95% O_2/5% CO_2) and radiation was tested in the FSaIIC tumor system.[100] Both the nitroimidazole drugs[91–93] and hyper-

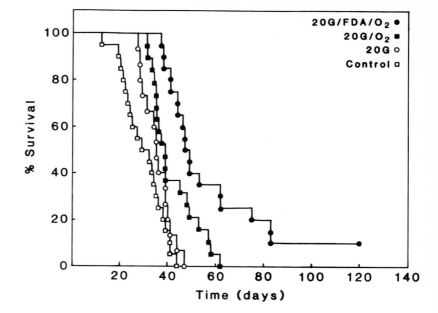

FIG. 3–5 Kaplan-Meier plot of the survival distribution for rats bearing intracranial 9L tumors. The groups shown are untreated controls (□); 20 Gy (0); 20 Gy with carbogen breathing for 1 hour prior to and during treatment (■); and 20 Gy preceded by Fluosol-DA with carbogen breathing for 1 hour prior to and during treatment (●). Reprinted from Teicher, Rose.[51]

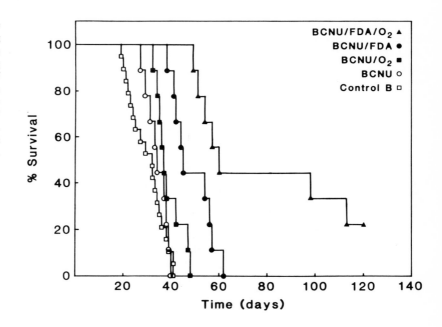

FIG. 3–6 Kaplan-Meier plot of the survival distribution for rats bearing intracranial 9L tumors. The groups shown are: untreated controls (□); BCNU (10 mg/kg) (0); BCNU (10 mg/kg) followed by 1 hour of carbogen breathing (■); BCNU (10 mg/kg) preceded by Fluosol-DA (●); and BCNU (10 mg/kg) preceded by Fluosol-DA and followed by 1 hour of carbogen breathing (Δ). Reprinted from Teicher, Rose.[51]

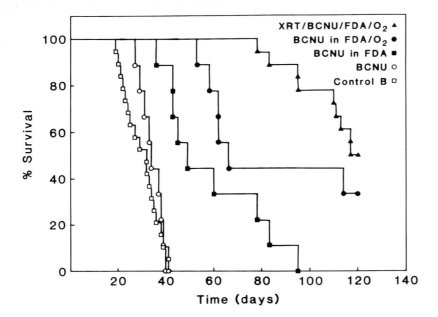

FIG. 3–7 Kaplan-Meier plot of the survival distribution for rats bearing intracranial 9L tumors. The groups shown are: untreated controls (□); BCNU (10 mg/kg) (0); BCNU (10 mg/kg) in Fluosol-DA (■); BCNU (10 mg/kg) in Fluosol-DA followed by 1 hour of carbogen breathing (●); and 20 Gy preceded by BCNU (10 mg/kg) and Fluosol-DA with 1 hour of carbogen breathing prior to and during radiation (▲). Reprinted from Teicher, Rose.[51]

thermia[101–103] produced additional tumor growth delays and tumor cell cytotoxicity when given with Fluosol-DA/carbogen, either prior to or after radiation (Figs. 3-8, 3-9, 3-10). For each of the modalities tested the dose-modifying effect was greater when that therapy preceded rather than followed radiation (misonidazole[103] 2.7 vs. 1.9, etanidazole[104–106] 2.4 vs. 1.7, hyperthermia[107] 4.0 vs. 1.7 relative to the effect of radiation alone). Since the nitroimidazole drugs must be present prior to radiation to exert their radiosensitizing effect, the increase in tumor growth delay observed when these hypoxic cell cytotoxic drugs were administered following Fluosol-DA/carbogen and radiation suggests that Fluosol-DA and carbogen was not able to fully oxygenate the tumors and that the nitroimidazole drugs were effectively toxic to residual hypoxic cells. The treatment Fluosol-DA/carbogen → hyperthermia → radiation produced a marked increase in tumor growth delay not seen with the sequence Fluosol-DA/carbogen → radiation → hyperthermia.[99] The results indicate that a treatment combination of radiation sensitizers may be more effective than radiation plus Fluosol-DA with oxygen breathing alone.

The cytotoxic effects of the addition of mitomycin C or porfiromycin on treatment with Fluosol-DA/carbogen breathing and radiation were also studied in the FSaIIC tumor system.[35] *In vitro* mitomycin C and porfiromycin are both preferentially cytotoxic toward hypoxic cells.[108–113] After *in vivo* exposure, however, the cytotoxicity of mito-

mycin C toward single cell tumor suspensions obtained from whole tumors was exponential over the dose range studied, but for porfiromycin a plateau in cell killings was observed.[35,114,115] With Fluosol-DA/carbogen breathing and single dose radiation, addition of either mitomycin C or porfiromycin increased the tumor cell kill achieved at 5 Gy by approximately 1.2 and 1.0 logs, respectively (Fig. 3-11). Less effect was seen with addition of the drugs at the 10 and 15 Gy radiation doses. In tumor growth delay experiments, the addition of either mitomycin C or porfiromycin increased the tumor cell kill achieved at 5 Gy by approximately 1.2 and 1.0 logs, respectively (Fig. 3-11). Less effect was seen with addition of delay experiments, the addition of either mitomycin C or porfiromycin to Fluosol-DA/carbogen breathing and radiation resulted in primarily an additive increase in tumor growth delay (Table 3-2).

Administration of the fluorescent dye Hoechst 33342 to tumor-bearing mice 20 minutes prior to sacrifice followed by the preparation of a single cell suspension from treated tumors allows separation of bright and dim cells by a fluorescently activated cell sorter. These separated populations can then be assayed for colony formation *in vitro*. Since the amount of dye present is a product of simple diffusion, bright cells were cells close to vessels (presumably well oxygenated) and dim cells were cells distant from vessels (presumably

(text continues on page 52)

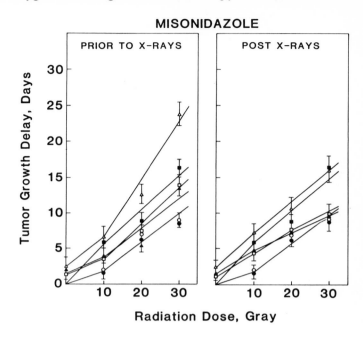

FIG. 3–8   Growth delay of the FSaIIC fibrosarcoma produced by radiation and misonidazole with Fluosol-DA with or without carbogen breathing. Misonidazole was administered either prior to or after irradiation. The treatment groups were: radiation (10, 20, or 30 Gy)/carbogen (●); Fluosol-DA (12 mL/kg) and radiation (■); Fluosol-DA/carbogen and radiation (■); misonidazole (1 g/kg) and radiation (▢); misonidazole/Fluosol-DA and radiation (▲); and misonidazole/Fluosol-DA/carbogen and radiation (△). Reprinted from Teicher, *et al.*[100]

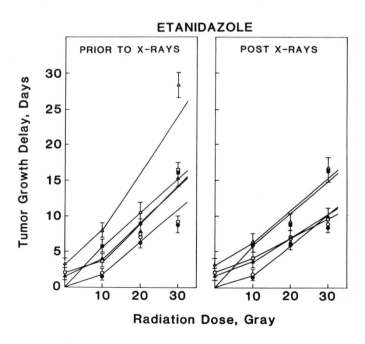

FIG. 3–9   Growth delay of the FSaIIC fibrosarcoma produced by radiation and etanidazole with Fluosol-DA with or without carbogen breathing. Etanidazole was administered either prior to or after irradiation. The treatment groups were radiation (10, 20, or 30 Gy)/carbogen (●); Fluosol-DA (12 mL/kg) and radiation (0); Fluosol-DA/carbogen and radiation (■); etanidazole (1 g/kg) and radiation (▢); etanidazole/Fluosol-DA and radiation (▲); and etanidazole/Fluosol-DA/carbogen and radiation (△). Reprinted from Teicher, *et al.*[100]

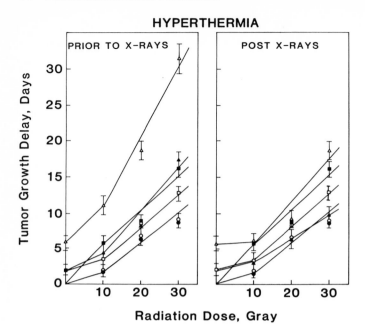

FIG. 3–10 Growth delay of the FSaIIC fibrosarcoma produced by radiation and hyperthermia with Fluosol-DA with or without carbogen breathing. Hyperthermia was administered either prior to or after irradiation. The treatment groups were radiation (10, 20, or 30 Gy)/carbogen (●); Fluosol-DA (12 mL/kg) and radiation (0); Fluosol-DA/carbogen and radiation (■); hyperthermia (43°C, 30 min) and radiation (▢); hyperthermia/Fluosol-DA and radiation (▲); and hyperthermia/Fluosol-DA/carbogen and radiation (△). Reprinted from Teicher, *et al.*[100]

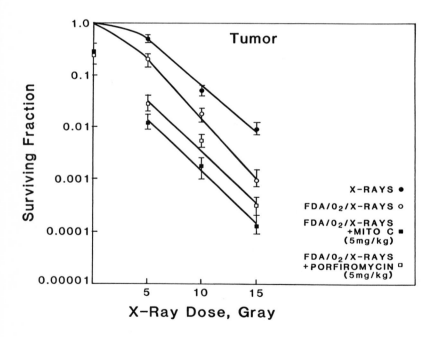

FIG. 3–11 Survival of cells from FSaIIC tumors treated with various doses of radiation alone or in combination with Fluosol-DA, carbogen or drugs. The treatment groups are x-rays with carbogen breathing for 1 hour prior to and during treatment (●); x-rays preceded by Fluosol-DA (12 mL/kg) and carbogen breathing for 1 hr. prior to and during treatment (■); x-rays preceded by Fluosol-DA (12 mL/kg) and carbogen breathing for 1 h prior to and during treatment followed by mitomycin C (5 mg/kg) (▢); and x-rays preceded by Fluosol-DA (12 mg/kg) and carbogen breathing for 1 hour prior to and during treatment followed by porfiromycin (5 mg/kg) (▢). Points, means of three independent experiments; bars, SE. Reprinted from Holden, *et al.*[35]

Table 3–2
Growth Delay of the FSaIIC Fibrosarcoma Produced by Treatment
with Fluosol-DA/Carbogen Breathing and Single Dose Radiation Combined
with a Hypoxic Cell Selective Drug.

Treatment Group	Hypoxic Cell Selective Drug[a]		
	None	Mitomycin C	Porfiromycin
Drug alone	—	5.4 ± 1.0	1.1 ± 0.5
Fluosol-DA[b] →	no effect	6.6 ± 1.2	4.8 ± 0.8
Fluosol-DA/carbogen[c] →	no effect	5.9 ± 1.0	4.5 ± 1.0
10 Gy[d] →	1.65 ± 0.5	7.4 ± 0.8	5.5 ± 1.0
20 Gy →	6.2 ± 1.0	8.5 ± 1.5	8.6 ± 1.1
30 Gy →	8.8 ± 1.0	11.4 ± 1.7	12.3 ± 1.5
Fluosol-DA/10 Gy →	2.9 ± 0.5	6.2 ± 1.0	6.1 ± 1.3
Fluosol-DA/20 Gy →	6.9 ± 1.0	9.2 ± 1.2	11.4 ± 1.5
Fluosol-DA/30 Gy →	9.1 ± 1.0	13.3 ± 1.5	15.3 ± 1.8
Fluosol-DA/carbogen/10 Gy →	5.8 ± 1.5	9.5 ± 1.2	10.0 ± 1.5
Fluosol-DA/carbogen/20 Gy →	8.8 ± 1.5	12.7 ± 1.5	13.5 ± 1.7
Fluosol-DA/carbogen/30 Gy →	16.3 ± 2.0	18.9 ± 1.9	19.6 ± 2.1

[a]A single dose of mitomycin C (5 mg/kg) or porfiromycin (5 mg/kg) was administered by i.p. injection immediately after radiation treatment.

[b]The dose of Fluosol-DA was 12 mL/kg (0.3 mL), administered i.v.

[c]Carbogen (95% O_2/5% CO_2) breathing was initiated immediately after Fluosol-DA administration and maintained for 1 hour prior to and during radiation delivery.

[d]Radiation was delivered as a single dose to the tumor-bearing limbs.

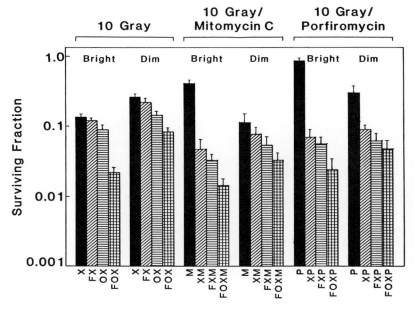

FIG. 3–12 Survival of subpopulations based on Hoechst 33342 fluorescence intensity of cells from FSaIIC tumors treated with a single dose of 10 Gray x-rays alone or in combination. The characters beneath the bars are X, 10 Gray of x-ray; F, Fluosol-DA (12 mL/kg); O, carbogen breathing for 1 hour prior to and during x-ray treatment; M, mitomycin C (5 mg/kg); and P, porfiromycin (5 mg/kg). Each experiment was repeated three times. Bars, SE. Reprinted from Holden, et al.[35]

hypoxic).[108,116–120] Unexpectedly, the survival of Hoechst 33342 dye-selected tumor cell subpopulations[108,116–120] indicated that Fluosol-DA/carbogen breathing increased the cytotoxicity of radiation (10 Gy) more in the bright cell subpopulation (fourfold) than in the dim cell subpopulation (twofold) resulting in an overall fourfold sparing of the dim subpopulation (Fig. 3-12). This may be because the Hoechst 33342 dye selected bright cells containing a significant number of acutely or intermittently hypoxic cells and Fluosol-DA/carbogen may not be most successful in the population of cells that are in flux relative to vascular perfusion. Mitomycin C and porfiromycin were both more toxic toward the dim cell subpopulations. Addition of mitomycin C or porfiromycin to Fluosol-DA/carbogen breathing and radiation 10 Gy) resulted in a primarily additive effect of the drugs and radiation killing in both tumor cell subpopulations. Thus, with mitomycin/Fluosol-DA/carbogen and radiation there was a twofold sparing of dim cells and with porfiromycin in the combined treatment a 1.6-fold sparing of the dim cell population. Our results indicate that treatment strategies directed against both intermittently and chronically hypoxic tumor subpopulations can markedly increase the tumor cell kill achieved by radiation.[35]

Clinical Aspects of Fluosol-DA/Oxygen Breathing in Radiation Therapy ■

In 1978, Makowski[121] reported on the infusion of Fluosol-DA into 7 decerebrate patients who had sustained severe head injury. He infused 1000 to 1500 mL of Fluosol-DA over a period of 60 to 70 minutes via a central venous line. Changes were noted in various cardiovascular parameters, all of which returned to normal within one hour. Ohyanagi and associates[122] reported on the infusion of Fluosol-DA in normal human volunteers. One mL of Fluosol-DA was infused intravenously and the patient observed for 60 minutes. Subjects were then infused at rates of 1 mL per minute for 20 to 500 mL total infusion. No changes were noted in blood pressure, pulse, or respiration. No significant changes were noted in blood count, liver enzymes, or renal function. Tremper and associates[123] subsequently reported on hemodynamic and oxygen transport effects of Fluosol-DA in an anemic patient who refused blood transfu-

sion and required pelvic surgery. No adverse effects were noted. Subsequently, Fluosol-DA was placed in clinical trials in Japan[124] and in the United States to be used in patients who were severely anemic and refused blood products and also required surgery. Tremper[125] demonstrated that a high fraction of inspired oxygen was necessary to raise the arterial oxygen pressure significantly. Recently, Spence and coworkers[126] reported an evaluation of Fluosol-DA as a blood substitute in the treatment of severe anemia. Fluosol-DA with oxygen breathing (FiO₂60–100%) significantly increased the dissolved component of oxygen content over 12 hours post Fluosol-DA administration.

A Phase I/II clinical study of adjuvant Fluosol-DA and oxygen was started in 1984 and the initial results reported by Rose and associates.[127] Additional patients were entered and further results have been reported by Lustig and coworkers.[128] Patients with advanced head and neck tumors were chosen as the initial patient population. These tumors are thought to contain a significant portion of hypoxic cells which contribute to the problem of local control. In addition, evidence exists that hyperbaric oxygen may be useful in improving local control. This study included Stage III and IV unresectable head and neck squamous cell carcinomas. Standard doses of radiation were used with daily fractions of 1.8 to 2 Gy per day and total doses of 60 to 74 Gy. Patients were infused once a week, generally on Monday, with doses of 7 mL or 8 mL/kg. As the study progressed, the total volume infused over the course of treatment increased from 40 mL to 56 mL/kg. Patients breathed 100% oxygen via nasal prongs and mask for at least one-half hour prior to and during radiation. Eleven of 45 patients who received Fluosol-DA experienced a reaction to the test dose of ½ mL given intravenously prior to the start of the infusion. This generally consisted of flushing, chest pain, nausea, or low back pain. These patients were treated with Benadryl and/or steroids and 37 were able to continue. Six of 42 patients experienced post transfusion reactions, most often consisting of fever, chills, headache, and low back pain. The exact cause of this allergic reaction is unknown but is much higher in cancer patients than in patients receiving Fluosol-DA in cardiac studies. A complement activation reaction has been postulated. Generally, these reactions are controlled with antihistamines or steroids.[129] While changes in hepatic enzymes were noted in most patients, none developed symptomatic hepatomegaly or became clinically hepatotoxic. All of their liver function studies returned to normal in a 1–60 month period. No significant changes in hematologic measurements were noted.

A total of 46 patients with squamous cell carcinoma of the head and neck were entered into this study. Thirty-seven patients were evaluable for response. Nine patients were Stage III, 20 patients Stage IV, and 8 patients had previous treatment with chemotherapy and/or surgery. Twenty-eight of 36 patients (76%) achieved a complete response.

At 1 year (Table 3-3), there were 27 patients evaluable with 18 alive free of disease, 5 dead with disease, and 4 dead of other causes. The absolute at 1 year was 67% and determinant survival was 78%. With follow-up of 3 to 27 months, 15 patients remained without evidence of disease, 6 were dead with disease, and 6 died of other causes with local control. Of those achieving a complete response, 75% have remained in remission.

In 1985, a Phase I/II study with adjuvant Fluosol-DA and oxygen was started for non-small cell carcinoma of the lung.[130] This study included Stage II, III, or IV patients without distant metastasis and a Karnofsky of 60 or greater. Radiation therapy doses ranged from 60 to 66 Gy at standard fractionation. Fluosol-DA was infused once weekly at 7 mL to 9 mL/kg for a total dose of 42 to 49 mL/kg. The total dose in this study was lower due to concern regarding pulmonary fibrosis. Forty-five patients started therapy and 34 completed treatment. Six subjects developed metastasis under treatment, three had disease-related death, and two patients were withdrawn. A high rate of Fluosol-DA reactions were noted in this study, with 36% reporting a reaction to the test dose on infusion and 40% having a post-infusion reaction. However, only four patients were withdrawn due to reactions. While abnormalities were again noted in the liver enzymes and a low white count reported in six patients and depressed platelets under 100,000 in two patients, all returned to normal within 3 to 6 months. In this study, 17 of

34 evaluable patients achieved a complete response. Thirteen patients remained alive at 12 to 20 months.

In 1987, a Phase I/II study was opened for the treatment of high-grade malignant gliomas with adjuvant Fluosol-DA and oxygen.[131] A weekly dose of 8 mL/kg of Fluosol-DA was used, given at weeks 1, 2, 3, 6, and 7 during radiation. Infusions were then increased to include 1 dose per week during the entire 7 weeks of therapy for a total dose of 56 mL/kg. Following attainment of this dose level, additional doses were given of 7 mL/kg on Wednesday or Thursday for up to 3 weeks of treatment. A total of 77 mL/kg will now be delivered over the radiation therapy treatment course, which consists of 65 Gy at standard fractionation. No significant toxicities have been reported. Of 18 evaluable patients at 1 year, 10 were alive for a 1-year survival of 56%. Five patients were alive free of disease from 65 to 96 weeks from diagnosis. No long term complications in the brain from this therapy had been observed. The above studies are summarized in Table 3-4. If only those patients that survive longer than one year are compared to a historical group of long-term survivors treated similarly but without Fluosol-DA, then a statistically significant improvement in survival (p<0.005) is obtained. The lack of toxicity and the increased therapeutic benefit argue for continued study of Fluosol-DA and high inspired oxygen tension as an adjuvant to radiation therapy for the

Table 3–3
Results of the Fluosol-DA/Radiation Phase I/II Head and Neck Clinical Study

Patient Status	Patient Number	
Evaluable	27	
Alive	18	
Dead with Disease	5	
Dead from Other Causes	4	
Absolute Survival	18/27	67%
Determinant Survival	18/23	78%

Table 3–4
Summary of the Fluosol-DA/Radiation Clinical Trials

Site/Stage	Evaluable Patients	RX Dose	Maximal Fluosol-DA Dose	CR	Absolute 1 Yr Survival
Head & Neck	37	66–74 Gy	56 mL/kg	76%	67%
Lung	34	60–66 Gy	49 mL/kg	50%	56%
Brain/Glioma	18	65 Gy	56 mL/kg	—	56%

management of patients with high-grade malignant brain tumors.

A clinical trial has started in locally advanced carcinoma of the cervix (personal communication, Dr. S. Bryant—Alpha Therapeutics). This trial will use weekly Fluosol-DA infusions with oxygen breathing during external radiation therapy and during radioactive implants. This will test the usefulness of Fluosol-DA during brachytherapy treatment.

The results of several Phase I studies of Fluosol-DA and oxygen breathing with single agent chemotherapy have been reported.[73–75] In a multi-center setting, 14 non-small cell lung cancer patients were treated with 1 of 3 incremental doses of Fluosol-DA/O_2 and cyclophosphamide to evaluate safety of the combination.[74] The mean age of the patients was 61 and their median KPS was 90%. The treatment schedule consisted of Fluosol-DA (150, 275, or 400 mL/m^2) followed by 100% O_2 for 5 hours plus 800 mg/m^2 cyclophosphamide administered $\frac{1}{2}$ hour after the start of oxygenation. Treatment was repeated every three weeks until disease progression or for six courses. When 28 courses had been completed (median two per patient), the cumulative mean dosage of Fluosol-DA was 398 mL/m^2 (range: 150–825). The cumulative mean dose of cyclophosphamide was 2867 mg (range: 1250-5384); the mean dose intensity was 269 mg/m^2/week. The nonhematologic toxicities included grade 1–3 nausea/vomiting (four patients), grade 1–2 fatigue (two patients), grade 1 anorexia (one patient), and grade 2 dehydration (one patient). The mean WBC nadir was 6970/mm^3 and the mean granulocyte nadir was 4920/mm^3. The mean platelet nadir was 280 × 10^3/mm^3. There were no dose delays or reductions. Fluosol-DA was well tolerated with few reactions including blood pressure changes (five patients), flushing (one patient), dyspnea (one patient), and diaphoresis and chills (one patient). Treatment continued at a Fluosol-DA dosage of 400 mL/m^2. In conclusion, Fluosol-DA/O_2 therapy can be safely combined with cyclophosphamide in the dosage ranges studied in advanced non-small cell lung cancer.

In another multicenter trial, 27 patients were assigned to 1 of 3 dosages of Fluosol-DA/O_2 with weekly 5-fluorouracil (600 mg/m^2) with Fluosol-DA (150, 275, or 400 mL/m^2) followed by 5 hours 100% O_2.[75] The mean patient age was 63 years and median KPS was 90%. A total of 179 courses of therapy was given (median 6, range 4–16). The median cumulative Fluosol-DA dosage was 2000 mL/m^2 (range 600–6400), the median 5-fluorouracil dosage was 3519 mg/m^2 (range 1803–9279) and the mean 5-fluorouracil dose intensity was 565 mg/m^2/wk (range 451–614). Ten patients required dose reduction while seven required dose delays. Three patients had grade 1–2 leukopenia and three had grade 1 thrombocytopenia. Nonhematological toxicities consisted of nausea/vomiting (six patients), anorexia, mild diarrhea (two patients), gastrointestinal bleeding and mild mucositis (one patient). Twelve patients experienced immediate Fluosol-DA related reactions: mild to severe back pain (five patients), chest tightness (five patients), mild to moderate body ache (three patients), mild chills (two patients), severe dyspnea and flushing, mild to moderate dizziness. These were ameliorated with diphenhydramine. The results indicated that Fluosol-DA can be combined with 5-fluorouracil without enhanced toxicity. Two partial and two minor responses were seen. This regimen had safely delivered the highest cumulative clinical Fluosol-DA doses at the time of its completion.

A Phase I/II trial was initiated in patients with residual or recurrent malignant glioma following surgery and radiation.[73] Fifty-one evaluable patients received Fluosol-DA (150–600 mL/m^2), O_2 (100% for 5 hours) and BCNU (200 mg/m^2 @ $\frac{1}{2}$ hour after start of O_2), every six weeks. The mean age of the patients was 45 years and their median KPS was 80%. One hundred sixty-six treatments were given. Fluosol-DA reactions included flushing (three patients), chest tightness, dyspnea, and nausea/vomiting (two patients each). Reversible liver enzyme elevations were observed in 30 patients. BCNU nonhematologic toxicity included mild to moderate nausea/vomiting (16 patients). Myelosuppression (WBC <2000, PLT <50,000, HBG <8.0) was seen in 7, 6, and 0 patients, respectively. Of 34 evaluable patients treated at recurrence, 12 patients had a partial response (35%, based on CT/MRI criteria, with steroids constant or decreasing), 13 patients had stable disease (38%), and 9 patients had progression (26%). Eight of 13 patients with glioblastoma multiforme treated at recurrence had stable or improved disease.

Future Directions ■

At this time, no proven benefit of Fluosol-DA and oxygen breathing as an adjuvant to radiation therapy has been demonstrated. While improved local control has been reported in the Phase II studies, a randomized trial is yet to be concluded. While the potential to increase tumor oxygenation exists in humans, many questions remain unanswered. The pharmacokinetics of Fluosol-DA in humans is poorly understood. The intravascular half-life as measured in the serum of patients in the head and neck study is quite variable. Most patients had some measurable fluorocarbons at 24 hours but few received Fluosol-DA doses sufficient to achieve maximum tumor oxygenation over a course of protracted radiation therapy is unknown. Currently studies are in progress to further evaluate the circulating half-life of the components of Fluosol-DA. The long-range goal is to provide maximum oxygenation of the tumor during all fractions of radiation. In this regard, fractionation schemes other than standard regimens may well be the most appropriate for Fluosol-DA and oxygen. Further results and clinical trials will be necessary to completely evaluate the place of Fluosol-DA in radiation therapy with chemotherapy.

Current and planned clinical protocols involving Fluosol-DA/oxygen will assess oxygen directly in tumors and identify parameters that correlate with hypoxia, and will be particularly designed to determine whether Fluosol-DA/oxygen breathing corrects tumor hypoxia and what doses and schedules of Fluosol-DA/oxygen are required to do this optimally. It is in that setting where hypoxia is corrected where the therapeutic advantage afforded by Fluosol-DA/oxygen to chemotherapy and to radiotherapy is likely to be optimized. In addition, several more concentrated emulsions are currently under development. These preparations may allow a higher concentration of perfluorochemicals to be administered more rapidly to patients, although the optimum dose rate of perfluorochemicals for these uses is also unknown.

References ∎

1. Vaupel P. Oxygenation of human tumors. Atrahlenther Onkol 1990;166:377–386.
2. Adams GE. The clinical relevance of tumour hypoxia. Eur J Cancer 1990;26(4):420–421.
3. Thomlinson RH, Gray LH. The histological structure of some human lung cancers and the possible implications for radiotherapy. Brit J Cancer 1955;9:539–549.
4. Jirtle R, Clifton KH. The effect of tumor size and host anemia on tumor cell survival after irradiation. Int J Radiat Oncol Biol Phys 1978;4:395–400.
5. Kjartasson I, Appelgren L, Peterson HJ, Rosengren B, Rudenstan CM, Lewis DH. Capillary blood flow, exchange and flow distribution in transplantable rat tumors. In: Seventh European Conference on Microcirculation. Aberdeen, Part II, Bibl Amat No. 12:519–526. Basel, Krager, 1978.
6. Eddy HA. Development of the vascular system in the hamster malignant neurilemoma. Microvasc Res1973; 6:63–82.
7. Endrich B, Antaglietta M, Reinhold HS, Gross JF. Hemodynamic characteristics in microcirculatory blood channels during early tumor growth. Cancer Res 1979;39: 17–23.
8. Tannock IF, Steel GG. Quantitative technique for the study of the anatomy and function of small blood vessels in tumors. J Natl Cancer Inst 1969;42:771–782.
9. Vaupel P. Hypoxia in neoplastic tissue. Microvas Res 1977;13:399–408.
10. Hirst DG. Oxygen delivery to tumors. Int J Radiat Oncol Biol Phys 1986;12:1271–1277.
11. Kennedy KA, Teicher BA, Rockwell SC, Sartorelli AC. The hypoxic tumor cell: a target for selective cancer chemotherapy. Biochem Pharmacol 1980;29:1–8.
12. Teicher BA, Sartorelli AC. Selective attack of hypoxic tumor cells. In: Fidler IJ, and White RJ, eds. Design of Models for Screening of Therapeutic Agents for Cancer. New York, Van Nostrand Reinhold, 1981:19–37.
13. Fowler JF. Chemical modifiers of radiosensitivity-theory and reality: a review. Int J Radiat Oncol Biol Phys 1986;11:665–677.
14. Reynard-Bougnoux A, Lespinasse F, Malaise EP, Guichard M. Partial hypoxia as a cause of radioresistance in a human tumor xenograft: its influence illustrated by the sensitizing effect of misonidazole and hyperbaric oxygen. Int J Radiat Oncol Biol Phys 1986;12:1283–1286.
15. Chaplin DJ, Durand RE, Olive PL. Acute hypoxia in tumors: implications for modifiers of radiation effects. Int J Radiat Oncol Biol Phys 1986;12:1279–1282.
16. Moulder JE, Rockwell S. Hypoxic fractions of solid tumors: experimental techniques, methods of analysis and a survey of existing data. Int J Radiat Oncol Biol Phys 1984;10:695–712.
17. Stanley JA, Shipley WV, Steel GG. Influence of tumor size on hypoxic fraction and therapeutic sensitivity of Lewis lung tumor. Br J Cancer 1977;36:105–113.
18. Vaupel P, Thews G. PO$_2$ distribution in tumor tissue of DS-carcinosarcoma. Oncology 1974;30:475–484.
19. Vaupel P, Frinak S, Bicher HI. Heterogenous oxygen partial pressure and pH distribution in C3H mouse mammary adenocarcinoma. Cancer Res 1981;41:2008–2013.
20. Vaupel P, Fortmeyer HP, Runkel S, Kallinowski F. Blood flow, oxygen consumption and tissue oxygenation of human breast cancer xenografts in nude rats. Cancer Res 1987;47:3496–3503.
21. Kallinowski F, Zander R, Hoeckel M, Vaupel P. Tumor tissue oxygenation as evaluated by computerized-pO$_2$-histography. Int J Radiat Oncol Biol Phys 1990;19:953–961.
22. Gatenby RA, Kessler HB, Rosenblum JS, Coia LR, Moldofsky PJ, Hartz WH, Broder GJ. Oxygen distribution in squamous cell carcinoma metastases and its relationship to outcome of radiation therapy. Int J Radiat Oncol Biol Phys 1988;14:831–838.
23. Sartorelli AC. Therapeutic attack of hypoxic cells of solid tumors: Presidential address. Cancer Res 1988; 48:775–78.
24. Teicher BA, Lazo JS, Sartorelli AC. Classification of

antineoplastic agents by their selective toxicities toward oxygenated and hypoxic tumor cells. Cancer Res 1981;41:73–81.

25. Teicher BA, Holden SA, Al-Achi A, Herman TS. Classification of antineoplastic treatments by their differential toxicity toward putative oxygenated and hypoxic tumor subpopulations in vivo in the FSaIIC murine fibrosarcoma. Cancer Res 1990;50:3339–3344.

26. Groebe K, Vaupel P. Evaluation of oxygen diffusion distances in human breast cancer xenografts using tumor-specific in vivo data: role of various mechanisms in the development of tumor hypoxia. Int J Radiat Oncol Biol Phys 1988;15:691–697.

27. Kallinowski F, Schlenger KH, Runkel S, Kloes M, Stohrer M, Okunieff P, Vaupel P. Blood flow, metabolism, cellular microenvironment and growth rate of human tumor xenografts. Cancer Res 1989;49:3759–3764.

28. Kallman RF, Rockwell S. In: Becker FF, ed. Cancer: A comprehensive treatise 6. New York, Plenum, 1977: 225.

29. Steel GG. Growth kinetics of tumors. Oxford, Clarendon, 1977:147–156.

30. Sutherland RM, Franko AJ. On the nature of the radiobiologically hypoxic fraction in tumors. Int J Radiat Oncol Biol Phys 1980;6:117–120.

31. Koch CJ, Meneses JJ, Harris JW. The effect of extreme hypoxia and glucose on the repair of potentially lethal and sublethal radiation damage by mammalian cells. Radiat Res 1977;70:542–551.

32. Bedford JS, Mitchell JB. The effect of hypoxia on the growth and radiation response of mammalian cells in culture. Brit J Radiol 1974;47:687–696.

33. Bush RS, Jenkin RDT, Allt WEC, Beale FA, Bean H, Dembo AJ, Pringle JF. Definitive evidence for hypoxic cells influencing cure in cancer therapy. Brit J Cancer 1978;37(Suppl III):302–306.

34. Herman TS, Teicher BA, Coleman CN. The interaction of SR-4233 with hyperthermia and radiation in the FSaIIC murine fibrosarcoma tumor system *in vitro* and *in vivo*. Cancer Res 1990;50:5055–5059.

35. Holden SA, Herman TS, Teicher BA. Addition of a hypoxic cell selective cytotoxic agent (mitomycin C or porfiromycin) to treatment with Fluosol-DA®/carbogen/radiation. Radiother Oncol 1990;18:59–70.

36. Teicher BA, Herman TS, Holden SA, Cathcart KNS. The effect of Fluosol-DA and oxygenation status on the activity of cyclophosphamide in vivo. Cancer Chemother Pharmacol 1988;21:286–291.

37. Martin DF, Porter EA, Rockwell S, Fischer JJ. Enhancement of tumor radiation response by the combination of a perfluorochemical emulsion and hyperbaric oxygen. Int J Radiat Oncol Biol Phys 1987;13:747–751.

38. Teicher BA, Rose CM. Perfluorochemical emulsion can increase tumor radiosensitivity. Science 1984;223:934–936.

39. Teicher BA, Herman TS, Jones SM. Optimization of perfluorochemical levels with radiation therapy. Cancer Res 1989;49:2693–2697.

40. Weissberg JB, On YH, Papac RJ, Sasaki C, Fischer DB, Lawrence R, Rockwell S, Sartorelli AC, Fischer JJ. Randomized clinical trial of mitomycin C as an adjunct to radiotherapy in head and neck cancer. Int J Radiat Oncol Biol Phys 1989;17:3–9.

41. Coleman CN. Hypoxia in tumors: a paradigm for the approach to biochemical and physiologic heterogeneity. J Natl Cancer Inst 1988;80:310–317.

42. Rose CM, Lustig R, McIntosh, N, Teicher BA. A clinical trial of Fluosol-DA® 20% in advanced squamous cell carcinoma of the head and neck. Int J Radiat Oncol Biol Phys 1986;12:1325–1327.

43. Lustig R, McIntosh-Lowe NL, Rose C, Has J, Krasnow S, Spaulding M, Prosnitz L. Phase I-II study of Fluosol-DA and 100% oxygen breathing as an adjuvant to radiation in the treatment of advanced squamous cell tumors of the head and neck. Int J Radiat Oncol Biol Phys 1989;16:1587–1594.

44. Lustig R, Lowe N, Prosnitz L, Spaulding M, Cohen M, Stitt S, Brannon R. Phase I/II study of fluosol and 100% oxygen breathing as an adjuvant to radiation in the treatment of unresectable non small cell carcinoma of the lung. Int J Radiat Oncol Biol Phys 1989;17s1:202.

45. Evans RG, Kimler BF, Morantz RA, Tribhawan SV, Gemer LS, O'Kell V, Lowe N. A Phase I-II study of the use of Fluosol®-DA 20% as an adjuvant to radiation therapy in the treatment of primary high-grade brain tumors. Int J Radiat Oncol Biol Phys 1989;17s1: 175.

46. Suit HD, Sedlacek RS, Silver G, Dosoretz D. Pentobarbital anesthesia and the response of tumor and normal tissue in the C3Hf/Sed mouse to radiation. Rad Res 1985;104:47–65.

47. Henk JM, Kinkler PB, Smith CW. Radiotherapy and hyperbaric oxygen in head and neck cancer. Lancet ii:1977;101–103.

48. Teicher BA, Rose CM. Oxygen-carrying perfluorochemical emulsion as an adjuvant to radiation therapy in mice. Cancer Res 1984;44:4285–4288.

49. Teicher BA, Rose CM. Effect of dose and scheduling on growth delay of the Lewis lung carcinoma produced by the perfluorochemical emulsion, Fluosol-DA. Int J Radiat Oncol Biol Phys 1986;12:1311–1313.

50. Teicher BA, Herman TS, Jones SM. Influence of scheduling dose and volume of administration of the perfluorochemical emulsion Therox®, on tumor response to radiation therapy. Int J Radiat Oncol Biol Phys 1991, in press.

51. Teicher BA, Herman TS, Rose CM. Effect of Fluosol®-DA on the response of intracranial 9L tumors to x-rays and BCNU. Int J Radiat Oncol Biol Phys 1988;15:1187–1192.

52. Lee I, Levitt SH, Song CW. Effects of Fluosol-DA and carbogen on the radioresponse of SCK tumors and skin of A/J mice. Radiat Res 1987;112:173–182.

53. Lee I, Lewitt SH, Song CW. Radiosensitization of Murine Tumors by Fluosol-DA 20%. Radiat Res 1990; 122:275–279.

54. Martin DF, Porter EA, Fischer JJ, Rockwell S. Effect of a perfluorochemical emulsion on the radiation response of BA 1112 rhabdomyosarcomas. Radiat Res 1987;112:45–53.

55. Moulder JE, Dutreix J, Rockwell S, Siemann DW. Applicability of animal tumor data to cancer therapy in humans. Int J Radiat Oncol Biol Phys 1988;14:913–927.

56. Moulder JE, Fish BL. Tumor sensitization by the intermittent use of perfluorochemical emulsions and carbogen breathing in fractionated radiotherapy, In: Fielden EM, Fowler JF, Hendry JH and Scott D, eds. Proceedings of the 8th International Congress of Radiation Research 1:299. London, Taylor and Francis, 1987.

57. Rockwell S, Mato TP, Irvin CG, Nierenburg M. Reactions of tumors and normal tissues in mice to irradiation in the presence and absence of a perfluorochemical

emulsion. Int J Radiat Oncol Biol Phys 1986;12:1315–1318.

58. Song CW, Lee I, Hasegawa T, Rhee JG, Levitt SH. Increase in pO$_2$ and radiosensitivity of tumors by Fluosol-DA (20%) and carbogen. Cancer Res 1987;47:442–446.

59. Song CW, Zhang WL, Pence DM, Lee I, Levitt SH. Increased radiosensitivity of tumors by perfluorochemicals and carbogen. Int J Radiat Oncol Bio Phys 1985; 11:1833–1836.

60. Teicher BA, Holden SA, Jacobs JL. Approaches to defining the mechanism of Fluosol-DA 20%/carbogen enhancement of melphalan antitumor activity. Cancer Res 1987;47:513–518.

61. Teicher BA, Holden SA, Rose CM. Differential enhancement of melphalan cytotoxicity in tumor and normal tissue by Fluosol-DA and oxygen breathing. Int J Cancer 1985;36:585–589.

62. Teicher BA, Crawford JM, Holden SA, Cathcart KNS. Effects of various oxygenation conditions on the enhancement by Fluosol-DA of melphalan antitumor activity. Cancer Res 1987;47:5036–5041.

63. Teicher BA, Holden SA. A survey of the effect of adding Fluosol-DA 20%/O$_2$ to treatment with various chemotherapeutic agents. Cancer Treat Rep 1987;71:173–177.

64. Teicher BA, McIntosh-Lowe NL, Rose CM. Effect of various oxygenation conditions and Fluosol-DA on cancer chemotherapeutic agents. Biomat Art Cells and Art Organs 1988;16:533–546.

65. Teicher BA, Holden SA, Rose CM. Effect of oxygen on the cytotoxicity and antitumor activity of etoposide. J Natl Cancer Inst 1985;75:1129–1133.

66. Teicher BA, Holden SA, Rose CM. Effect of Fluosol-DA/O$_2$ on tumor cell and bone marrow cytotoxicity of nitrosoureas in mice bearing FSaII fibrosarcoma. Int J Cancer 1986;38:285–288.

67. Teicher BA, Lazo JS, Merrill WW, Filderman AE, Rose CM. Effect of Fluosol-DA/O$_2$ on the antitumor activity and pulmonary toxicity of bleomycin. Cancer Chemother Pharmacol 1986;18:213–218.

68. Teicher BA, Holden SA, Crawford JM. Effects of Fluosol®-DA and oxygen breathing on adriamycin antitumor activity and cardiac toxicity in mice. Cancer 1988;61:2196–2201.

69. Teicher BA, Holden SA, Cathcart KNS, Herman TS. Effect of various oxygenation conditions and Fluosol®-DA on the cytotoxicity and antitumor activity of bleomycin. J Natl Cancer Inst 1988;80:599–603.

70. Teicher BA, Bernal SD, Holden SA, Cathcart KNS. Effect of Fluosol-DA/carbogen on etoposide/alkylating agent antitumor activity. Cancer Chemother Pharmacol 1988;21:281–285.

71. Martin DF, Kimler BF, Evans RG, Morantz RA, Vats TS. Potentiation of rat brain tumor therapy by Fluosol and carbogen. NCI Monogr 1988;6:119–122.

72. Kim GE, Song CW. The influence of Fluosol-DA and carbogen breathing on the antitumor effects of cyclophosphamide *in vivo*. Cancer Chemother Pharmacol 1989;25:99–102.

73. Gruber M, Prados M, Russel C, Hochberg F, Cook P, Weissman D, Evans R, Burton G, Allen D, Brannon R. Phase I/II study of Fluosol®/O$_2$ in combination with BCNU in malignant glioma. Proc Amer Assoc Cancer Res March 1990;31:190.

74. Garewal H, Skarin A, Kessler J, Smith R, Hedberg J. Fluosol®/oxygen in combination with cyclophosphamide in advanced non-small cell lung carcinoma

(NSCLC): phase I results. Proc Amer Assoc Cancer Res March 1989;30:271.

75. Meyers F, Alberts D, Spaulding M, Garewal H, Flam M, Allen D. Phase I/II study of Fluosol®/oxygen in combination with weekly 5-fluorouracil (5FU) in metastatic colorectal carcinoma. Proc Amer Assoc Cancer Res March 1989;30:256.

76. Clark LC, Gollan F. Survival of mammals breathing organic liquids equilibrated with oxygen at atmospheric pressure. Science 1966;152:1755–1756.

77. Sloviter HA, Kamimoto T. Erythrocyte substitute for perfusion of brain. Nature 1967;216:458–460.

78. Geyer RP. Substitutes for blood and its components. In: Jamieson GA and Greenwalt (eds): Blood Substitutes and Plasma Expanders, 19:1021. New York, AR Liss, 1978.

79. Riess JG, LeBlanc M. Solubility and transport phenomena in perfluorochemicals relevant to blood substitution and other biomedical applications. Pure and Appl Chem 1982;54:2383–2406.

80. Riess JG. Reassessment of criteria for the selection of perfluorochemicals for second-generation blood substitutes: analysis of structure/property relationships. Art Organs 1984;8:44–56.

81. Song CW. Increase in pO$_2$ and radiosensitivity of tumors by Fluosol-DA (20%) and carbogen. Cancer Res 1987;47:442–446.

82. Hasegawa T, Rhee JG, Levitt SH, Song CW. Increase in tumor pO$_2$ by perfluorochemicals and carbogen. Int J Radiat Oncol Biol Phys 1987;13:569–574.

83. Hiraga S, Klubes P, Owens ES, Cysack RL, Blasberg RG. Increases in brain tumor and cerebral blood flow by blood-perfluorochemical emulsion (Fluosol-DA) exchange. Cancer Res 1987;47:3296–3302.

84. Klubes P, Hiraga S, Cysyk RL, Owens ES, Blasberg RG. Attempts to increase intratumoral blood flow in the rat solid Walker 256 tumor by the use of the perfluorocarbon emulsion Fluosol-DA. Eur J Cancer Clin Oncol 1987;23(12):1859–1867.

85. Teicher BA, McIntosh NL. Optimization of Fluosol-DA administration during a fractionated radiation protocol in the Lewis lung carcinoma. 35th Mtg Radiat Res Soc abstract Em-1, Atlanta, 1987.

86. Rockwell S. Use of perfluorochemical emulsion to improve oxygenation in a solid tumor. Int J Radiat Oncol Biol Phys 1985;11:97–103.

87. Moulder JE, Fish BL. Intermittent use of a perfluorochemical emulsion (Fluosol-DA 20%) and carbogen breathing with fractionated irradiation. Int J Radiat Oncol Biol Phys 1988;15:1193–1196.

88. West L, McIntosh N, Gendler S, Seymour C, Wisdom C: Effects of intravenously infused Fluosol-DA 20% in rats. Int J Radiat Oncol Biol Phys 1986;12:1319–1323.

89. Fischer JJ, Rockwell S, Martin DF. Perfluorochemicals and hyperbaric oxygen in radiation therapy. Int J Radiat Oncol Biol Phys 1986;12:95–102.

90. Teicher BA, Waxman DJ, Holden SA, Wang Y, Clarke L, Alvarez Sotomayer E, Jones SM, Frei E III. Evidence for enzymatic activation and oxygen involvement in cytotoxicity and antitumor activity of N,N′, N″-triethylenethiophosphoramide. Cancer Res 1989;49:4996–5001.

91. Adams GE, Ahmed I, Sheldon PW, Stratford IJ. Radiation sensitization and chemopotentiation: RSU-1069, a compound more effective than misonidazole *in vitro* and *in vivo*. Br J Cancer 1984;49:5571–5577.

92. Chaplin DJ, Durand RE, Stratford IJ, Jenkins TC. The radiosensitizing and toxic effects of RSU-1069 on hypoxic cells in a murine tumor. Int J Radiat Oncol Biol Phys 1986;12:1091–1095.

93. Frank AJ. Misonidazole and other hypoxia markers. Metabolism applications. Int J Radiat Oncol Biol Phys 1986;12:1195–1202.

94. Hill RP. Sensitizers and radiation dose fractionation. Results and interpretations. Int J Radiat Oncol Biol Phys 1986;12:1049–1054.

95. Clement JJ, Gorman MS, Wodinsky I, Catanc R, Johnson RK. Enhancement of antitumor activity of alkylating agents by the radiation sensitizer misonidazole. Cancer Res 1980,50:4165.

96. Teicher BA, Herman TS, Tanaka J, Eder JP, Holden SA, Bubley G, Coleman CN, Frei E III. Modulation of Alkylating Agents by Etanidazole and Fluosol-DA/carbogen in the FSaIIC fibrosarcoma and EMT6 mammary carcinoma. Cancer Res 1991;51:1086–1091.

97. Kokunai T, Kuwamura K. Effect of perfluorochemicals on BCNU chemotherapy: preliminary study in a rat brain tumor model. Surg Neurol 1982;18:258–261.

98. Kuwamura K, Kokunai T, Tamaki N, Matsumoto S. Synergistic effect of perfluorochemicals on BCNU chemotherapy: experimental study in a 9L rat brain-tumor model. J Neurosurg 1982;57:467–471.

99. Morton JD, Porter E, Yabuki H, Nath R, Rockwell S. Effects of a perfluorochemical emulsion on the response of BA1112 rhabdomyosarcomas to continuous low dose rate irradiation. Rad Res 1990;124:178–182.

100. Teicher BA, Herman TS, Holden SA, Jones SM. Addition of misonidazole, etanidazole or hyperthermia to treatment with Fluosol-DA®/carbogen/radiation. J Natl Cancer Inst 1990;12:929–934.

101. Herman TS, Teicher BA, Jochelson M, Clark J, Svensson G, Coleman CN. Rationale for use of local hyperthermia with radiation therapy and selected anticancer drugs in locally advanced human malignancies. Int J Hyperthermia 1988;4:143–158.

102. Hofer KG. Heat potentiation of radiation damage versus radiation potentiation of heat damage. Radiat Res. 1987;110:450–457.

103. Dewey WC. Interaction of heat with radiation and chemotherapy. Cancer Res. 1984;44:4714S–4720S.

104. Coleman CN, Halsey J, Cox RS, Hirst VK, Blasche T, Howes AE, Wasserman TH, Urtasun RC, Pajak T, Hancock S, Phillips TL, Noll L. Relationship between the neurotoxicity SR-2508 and the pharmacokinetic profile. Cancer Res. 1987;47:319–322.

105. Coleman CN, Wasserman TH, Urtasun RC, Halsey J, Hirst VK, Hancock S, Phillips TL. Phase I trial of the hypoxic cell radiosensitizer SR-2508: the results of the five to six week drug schedule. Int J Radiat Oncol Biol Phys 1986;12:1105–1108.

106. Dische S, Saunders MI, Dunphy EP, Bennett MH, Des Rochers C, Stratford MRL, Minchinton AI, Orchard RA. Concentration achieved in human tumors after administration of misonidazole, SR-2508 and Ro-03-8799. Int J Radiat Oncol Biol Phys 1981;12:1109–1111.

107. Herman TS, Teicher BA, Holden SA, Collins LC. Interaction of hyperthermia and radiation: hypoxia and acidosis in vitro, tumor subpopulations in vivo. Cancer Res 1989;49:3338–3343.

108. Kennedy KA, McGurl JD, Leonardis L, Alabaster O. pH dependence of mitomycin C-induced cross-linking activity in EMT6 tumor cells. Cancer Res 1985; 45:3541–3547.

109. Kennedy KA, Mimnaugh EG, Trush MA, Sinha BK. Effects of glutathione and ethylxanthate on mitomycin C activation by isolated rat hepatic on EMT6 mouse mammary tumor nuclei. Cancer Res 1985;45:4071–4076.

110. Keyes SR, Fracasso PM, Heimbrook DC, Rockwell S, Sligar SG, Sartorelli AC. Role of NADPH: cytochrome C reductase and DT-diaphorase in the biotransformation of mitomycin C. Cancer Res 1984;44:5638–5643.

111. Keyes SR, Rockwell S, Sartorelli AC. Enhancement of mitomycin C cytotoxicity to hypoxic tumor cells by dicumarol in vivo and in vitro. Cancer Res 1985;45:213–216.

112. Marshall RS, Rauth AM. Modification of the cytotoxic activity of mitomycin C by oxygen and ascorbic acid in Chinese hamster ovary cells and a repair-deficient mutant. Cancer Res 1986;46:2709–2713.

113. Rauth AM, Mohindra JK, Tannock IF. Activity of mitomycin C for aerobic and hypoxic cells in vitro and in vivo. Cancer Res 1983;43:4154–4158.

114. Rockwell S. Effects of mitomycin C alone and in combination with x-rays on EMT6 mouse mammary tumors in vivo. J Natl Cancer Inst 1983;71:765–771.

115. Rockwell S, Mierenburg M, Irvin CG. Effects of the mode of administration of mitomycin on tumor and marrow response and on the therapeutic ratio. Cancer Treat Rep 1987;71:927–934.

116. Chaplin DJ, Durand RE, Olive PL. Cell selection from a murine tumor using the fluorescent probe Hoesch 33342. Br J Cancer 1985;51:569.

117. Chaplin DJ, Olive PL, Durand RE. Intermittent blood flow in a murine tumor: radiobiological effects. Cancer Res 1987;47:597–601.

118. Siemann DW, Keng PC. Cell cycle-specific toxicity of the Hoechst 33342 stain in untreated or irradiated murine tumor cells. Cancer Res 1986;46:3556–3559.

119. Siemann DW, Keng PC. Characterization of radiation resistant hypoxic cell subpopulation in KHT sarcomas. (ii)Cell Sorting. Brit J Cancer 1988;58:296–300.

120. Teicher BA, Herman TS, Holden SA. Combined modality therapy with bleomycin, hyperthermia and radiation. Cancer Res 1988;48:6291–6297.

121. Makowski H, Tentshev P, Frey P, Necek ST, Bergmann H, Blauhut B. Tolerance of an oxygen-carrying colloidal plasma substitute in human beings. Proc 4th Int Symp Perfluorochemical Blood Substitutes, Kyoto, Japan, 1978:47–52.

122. Ohyanagi H, Tosha K, Sekita M, Okamoto M, Itoh T, Mitsuno T. Clinical studies of perfluorochemical whole blood substitutes: safety of Fluosol-DA (20%) in normal human volunteers. Clin. Ther 1979;2(4):306–312.

123. Tremper K, Lapin R, Levine E, Friedman A, Shoemaker W. Hemodynamic oxygen transport effects of a perfluorochemical blood substitute, Fluosol-DA 20%. Critical Care Medicine 1989;8(12):738–741.

124. Mitsuno T, Ohyanagi H, Naito R. Clinical studies of a perfluorochemical whole blood substitute, Fluosol-DA: a summary of 186 cases. Annals of Surgery 1982;1:60–69.

125. Tremper K, Friedman A, Levine E, Labin R, Camarillo D. The preoperative treatment of severe anemia patients with a perfluorochemical oxygen transport fluid, Fluosol-DA. New England J Med 1982;307:277–282.

126. Spence RK, McCoy S, Costabile J, Norcross ED, Pello MJ, Alexander JB, Wisdom C, Camishion RC. Fluosol DA-20 in the treatment of severe anemia: randomized, controlled study of 46 patients. Critical Care Med 1990;18(11):1227–1230.

127. Rose C, Lustig R, McIntosh N, Teicher BA. A clinical trial of Fluosol-DA in advanced head and neck cancer. Int J Radiat Oncol Biol Phys 1986;12:1325–1327.

128. Lustig R, McIntosh-Lowe N, Rose C, Haas J, Krasnow S, Spaulding M, Prosnitz L. Phase I/II study of Fluosol-DA and 100% oxygen as an adjuvant to radiation in the treatment of advanced squamous cell carcinoma of the head and neck. Int J Radiat Oncol Biol Phys 1989; 16(6):1587–1593.

129. Vercellottie G, Hammerschmidt D, Craddock P, Jacob H. Activation of plasma compliment by perfluorocarbon artificial blood: probable mechanism of adverse pulmonary reactions in treatment patients and rationale for corticosteroid prophylaxis. Blood 1982;59:1299–1304.

130. Lustig R, Lowe N, Prosnitz L, Spaulding M, Cohen M, Stitt J, Brannen R. Phase I/II study of Fluosol-DA and 100% oxygen breathing as an adjuvant to radiation in the treatment of unresectable non small cell carcinoma of the lung. Int J Radiat Oncol Biol Phys 1990;19:97–102.

131. Evans RG, Kimler BF, Morantz RA, Vats TS, Gemer LS, Liston V, Lowe N. A Phase I/II study of the use of Fluosol as an adjuvant to radiation therapy in the treatment of primary high-grade brain tumors. Int J Radiat Oncol Biol Phys 1990;19:415–420.

Olivera J. Finn

Pancreatic Tumor Antigens: Diagnostic Markers and Targets for Immunotherapy

4

Ever since it was first shown that mice could be immunized to reject syngeneic chemically induced tumors,[1,2] the search has been on for antigens on animal and human tumors capable of inducing an immune response. Early studies (review[3,4]) demonstrated the existence of tumor specific immunity in tumor-bearing animals and in patients with certain types of tumors, and showed that cell-mediated effector mechanisms, rather than antibody-mediated immunity, were of primary importance in rejection of solid tumors.[5–8] Isolation of immune cells with autologous tumor reactivity from patients with a variety of tumor types provides the best current evidence that at least some human tumors elicit a cell-mediated immune response in the host. Lymphocytes with antitumor reactivity have been derived from peripheral blood,[9–14] malignant effusions,[15] tumor-draining lymph nodes,[16–18] and tumors themselves (tumor-infiltrating lymphocytes, TILs).[19–23] While most tumor-reactive lymphocytes studied to date are from patients bearing melanoma, several studies have dealt with tumors of other histologic origin: by us and others in breast carcinomas,[15,22,24] by others in colon carcinomas,[25] ovarian carcinomas,[26] renal cell carcinomas,[27,28] lymphomas,[29] osteosarcomas,[13] and by us in pancreatic carcinomas.[16,30,31] Clonal analysis of these populations showed involvement of CD4+

as well as CD8+ T-cells, although the vast majority of tumor specific clones were CD8+ CTL.

Identification in animal models and human tumors of cytotoxic T-cells which *in vitro* exhibit strong antitumor reactivity has led to experiments testing their *in vivo* ability to eradicate tumors. Transfer of CD8+ CTL into tumor-bearing mice has been repeatedly shown to lead to tumor eradication, providing the T-cell inoculum is large and the tumor burden small.[32–36] Several studies showed that adoptive transfer of noncytolytic CD4+ T-cells can also lead to tumor elimination, presumably through delayed type hypersensitivity (DTH)-like mechanisms.[37,38] Adoptive transfer of tumor specific T-cells has recently been tried in patients, with limited but encouraging results. The best results have been obtained in melanoma and renal cell carcinoma patients treated with TILs, IL-2, and cyclophosphamide.[23,39]

The most useful, both from the point of understanding the basic mechanisms of cellular immunity as well as immunotherapy, have been animal models which have dealt with tumors with known tumor specific antigens.[35,38,40,41] Even though tumor-specific antigens have been postulated in a variety of human tumors, no specific antigen, with the exception of the mucin antigen characterized by us[31] and described below, has as yet been as-

61

sociated with human immune responses. Many other attempts are under way, with the most promising results being reported for melanomas.[10,42]

This chapter will review the progress made in identifying tumor-specific antigens and epitopes on human pancreatic carcinomas, and will present a possibility of utilizing an epithelial cell-specific molecule with an apparent tumor-specific epitope for induction of immunity and realization of specific immunotherapy.

Pancreatic Tumor Antigens ■

Over the years numerous attempts were made to identify antigens on pancreatic tumors, which may be useful in early diagnosis of this disease, monitoring of effects of the treatment, and ultimately designing immunotherapy approaches. Even though a number of different molecules or different epitopes on the same molecule were identified, and will be described below, their usefulness was limited by the fact that the reagents used for their identification were either rabbit or mouse antibodies. This showed that these antigens were indeed capable of inducing an immune response in those species, without providing any indication that the human immune system would recognize these same antigens, which may have just as easily been seen as autoantigens. Similarly, none of these epitopes were expected to be recognized by T-cells, known to be crucial in tumor rejection. The fact that the antibodies were frequently of the IgG isotype spoke in favor of the existence of epitopes recognized by helper T-cells, but those have remained unidentified. In spite of these limitations, some of these antigens and the antibodies which recognize them have provided information about the biology of pancreatic carcinomas that may be useful in designing therapeutic approaches using other reagents.

Recent progress in cellular immunology and in molecular oncology has illuminated several new paths for searching for tumor-specific antigens capable of stimulating cellular immunity. Protein products of mutated genes in tumor cells are now known to be potential antigens. Transformation-specific mutations in pancreatic tumors and the role of the mutated products as tumor-specific antigens have not yet been fully explored.

Antibody Defined Pancreatic Tumor Antigens ■

The search for tumor-specific antigens was initially performed using polyclonal sera, usually rabbit, derived by immunization with human pancreatic tumors. Even though many molecules on the immunizing cells were capable of stimulating rabbit antibody production, none were exclusively expressed on the tumor or on the corresponding normal tissues. Very often the antibodies would broadly cross react with other tissues, showing not only the paucity of tumor-specific antigens, but also the difficulty in establishing the existence of tissue-specific antigens. Some exceptions now, over 10 years later, hold considerable interest because they can be viewed as precursors to the current observations which, given the molecular techniques of today, can be carried further and described fully.

The more notable early efforts resulted in the description of several molecules whose full characterization was hampered by the technology of that period, but whose partial characterization provided impetus to continue the search. In 1979 Kuntz and Archer immunized rabbits with saline extracts of pancreatic tumors and obtained antiserum which, after proper absorption with various normal tissues including pancreas, reacted in gel diffusion tests with pancreatic tumor cell extract, but not with normal pancreas cell extract.[43] The reactive molecule was found in the void volume of a Sephadex G-200 column, suggesting a molecular weight over 380,000 daltons.

An apparently similar molecule was identified that same year by Shultz and Yunis,[44] who immunized rabbits with the human pancreatic cell line MIA PaCa-2. Following absorption with normal pancreatic tissue, the antisera defined an antigen with a molecular weight in excess of 900,000 daltons. In addition to the tumor, the antigen was also expressed on fetal pancreas and could be detected in sera of patients with pancreatic carcinoma.

A third high molecular weight antigen defined by rabbit antibodies was named pancreas cancer associated antigen (PCAA) and resulted from immunization with pancreatic cancer patient ascites.[45] After absorption with normal human plasma, the rabbit antisera were used to monitor antigen purification by chromatography, localizing the reactive molecule in the fraction of a molecular weight greater than 1×10^6 daltons.

As will be discussed later in the chapter, a family of molecules known as mucins, in that same molecular weight range, is now known to be expressed by pancreatic tumors, to be very immunogenic, and to contain tumor-specific epitopes. Monoclonal antibodies reactive with the protein core of these molecules have been used to isolate the genes encoding these molecules, and the deciphering of their molecular structure has led to a new understanding of how tumor-specific epitopes may be generated.

The development of hybridoma technology[46] held promise of increased specificity and the possibility of defining unique epitopes that may be either tissue-specific, differentiation-stage-specific, or transformation-specific, any of these potentially useful in defining and managing the malignant phenotype. This technology was immediately applied to looking for tumor-specific antigens in many different human malignancies. Several antigens were defined with antibodies generated following immunization of mice with tumors other than pancreatic but which reacted with the pancreatic carcinomas as well. Even though none of them was tumor-specific, they had some of the desired properties: reexpression or increased expression in tumors vs. normal tissue, and increased levels of expression in patients' blood, which could be used for early diagnosis of that malignancy. Table 4-1 lists a number of the molecules that have been best characterized to date, most of which have been tested as targets for either diagnosis or therapy of malignancies that express them.

Oncofetal antigens, as their name implies, are characterized by expression which is limited to fetal tissue, not the corresponding adult tissue, and reexpression following malignant transformation. Several oncofetal pancreatic antigens have been described and their expression in pancreatic malignancies monitored. In 1974 Banwo and associates[47] found increased levels of pancreatic oncofetal antigen (POA) in 29 out of 30 patients with pancreatic malignancies, but none in patients with other malignancies or benign pathological conditions, such as pancreatitis. The antigen was purified by Gelder and colleagues[48] from fetal pancreas, but when further tests were run to measure serum levels in pancreatic cancer patients, very few patients had elevated levels. In addition, patients with diseases of the liver and biliary tract also showed greatly elevated levels of this antigen in the serum, thereby diminishing the initially very promising utility of this molecule in the diagnosis and monitoring of pancreatic cancer.

Another oncofetal pancreatic antigen (OPA) was affinity purified from the blood of patients with pancreatic cancer, using antibodies generated against human fetal pancreas.[49] It was found to be a protein of 40,000 daltons molecular weight, distinct from other oncofetal antigens. The presence of this antigen was examined in the serum of 700 individuals with a variety of conditions. Even though 42 of 48 (88%) pancreatic cancer patients had elevated levels of this antigen in their serum, the significance of this finding was lessened by the fact that elevated levels of OPA were also found in many other benign and malignant conditions.

The serum diagnostic value of yet another oncofetal antigen, fetoacinar pancreatic protein (FAP), was tested in 201 patients with pancreatic and extrapancreatic malignancies.[50] This molecule was defined by a murine monoclonal antibody which recognized a glycoprotein of 110,000 daltons molecular weight.[51] The highest expression of this molecule was associated with fetal acinar cells at around 20 weeks of gestation. It remained at a very low level in the normal adult pancreas[52] and was found to be reexpressed strongly in pancreatic carcinomas. FAP protein was detected in the majority of sera from patients with cancer of the pancreas, but as in the case of other antigens above, it could also be detected in benign diseases of the pancreas, for example, pancreatitis.[53]

The development of a new monoclonal antibody, PA8-15, was recently reported,[54] generated against the pancreatic cell line SUIT-2, and reactive with gastrointestinal cancers, especially those of the pancreatico-biliary tract. Expression of this antigen in fetal pancreas qualifies it as an oncofetal antigen, even though some preliminary attempts at its molecular characterization suggest that it may be an epitope on a mucin-like molecule and dependent on the presence of sialic acid for its expression. Very high levels of this antigen were detected in sera of patients with pancreatic and other gastric malignancies, and resection of the tumor lowered the serum antigen level, while without resection the levels continued to rise. Even though detectable in various benign diseases, such as liver cirrhosis, hepatitis, and pancreatitis, these levels of the PA8-15 antigen were considerably lower, making the distinction between a malignant and a benign state possible. Further characterization of this antigen, the molecule which expresses it, and its utility in diagnosis of pancreatic cancer is forthcoming.

Perhaps the best known oncofetal antigen is the

Table 4–1
Antigens on Pancreatic Tumors Detected by Antibodies

Antigen	Immunizing Tissue	Antibody	Reference
Oncofetal			
OPA	Fetal pancreas	Rabbit, polyclonal	Knapp, 1981[49]
CEA	Colon cancer and other tissues	Rabbit, sheep, monkey, polyclonal	Burtin and Gold, 1978[55]
POA	Fetal pancreas	Rabbit, polyclonal	Gelder, *et al,* 1978[48]
FAP	Fetal pancreas	Mouse, MAb J28	Escribano and Albers, 1986[51]
PA8-15	Pancreatic cancer cell line SUIT-2	Mouse, MAb PA8-15	Arai, *et al,* 1991[54]
Mucin			
CA 50	Colorectal carcinoma cell line	Mouse MAb C 50	Lindholm, *et al,* 1983[57]
CA 19-9	Colon carcinoma cell line SW1116	Mouse MAb 19-9	Koprowski, *et al,* 1979[58]
CA 242	Colorectal carcinoma cell line COLO 205	Mouse MAb C 242	Haglund, *et al,* 1989[59]
CAR-3	Epidermoid carcinoma cell line A 431	Mouse MAb AR-3	Prat, *et al,* 1989[60]
DU-PAN-2	Pancreatic carcinoma cell line HPAF	Mouse MAb DU-PAN-2	Lan, *et al,* 1987[61]
Ypan-1	Pancreatic carcinoma cell line SW1990	Mouse MAb Ypan-1	Yvan, *et al,* 1985[62]
Span-1	″	Mouse MAb Span-1	″
BW494	Pancreatic tumor tissue	Mouse MAb BW494	Bosslet, *et al,* 1986[63]
Other			
MUSE 11	Gastric cancer ascites fluid	Mouse MAb MUSE 11	Ban, *et al,* 1989[69]

carcinoembrionic antigen (CEA) of the human digestive system, which is an epitope expressed on a family of acid glycoproteins of around 200,000 daltons molecular weight and considerable molecular heterogeneity.[55] Like the previously mentioned antigens, it is shed into circulation and consequently could be considered as a potential tumor marker. Unfortunately it has been found to have very low sensitivity and poor specificity and may have limited usefulness only in sequential monitoring of already diagnosed malignancies.[56]

It is now clear that immunization of mice with tumors of epithelial cell origin, such as colon tu-

mors, pancreatic and breast tumors, and gastric tumors, resulted in antibodies recognizing a large number of epitopes, most of which were carbohydrate in origin and expressed by very high molecular weight glycoproteins. Further characterization of these molecules indicated that they were all members of the mucin family. As will be discussed later in the chapter, recent molecular cloning of several mucin genes from different organ sites indicated that the protein structure may be considerably different but that great similarity exists in the O-linked carbohydrate chains and the presence of sialic acid residues in all the molecules. A partial list of pancreatic mucin antigens and antibodies that detect them is given in Table 4-1. CA 50, CA-19-9, and CA 242[57-59] were defined with antibodies generated against colon carcinomas and CAR-3[60] against human epidermoid cell line, and yet they are expressed on pancreatic tumors in levels comparable to the levels of DU-PAN 2, Ypan-1, Span-1, and BW494 epitopes defined with antibodies generated against pancreatic tumors.[61-63]

Mucin molecules carrying these epitopes are found in very high levels in the circulation of tumor-bearing patients and thus have been used and compared to each other for sensitivity and tumor specificity.[64-68] Although these markers as a group appear superior to previously used markers like CEA, and even more so when used in combination with one another, they suffer the same disadvantage of the previous markers in that they are also elevated in certain benign diseases. Additionally, expression of these individually distinct carbohydrate epitopes on mucin molecules from different organ sites diminishes their tumor specificity.

The recently described pancreatic antigen MUSE11[69] does not appear to be a member of either the oncofetal group or the mucin group of antigens. MUSE11 epitope is found on a glycoprotein of 300,000 daltons molecular weight. The epitope is peptide in nature, which may account for a higher degree of tumor specificity seen with the MUSE11 antibody. The molecule is found in sera of patients with pancreatic and gastric cancer and not with pancreatitis, suggesting that it may be useful as a tumor marker for early diagnosis.

Mutated Oncogene Products as Pancreatic Tumor Antigens ■

Transformation of normal cells to malignant cells is often accompanied or, in some instances, caused by mutations of somatic cell genes. Those genes that can be shown to be involved in the transforming process were termed oncogenes, having been originally identified as genetic material of oncogenic viruses.[70] Protein products of "proto-oncogenes," normal cellular counterparts of oncogenes, play an important role in cell division, signal transduction, and differentiation. Rearrangements, mutations, and/or amplifications of the normal genes lead to their activation and contribution to the malignant phenotype of a cell. As many as 40 different oncogenes have been identified to date, several of which are consis-

tently found activated in human tumors of various organ sites. In addition to providing some clues regarding the mechanism of transformation in certain human malignancies, predicted activation of oncogenes associated with a particular tumor type also suggests synthesis of a mutated oncogene product that will be different from the proto-oncogene product in normal cells and an ideal candidate for a tumor-specific molecule. Those oncogene products encoding cell surface molecules could be targeted by antibodies for diagnosis as well as therapy of the tumor. Other oncogene products that are strictly nuclear or cytoplasmic proteins would be expected to appear on the surface of the tumor as peptides bound to class I HLA molecules, and to be recognized by the patient's T-cells. More importantly, immunotherapy protocols could be designed to specifically generate, *in vivo* or *in vitro,* large numbers of T-cells specific for oncogene encoded peptides, expressed only on the tumor and not on normal cells.

Two oncogenes have been found associated with pancreatic tumors, the neu (c-erbB-2) and c-K-ras. The first encodes a cell surface protein, while the second encodes a cytoplasmic protein. The protein encoded by c-erbB-2 is a 190,000 daltons transmembrane putative growth factor receptor, closely related to the epidermal growth factor receptor (EGF).[71,72] It has been found amplified and overexpressed in a number of different human adenocarcinomas, including carcinoma of the pancreas.[73-75] This expression is easily detected by antibodies generated against various peptides on this molecule. It is not clear yet what is the mechanism of activation of this oncogene in human adenocarcinomas. The single point mutation which has been previously described in the transmembrane region of the rat c-erbB-2 gene[76] has not been found in the homologous region of the human gene. However, this does not exclude mutations at other, not yet identified sites, as the activating mechanism. One case of an amplified and rearranged c-erb-B gene has been reported in a human gastric adenocarcinoma.[77]

Expression of the c-erbB-2 oncogene product on the tumor cell surface provides an attractive target for immunotherapy. The results obtained in animal models with cells transformed with the rat oncogene established the precedent that tumors which express an oncogene product on the cell surface can be targeted effectively and therapeutically with antibodies reactive with epitopes on the external domain of that oncogene product.[78-80] The c-erbB-2 transformed NIH-3T3 cells rapidly grow as subcutaneous fibrosarcomas in nude mice. However, intravenous injection of a monoclonal antibody reactive with the c-erbB-2 product, immediately or seven days after tumor implantation, inhibited tumor cell growth. Injection of two antibodies, reactive with different epitopes on the c-erbB-2 protein, showed a synergistic effect and cured half of the injected mice. The antibodies had a similar inhibitory effect on the growth of a c-erbB-2 expressing rat neuroblastoma in syngeneic rats. *In vitro* and *in vivo* experiments showed this effect to be mediated by down-regulation of the oncogene product, apparently obligatory for the maintenance of tumor growth.

The product of this same oncogene was also used in animal models of immune mediated tumor cell regression.[81] A cDNA clone of the c-erbB-2 oncogene was incorporated into a recombinant vaccinia virus and the construct used to immunize mice to the oncogene product. Infection of mice with the recombinant vaccinia virus resulted in the production of high titers of antisera reactive with the oncogene product. Moreover, when recombinant vaccinia immunized mice were injected with tumor cells expressing the c-erbB-2 oncogene product on their surface, no tumor growth was observed. Immunization with a single oncogene-encoded product was, in this case, sufficient for induction of protective immunity against tumor cells expressing that product. It is not unreasonable to postulate that similar types of responses might be achieved against human tumors, providing our full understanding of the ability of the human immune repertoire to recognize mutated oncogene products, and more importantly, respond against them in the environment of an already established tumor.

While c-erbB-2 was found to be overexpressed in only a fraction of pancreatic adenocarcinomas, activation of another oncogene, c-K-ras, has been reported in over 90% of human pancreatic tumors. This oncogene is a member of a ras gene family whose products are membrane bound guanine nucleotide binding proteins involved in signal transduction across the membrane (review [82]). The ras oncogenes are activated by single nucleotide substitutions at codons 12, 13, or 61, and their role in tumorigenesis has been well documented in animal tumor model systems.[82] They have also been implicated in human tumorigenesis by virtue of the presence of activated ras genes in a significant percentage of human tumors from different tissue and organ sites (review [83]). The most striking observation is the presence of activated c-K-ras onco-

gene in the majority of human pancreatic adenocarcinomas. In numerous studies performed to date, between 75% and 90% of pancreatic tumors were found to contain this oncogene mutated in codon 12.[84–89] The amino acid that is encoded in this position in the proto-oncogene is substituted without any evidence for a predominant nucleotide transition. A single exception is a report of a predominant glycine to aspartic acid mutation in 24 out of 25 cases of human pancreatic cancer in Japan,[90] which may indicate possible genetic or nongenetic factors in determining preferential substitutions at this codon, not observed in European samples.

The finding of this oncogene mutation in human pancreatic cancer is very exciting, as it again offers an opportunity to explore the possibility of generating an immune response to a truly tumor-specific antigen. Moreover, since the T-cell component of the immune system is particularly efficient in discriminating between epitopes resulting from single amino acid substitutions, the predominant immune response expected would be T-cell mediated. This would be a desired outcome considering the overwhelming evidence that T-cells are the main antitumor effector cells. What has been a working hypothesis of tumor immunologists for a number of years has recently become an established fact: mutations throughout the human genome generate new antigenic peptides that can be recognized by T-cells. Thus any mutation in a tumor cell is a putative tumor-specific antigen.[91] Inasmuch as their variation can be infinite, it may be most efficient to focus the efforts of tumor immunologists on the more predictable mutations, such as those found in activated oncogenes.

The ability of the oncogenic form of the ras protein to induce T-cell immunity has already been tested in mice.[92] Immunization with short synthetic peptides containing the mutated amino acid at codon 12 was shown to elicit T-cell immunity to the mutated ras protein. Whether or not human T-cells will be able to recognize mutated oncogene products will depend on many factors including (1) the existence in the peripheral T-cell repertoire of CD4+ as well as CD8+ T-cells capable of recognizing the mutated epitopes; (2) the ability of the patient's HLA molecules on tumors and on antigen presenting cells to bind and present mutated peptides; and (3) the level of expression of the oncogene protein in the tumor cells. The predictable activation of c-K-ras oncogene in pancreatic carcinomas, and the opportunity it provides for designing tumor antigen-specific T-cell therapy for this otherwise incurable cancer, make this direction of research compulsory.

Studies Directed Towards Immunotherapy of Pancreatic Cancer ■

Development of new reagents and increased understanding of the requirements for growth of human T-cells *in vitro* provided a renewed opportunity to examine the human T-cell repertoire for the presence of cells capable of specifically recognizing human tumors. In addition to yielding information on the ability of the cellular component of the immune system to recognize autologous tumors, propagation of tumor-specific T-cell clones *in vitro* provides a new set of reagents for identification of T-cell-stimulatory, tumor-specific molecules and epitopes, and a potential to generate a large number of tumor-specific T-cells that may be administered back to the patient to increase the effector cell/tumor cell ratio and thus the tumor fighting capacity of the patient.

Peripheral blood, although the most accessible source, has proved to have very low numbers of tumor reactive cells, which has been interpreted to mean that any accumulation of tumor reactive cells at the tumor site may actually lead to a depletion of these cells from the periphery. Clearly, cells found to infiltrate excised tumors (named TIL for tumor-infiltrating lymphocytes) would appear to be likely candidates for tumor reactive cells. Many tumors, however, exert a growth inhibitory effect on these cells, which is difficult to overcome *in vitro,* making their propagation problematic. In addition, many tumors (e.g., pancreas) are not resectable and consequently lymphocytes infiltrating those tumors are not accessible.

In our attempts to identify T-cells reactive with pancreatic tumors, we chose what we consider the superior source of tumor-specific T-cells, tumor-draining lymph nodes. These lymph nodes very often contain large numbers of tumor cells, are expected to trap whatever molecules are being secreted or shed by the tumor, and are lymphoid organs with cellular scaffolding uniquely designed to facilitate the interaction of antigen and antigen presenting cells with lymphocytes.

Our initial attempts resulted in specific expansion of pancreatic tumor reactive T-cells in 14:14 pancreatic cancer patients.[16] Recently similar results were reported by another group in 16:16 pancreatic cancer patients.[93] Extensive studies by us positively identified the mucin molecule as the target of that immunity.[30,31] The significance of these findings was twofold. (1) An antigen was identified for the first time on human tumors capable of stimulating T-cell immunity and, even more importantly, (2) this antigen was known to be expressed by a large number of human tumors from various sites, all of epithelial cell origin. The list includes, in addition to pancreatic cancer, breast carcinomas, colon carcinomas, cervical carcinomas, ovarian carcinomas, renal cell carcinomas, and some lung carcinomas. This list suggested that similar T-cell responses could be elicited by mucin antigens on all of these tumors, making mucins the long-sought "shared tumor antigens," potentially useful for immunotherapy.

Biochemical and Molecular Characteristics of Mucins ■

Mucins are glycoproteins abundantly present at the luminal side of ductal epithelial cells and on tumors derived from this cell type. They are molecules of very high molecular weight, greater than 50% of that weight being attributed to long carbohydrate side chains attached to the protein backbone by O-glycoside linkages to threonine and serine residues.

Numerous mucin-specific antibodies have been derived following immunization of animals with normal or malignant epithelial cells. They were initially thought to recognize different molecules, but in most instances were determined to react with various carbohydrate mucin epitopes (selected examples shown in Table 4-1). Heterogeneity of mucin molecules, as defined by carbohydrate epitope-specific antibodies, appeared to be very extensive. The reported antibodies reacted with both normal and tumor mucins—some exhibited apparent tumor specificity, some showed organ specificity, some reacted with mucins from most organ sites. The most discriminating were antibodies that reacted with protein epitopes on the mucin polypeptide core. Some of those antibodies were generated by using deglycosylated protein core as immunogen, while others came out of immunizations with whole mucins or epithelial tumor cells. The latter provided the first evidence that some protein epitopes must be exposed on this highly glycosylated molecule.[94–97]

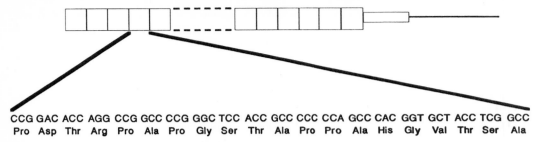

CCG	GAC	ACC	AGG	CCG	GCC	CCG	GGC	TCC	ACC	GCC	CCC	CCA	GCC	CAC	GGT	GCT	ACC	TCG	GCC
Pro	Asp	Thr	Arg	Pro	Ala	Pro	Gly	Ser	Thr	Ala	Pro	Pro	Ala	His	Gly	Val	Thr	Ser	Ala

FIG. 4–1 This schematic representation of the highly repetitive structure of the mucin cDNA shows the amino acid sequence of one of the tandem repeats.

The nature of mucins produced by different organs, as well as possible differences between tumor-derived and normal epithelial cell-derived mucins became clear only recently, following isolation of cDNA clones for breast,[98–102] pancreas,[103] and small intestine/colon mucins.[104,105] Comparison of the cDNAs indicated important similarities in the overall structure of the molecule, but also showed that at least three different genes located on different chromosomes encode mucin molecules, and that the expression of these genes can be tissue-specific. The sequences of all the genes cloned from breast adenocarcinomas were nearly identical, and those in turn were nearly identical to the sequence of the gene cloned from a pancreatic adenocarcinoma. The genes and the encoded mucins were named MUC 1. Two genes isolated from a small intestine cDNA library and expressed in colon adenocarcinomas were distinct from one another and from the breast and pancreatic mucin genes. They were named MUC 2 and MUC 3.

The most unifying feature of all the mucin genes is the presence of numerous (between 40 and 100) tandem repeats that comprise approximately two-thirds of the protein. The amino acid sequence of the repeats is abundant in serines and threonines, sites of O-linked glycosylation. The amino terminus consists of a putative signal peptide followed by degenerate tandem repeats, and the carboxyl terminus contains degenerate tandem repeats and unique transmembrane sequence and a cytoplasmic tail. Figure 4-1 shows the tandem repeat structure of the breast and pancreas mucin cDNA (MUC 1). It consists of 60 nucleotides encoding a polypeptide of 20 amino acids in length. Five O-linked glycosylation sites (2 serines and 3 threonines) are present per repeat.

Table 4-2 compares the tandem repeat amino acid sequence encoded by the three genes. It is clear that the presence of many serines and threonines in all the repeats directs similar glycosylation; antibodies directed to carbohydrate structures would be expected to cross react with all of these mucins. On the other hand, antibodies directed to a linear amino acid sequence, or T-cells that would be expected to recognize such a sequence, would be expected to be exquisitely specific for the individual mucins. This indeed is the case for a number of core specific antibodies and for pancreatic mucin-specific T-cells, as will be discussed below.

Table 4–2
Repetitive Sequences in Human Mucins

Mucin	Amino Acid Residues	Reference
MUC 1 (chromosome 1)	PDTRPAPGSTAPPAHGGVTSA	Gendler, *et al*, 1987[98] Siddiqui, *et al*, 1988[100] Ligtenberg, *et al*, 1990[101] Wreschner, *et al*, 1990[102] Lan, *et al*, 1990[103]
MUC 2 (chromosome 11)	PTTTPITTTTTVTPTPTPTGTTQT	Gum, *et al*, 1989[104]
MUC 3 (chromosome 7)	HSTPSFTSSITTTETTS	Gum, *et al*, 1990[105]

Tumor Specific Epitopes on Mucin Molecules ■

In order for mucins to qualify as tumor-specific antigens it must be supposed that mucins made by tumor cells are in some way distinct from mucins made by normal cells. While many mucin-specific antibodies react with mucins expressed on the tumor cells and found in the circulation of tumor-bearing patients, they also recognize their respective epitopes on mucins expressed on normal ductal epithelial cells. Since those epitopes could be considered self-antigens, tolerance rather than reactivity towards those antigens would be expected of the immune system. On the other hand, normal expression of mucins is limited to the luminal surfaces of ductal cells, and it is possible that this molecule, although always present, is never presented to the immune system, and tolerance has not been established. Consequently, even if tumor mucins are identical to normal mucins, their mere presence on the tumor mass, which has lost its normal architectural constraints, or in serum may be sufficient to initiate an immune response. The majority of mucin core specific antibodies react equally well with normal and tumor mucins, indicating identity of these two molecules on the protein level. A very different picture is seen with antibodies to carbohydrate determinants, and several protein core specific antibodies with unique tumor mucin reactivity. They indicate that mucins are expressed on tumors in an aberrantly glycosylated form. The carbohydrate side chains of the tumor-produced mucins are shorter than the side chains of mucins produced by normal cells. There is also an indication that in tumor mucins not all the potential glycosylation sites are used. This results in unmasking of protein core epitopes on tumor mucins (tumor-specific antigens), the same epitopes being concealed in normal mucins by complete glycosylation.[106]

Unique Aspects of Mucin-Specific T-Cell Immunity Correlated With Unique Aspects of Mucin Structure ■

MCH-RESTRICTED AND UNRESTRICTED RECOGNITION □

Figure 4-2 outlines the cardinal features of the interaction of mucin-specific T-cells with the mucin molecule. Whole mucin purified from pancreatic tumors (represented in the figure as a chain of tandem repeat peptides) was able to stimulate proliferation of cytotoxic CD8+ T-cells and to serve as a target for tumor lysis, apparently without the requirement for the presence of antigen presenting cells or autologous HLA antigens on the tumor targets. (See original data [31].) As a result, every pancreatic adenocarcinoma expressing detectable levels of mucin was efficiently lysed by the T-cells derived from pancreatic cancer patients. This was a startling observation, considering that most T-cell responses are MHC (HLA) restricted. MHC-unrestricted activation of T-cells, although uncommon, is not unique to mucins, but rather it may be a property of molecules and epitopes of certain de-

FIG. 4–2 Activation of mucin-specific T-cells. (T) T-cell; (TCR) T-cell receptor; (HLA) human major histocompatibility complex molecules; (APC) antigen presenting cells; (oooooo) whole mucin; (o) a single mucin core peptide.

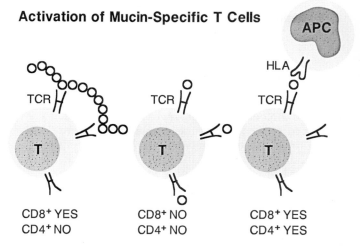

Activation of Mucin-Specific T Cells

CD8+ YES
CD4+ NO

CD8+ NO
CD4+ NO

CD8+ YES
CD4+ YES

fined characteristics (review [107]). A T-cell is activated through its antigen receptor either by antigen or antireceptor antibody. Activation with antireceptor antibody shows the need for receptor crosslinking in order for an efficient signal to be delivered to the T-cell. Multiple engagements and crosslinking of the TCR are highly unlikely events for most antigens. An efficient signal through a single receptor is thus delivered trough the trimolecular, TCR/antigen/MHC complex, but only when that complex is made more stable by the accessory interactions of the CD4 and CD8 molecules with their MHC ligands. Most antigens alone do not, under normal circumstances, bind to the TCR with the sufficient affinity to trigger T-cell response. Situations when this can be expected and has been seen to occur are: (1) when the density of the antigen on the cell is very high so that multiple T-cell receptors can simultaneously engage, and (2) when the antigen is sufficiently large and highly multivalent, again allowing simultaneous binding of multiple receptors to multiple identical epitopes.

Mucin molecules fulfill both of these requirements by being abundantly expressed on the tumor cell and by being large and highly repetitive structures with the potential of containing many identical T-cell epitopes.

While CD8+ CTL could be stimulated by a whole molecule in an MHC-unrestricted fashion, CD4+ mucin-specific T-cells reacted with synthetic peptides corresponding to a single mucin tandem repeat only when the peptide was presented on self-MHC (HLA) molecules (Barnd and Finn, unpublished observations). The CD8+ cells could also be stimulated in this way. A single peptide alone, as expected, was unable to stimulate either cell population.

ORGAN SPECIFICITY □

Identity of sequence between breast and pancreatic mucins, and their difference from colon mucins was also reflected in the T-cell reactivity with these molecules. Mucin-specific CD8+ CTL established from pancreatic cancer patients were unable to distinguish between pancreatic and breast tumor targets and killed both equally well, while they had no recognition of mucin-producing colon tumors. Mucin-specific CTL established from breast cancer patients exhibited identical reactivity by killing pancreatic and breast tumors and not colon tumors.[24,31,108] This pattern of reactivity is to be expected of T-cells that recognize

linear amino acid sequence epitopes, since those epitopes would clearly be the same in breast and pancreatic mucins and different in colon mucins (see Table 4-2).

TUMOR SPECIFICITY □

Figure 4-3 illustrates the ability of mucin-specific T-cells derived from a pancreatic cancer patient to recognize and kill mucin-producing pancreatic and breast tumor cell lines and not mucin-producing normal epithelial cell lines. The clue to that specificity has been provided by a mouse monoclonal antibody SM-3, which has been raised to deglycosylated mucin core protein and reacts with the epitope comprised of the first five amino acids of the tandem repeat. Moreover, the epitope recognized by SM-3 is exposed only in tumors due to incomplete glycosylation of the mucin.[97] All tumor cells in Figure 4-3, which are shown to be killed by the CTL, express the SM-3 epitope abundantly, while the normal epithelial cell lines, which are not killed, do not. We previously reported that this antibody blocks recognition of tumor cells by mucin-specific T-cells,[31] suggesting close spatial relationship between the T-cell epitope and the SM-3 epitope. Other antibodies (e.g., BC-1, BC-2,

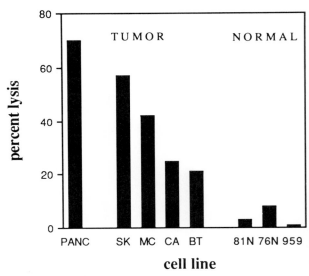

FIG. 4–3 Specific recognition of tumor cells and not normal ductal epithelial cells. Chromium release assay was employed using cytotoxic T-cells established from a pancreatic cancer patient as effector cells, at 10:1 effector to target cell ratio. (PANC) pancreatic carcinoma cell line; (SK, MC, CA, BT) breast carcinoma cell lines; (81N, 76N, 959) normal epithelial cell lines.

BC-3), reactive with different epitopes on the repeat peptide expressed on normal mucins as well,[96] do not affect the function of the CTL. Combined, these data indicate that the CTL also depend on the incomplete or aberrant glycosylation of the mucin molecules by the tumor cell for the recognition of the specific epitope.

Figure 4-4 is a proposed model for recognition of the mucin core of the tumor-specific CTL. Two tandem repeats are represented. The portion of the core predicted by the program AMPHI[109] to form an amphipathic α-helix reaches from the proline at position 7 to the threonine at position 3 of the next repeat. This region is roughly bisected by the binding site for SM-3 (residues 1–15, the first 5 comprising the minimal peptide epitope). Since the BC antibodies do not affect the reactivity of the CTL, we propose that amino acids 7–15 form the T-cell epitope. It is conceivable that glycosylation of residues 9 and 10, and possibly residue 3, would profoundly affect the ability of the CTL to bind and that those residues are likely to be incompletely glycosylated in tumors, allowing tumor-specific expression of the core epitopes.

The fortuitous deficiency in the function of tumor cell glycosyltransferases and/or glycosidases, which is likely responsible for unmasking of tumor-specific epitopes on MUC 1 molecules, and the presence in the human peripheral T-cell repertoire of cells that can recognize this epitope may be a unique situation for the MUC 1 antigens. The potential of generating similar tumor-specific protein epitopes on the MUC 2 and MUC 3 molecules

has not yet been examined. Of all three tandem repeats the MUC 1 repeat has the smallest number of glycosylation sites (5), while MUC 2 and MUC 3 have 14 and 11 respectively, and thus a much greater potential for concealing the protein core. Polyclonal antisera generated to partially and completely deglycosylated colon mucins have been able to detect protein epitopes on precursor molecules in the cytoplasm of tumor cells but not on their surface.[110] While this may be a problem for antibodies, T-cells would still be able to recognize these epitopes when they are transported out of the cytoplasm as HLA bound peptides.

Potential Application of Tumor Mucins in Immunotherapy of Epithelial Tumors ■

The finding that tumor-specific epitopes can elicit immune responses to human tumors foreshadows an era of immune manipulation of tumor growth and eventual recruitment of the immune system in the process of tumor destruction. The success of immunotherapy depends on further understanding of the multitude of reasons why the observed antitumor response is seldom efficient. At the root of that understanding is the need to know the target antigen on the tumor cell. Mucin molecules expressed by a variety of human solid tumors clearly have the potential of expressing tumor-specific epitopes recognized by the human immune system.

FIG. 4–4 A proposed model for the recognition of the mucin core by tumor-specific cytotoxic T-cells.

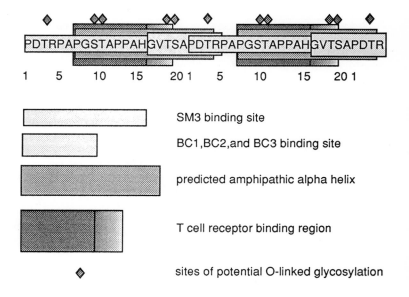

How can that potential now be utilized in designing novel approaches for immunotherapy of mucin expressing carcinomas?

Knowing the specific antigen facilitates expansion *in vitro* of T-cells with specific reactivity. We have utilized purified mucins, recombinant mucin molecules synthesized in *E. coli* and therefore unglycosylated, as well as synthetic peptides corresponding to the tandem repeat, to stimulate expansion of mucin specific T-cells *in vitro*. The effectiveness of adoptive immunotherapy with mucin specific T-cells will now be evaluated.

The knowledge of the target antigen is also requisite for designing approaches for eliciting and maintaining tumor-specific immune responses *in vivo*, in the tumor-bearing patient. Our efforts will be directed towards generation of mucin containing vaccines, which will fulfill these two important requirements: (1) express the tumor-specific T-cell stimulatory epitopes, and (2) be able to stimulate both CD4+ helper T-cells and CD8+ cytotoxic T-cells.

The most likely candidate would be a recombinant mucin synthesized in *E. coli*. We have already obtained this product and know that it reacts very well with the tumor-specific antibody SM-3 (Kirk and Finn, unpublished observations). The possible disadvantage of this molecule as a vaccine is that it is expected to be taken up by antigen presenting cells and processed via the exogenous antigen presenting pathway, which results in the presentation of the antigenic peptides on HLA Class II molecules.[111] This may preferentially stimulate CD4+ T-cells, and our *in vitro* experiments show that the tumor cytotoxic T-cells are mostly CD8+.

A similar problem might be expected following immunization with a soluble peptide encompassing the tumor-specific epitope. However, successful immunization protocols with soluble peptides, leading to generation of specific cytotoxic T-cells have been reported recently.[112] Success of this approach will depend on determining the right peptide and the correct length that will allow it to bind to Class I molecules on the surface of antigen presenting cells for efficient stimulation of CD8+ cytotoxic T-cells.

Our approach of choice, however, is to express the mucin molecules by gene transfer into the patient's antigen presenting (e.g., skin fibroblasts) cells and use the transfected cells as immunogen. The cells would be expected to present endogenously synthesized mucin peptides on Class I molecules for recognition by CD8+ CTL.[111] The whole mucin molecules expressed on the surface or secreted by the transfected cells would be internalized either by those same cells or other antigen presenting cells in the vicinity, for processing and presentation on Class II molecules to the CD4+ helper T-cells.

To begin to test this approach *in vitro*, we chose patients' Epstein-Barr (EBV) virus-immortalized B lymphoblastoid cell lines for transfection. EBV readily transforms human B-cells into established cell lines. The expression vector we selected for their transfection is shown in Figure 4-5. A fragment of EBV DNA (EBV oriP) was added to the vector to assure its replication as an unintegrated plasmid in multiple copies in B-cells containing EBV DNA.[113] The β-actin promoter/enhancer sequences were added to ensure high-level expression of the mucin cDNA. The gene for neomycin resistance was also included for easy selection of transfected cells.

Transfection of this vector into EBV immortalized B-cells resulted in a high level of expression of mucin molecules, but they were fully glycosylated and did not express tumor specific epitopes. Interestingly, the Burkitt lymphoma cell line RAJI also expressed high levels of transfected mucin, but, just as in pancreatic tumors, these molecules were abundant with underglycosylated tumor-specific epitopes (Table 4-3). Since the EBV immor-

FIG. 4-5 Mucin cDNA expression vector used for transfection of EBV immortalized B-cells.

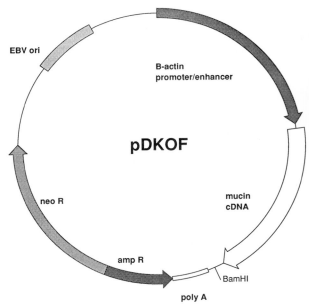

Table 4–3
Expression of Tumor Specific Epitopes on Transfected Cells[a]

Cells	Antigen Expression (% positive)	
	BC-3[b]	SM-3[c]
ClSm-EBV (untransfected)	8.1	2.5
ClSm-EBV (transfected)	88.4	7.6
RAJI (untransfected)	3.0	1.4
RAJI (transfected)	71.3	77.4

[a]Analyzed by flowcytometry

[b]Epitopes expressed on normal and tumor mucins

[c]Epitopes expressed preferentially on tumor mucins

talized cells and the Burkitt lymphoma line RAJI are both B-cells, the inability to fully glycosylate the mucin is not cell specific but appears to be transformation related.

Considering that the success of the immunization will depend on the presence of the tumor-specific epitope, and that transfection of normal cells does not produce this epitope, we have resorted to short term treatments of transfected cells with reagents that inhibit O-linked glycosylation.[114] Table 4 shows that inhibition of glycosylation results in the expression of a significant number of tumor-specific epitopes as measured by reactivity of tumor-specific antibody SM-3. Transfected normal cells, treated for 24 hours with O-linked glycosylation inhibitors, are at the moment considered ideal stimulators of mucin-specific T-cells, and their effectiveness *in vitro* as well as *in vivo* will be evaluated.

A number of other vectors may be ultimately selected when using the mucin vaccine *in vivo*. Recombinant DNA technology has made possible expression of a variety of heterologous genes in several animal viruses that have been either attenuated or genetically disabled, but are still capable of transferring a desired genetic information into a host cell.[115] Recombinant vaccinia virus vector has already been utilized to explore the possibility of a vaccine made against the human melanoma antigen p 97[42], and it may also prove to be the vector of choice for mucin-specific vaccines.

Further studies will be necessary to ensure that immunization with mucin core sequences elicits only antitumor immunity, and not undesired autoimmunity against normal ductal tissues. Our findings that mucins can serve as immunostimulatory, tumor-specific molecules in pancreatic and breast cancer raises hope that similar responses may be initiated against other mucin producing carcinomas.

Many obstacles stand in the way of a successful immunotherapy approach to the treatment of human cancer. The knowledge of a tumor-specific antigen is a powerful tool with which to begin to overcome some of these obstacles.

Acknowledgments. I am indebted to my graduate students and fellows, Donna Barnd, Keith Jerome, Allan Kirk and Da Wen Bu, whose work and ideas shaped the ideas presented here. This work was supported by National Institutes of Health grants RO1-CA-56103 and RO1-AI-26935, a grant from Cytogen Corporation, and a gift from Ellen and Gerry Siegel. I thank Elizabeth Hubbard, Director of the Pittsburgh Cancer Institute Information Resource Center for her assistance. It was not the intention of this manuscript to provide a comprehensive review of the pancreatic tumor antigens literature, and I apologize to those whose work was not cited here.

Table 4–4
Expression of the SM-3 Epitope Following Treatment of Transfected Cells with 5mM Phenyl-α-GalNAc[a]

Cells	Antigen Expression (% positive)[b]	
	BC-3[c]	SM-3[d]
ClSm (untreated)	91.1	2.0
ClSm (treated)	86.5	36.6

[a]Inhibitor of O-linked glycosylation

[b]Analyzed by flowcytometry

[c]Epitopes expressed on normal and tumor mucins

[d]Epitopes expressed preferentially on tumor mucins

References ∎

1. Foley EJ. Antigenic properties of methylcholantrene-induced tumors in mice of the strain of origin. Cancer Res 1953;13:835.
2. Prehn R, Main D. Immunity to methylcholantrene-induced sarcomas. J Natl Cancer Inst 1957;18:768.
3. Hellstrom KE, Hellstrom I. Cellular immunity against tumor antigens. In: Advances in cancer research. New York: Academic Press, 1969:167.
4. Hellstrom I, Hellstrom KE. Cell mediated reactivity to human tumor-type associated antigens: does it exist? J Biol Response Modif 1968;2:1352.
5. Hellstrom KE, Hellstrom I. Lymphocyte mediated cytotoxicity and blocking serum activity to tumor antigens. Adv Immunol 1974;18:209.
6. Baldwin RW, Robins RA. Factors interfering with the

immunologic rejection of tumors. Br Med Bull 1976; 32:118.

7. North RJ. The murine anti-tumor immune reaction and its therapeutic manipulation. Rev Immunol 1984;35:89.

8. Robins RA, Baldwin RW. T-cell subsets in tumor rejection responses. Immunol Today 1985;6:55.

9. Mukherji B, MacAlister TJ. Clonal analysis of cytotoxic T-cell response against human melanomas. J Exp Med 1983;158:240.

10. Knuth A, Wolfel T, Klehmann E, Boon T, Meyer zum Buschenfelde KH. Cytolytic T-cell clones against an autologous human melanoma: Specificity study and definition of 3 antigens by immunoselection. Proc Natl Acad Sci. USA 1989;86:2804.

11. DeVries JE, Spits H. Cloned human cytotoxic lymphocyte(CTL) lines reactive with autologous melanoma cells. J Immunol 1984;132:510.

12. Anichini A, Fossati G, Parmiani G. Clonal analysis of cytotoxic T-lymphocyte response to autologous human metastatic melanoma. Int J Cancer 1985;35:683.

13. Slovin SF, Lackman RD, Ferrone S, Kiely PE, Mastrangelo M. Cellular immune response to human sarcomas: cytotoxic T-cell clones reactive with autologous sarcomas. I. Development, phenotype and specificity. J Immunol 1986;137:3042.

14. Hersey P, MacDonald M, Schibeci S, Burns C. Clonal analysis of cytotoxic T lymphocytes(CTL) against autologous melanoma. Cancer Immunol Immunother 1986;22:15.

15. Sato T, Sato N, Takahashi S, Koshiba H, Kikuchi K. Specific cytotoxicity of a long-term cultured T-cell clone on human autologous mammary cancer cells. Cancer Res 1986;46:4384.

16. Barnd DL, Kerr LA, Metzgar RS, Finn OJ. Tumor-specific cytotoxic T-cell lines generated from tumor-draining lymph node infiltrate. Transpl Proc 1988; 20:339.

17. Cozzolino F, Torcia M, Carrossino AM, Giordani R, Selli C, Talini G, Reali E, Novelli A, Pistoia V, Ferrarini M. Characterization of cells from invaded lymph nodes in patients with solid tumors: Lymphokine requirement for tumor-specific lymphoproliferative response. J Exp Med 1987;166:303.

18. Mukherji B, Guha A, Chakrabarty N, Sivandham M, Nafhed A, Sporn J, Ergin M: Clonal analysis of cytotoxic and regulatory T-cell responses against human melanoma. J Exp Med 1989;169:1961.

19. Slovin SF, Lackman RD, Ferrone S, Kiely PE, Mastrangelo M. Cellular immune response to human sarcomas: Cytotoxic T-cell clones reactive with autologous sarcomas. J Immunol 1986;137:3042.

20. Muul LM, Spiess PJ, Director EP, Rosenberg SA. Identification of specific cytolytic immune responses against autologous tumor in humans bearing malignant melanoma. J Immunol 1987;138:989.

21. Topalian SL, Solomon D, Rosenberg SA. Tumor-specific cytolysis by lymphocytes infiltrating human melanomas. J Immunol 1989;142:3714.

22. Whiteside TL, Miescher S, Hulimann J, Moretta L, Von Hiedner U. Clonal analysis and in situ characterization of lymphocytes infiltrating human breast carcinomas. Cancer Immunol Immunother 1986;23:169.

23. Rosenberg SA. Use of tumor-infiltrating lymphocytes and interleukin-2 in the immunotherapy of patients with metastatic melanoma. New Engl J Med 1988;319:1676.

24. Jerome KR, Barnd DB, Boyer CM et al. Adenocarcinoma reactive cytotoxic T-lymphocytes recognize an epitope on the protein core of epithelial mucin molecules. In: Cellular Immunity and the Immunotherapy of Cancer. UCLA Symposium on Molecular and Cellular Biology, New Series, Lotze MT and Finn OJ, eds. New York, Wiley Liss, 1990:321.

25. Vose BM, White W. Tumor reactive lymphocytes stimulated in mixed lymphocyte and tumor culture. Cancer Immunol Immunother 1983;15:227.

26. Ferrini S, Biassoni R, Moretta A, Bruzzone M, Nicolini A, Moretta L. Clonal analysis of T-lymphocytes isolated from ovarian carcinoma ascitic fluid. Phenotypic and functional characterization of T-cell clones capable of lysing autologous carcinoma cells. Int J Cancer 1985;36:337.

27. Roberts TE, Shipton V, Moore M. Proliferation and cytotoxic responses of human peripheral blood lymphocytes to autologous malignant effusions. Cancer Immunol Immunother 1986;22:107.

28. Belldegrun D, Muul LM, Rosenberg SA. Interleukin-2 expanded tumor-infiltrating lymphocytes in human renal cell cancer: isolation, characterization and antitumor activity. Cancer Res 1988;48:206.

29. Yssel H, Spits H, deVries JE. A cloned human T-cell line cytotoxic for autologous and allogeneic B lymphoma cells. J Exp Med 1984;160:239.

30. Finn OJ, Barnd DL, Kerr LA, Miceli CM, Metzgar RS. Specific recognition of tumor target antigens by non-MHC-restricted CTL. In: Human Tumor Antigens and Specific Tumor Therapy. UCLA Symposium on Molecular and Cellular Biology, New Series, Metzgar RS, Mitchel MS, eds. New York, Liss, 1989;99:157.

31. Barnd DL, Lan MS, Metzgar RS, Finn OJ. Specific, MHC-unrestricted recognition of tumor associated mucins by human cytotoxic T cells. Proc Natl Acad Sci USA 1989;86:7159.

32. Mills CD, North RJ. Expression of passively transferred immunity against an established tumor depends on generation of cytolytic T-cells in recipient. J Exp Med 1983;157:1448.

33. Rosenstein M, Elberlein TJ, Rosenberg SA. Adoptive immunotherapy of established syngeneic solid tumors: role of T-lymphoid populations. J Immunol 1984;132: 2117.

34. Yamasaki T, Hanada H, Yamashita J, Watanabe Y, Namba Y, Hanaoka M. Specific adoptive immunotherapy with tumor-specific cytotoxic T-lymphocyte clone for murine malignant gliomas. Cancer Res 1986;44: 1776.

35. Chen W, Reese VA, Cheever MA. Adoptively transfered antigen-specific T-cells can be grown and maintained in large numbers in vivo for extended periods of time by intermittent restimulation with specific antigen plus IL-2. J Immunol 1990;144:3667.

36. Dailey MD, Pillimer E, Weissman IL. Protection against syngeneic lymphoma by a long-lived cytotoxic T-cell clone. Proc Natl Acad Sci USA 1982;79:5384.

37. Fujiwara H, Fukuzawa M, Yoshiba T, Nakajima H, Hamaoka T. The role of tumor-specific Lyt1 + 2 − T-cells in erradicating tumor cells in vivo. J Immunol 1984; 133:1671.

38. Greenberg PD, Kern DE, Cheever MA. Therapy of disseminated murine leukemia with cyclophosphamide and immune Lyt1 + 2 − T-cells. Tumor erradication does not require participation of cytotoxic T-cells. J Exp Med 1985;161:1122.

39. Lotze MT, Tomita S, Rosenberg SA. Human tumor antigens defined by cytotoxic and proliferative T-cells. In: Human Tumor Antigens and Specific Tumor Therapy. UCLA Symposium on Molecular and Cellular Biology, New Series, Metzgar RS, Mitchel MS, eds. New York, Liss, 1989:167.

40. Lurquin C, Van Pel A, Mariame B et al. Structure of the gene of tum- transplantation antigen P91A: The mutated exon encodes a peptide recognized with Ld by cytotoxic T-cells. Cell 1989;58:293.

41. Kast WM, Offringa R, Peters PJ et al. Erradication adenovirus E1-induced tumors by E2A-specific cytotoxic T-lymphocytes. Cell 1989;59:603.

42. Estin CD, Stevenson US, Plowman GD et al. Recombinant vaccinia virus vaccine against the human melanoma antigen p97 for use in immunotherapy. Proc Natl Acad Sci USA 1988;85:1052.

43. Kuntz DJ, Archer SJ. Extraction and identification of a human pancreatic-tumor-associated antigen. Oncology 1979;36:134.

44. Schulz DR, Yunis AA. Tumor-associated antigen in human pancreatic cancer. JNCI 1979;62:777.

45. Schimano T, Loor RM, Papsidero LD, et al. Isolation, characterization and clinical evaluation of a pancreas cancer-associated antigen. Cancer 1981;47:1602.

46. Kohler M, Milstein C. Continuous cultures of fused cells secreting antibody of predefined specificity. Nature 1975;256:494.

47. Banwo O, Versey J, Hobbs JR. New oncofetal antigen from human pancreas. Lancet 1974;1:643.

48. Gelder FB, Reese CJ, Moossa AR, Hall T, Hunter R. Purification, partial characterization, and clinical evaluation of a pancreatic oncofetal antigen. Cancer Res 1978;38:313.

49. Knapp ML. Partial characterization of an oncofetal pancreatic antigen. Ann Clin Biochem 1981;18:131.

50. Fujii Y, Albers GHR, Carre-Llopis A, Escribano MJ. The diagnostic value of the fetoacinar pancreatic (FAP) protein in cancer of pancreas; a comparative study with CA19/9. Br J Cancer 1987;56:495.

51. Escribano MJ, Albers GHR. Differentiation antigens in fetal human pancreas, reexpression in cancer. Int J Cancer 1986;38:155.

52. Albers GHR, Escribano MJ, Gonzalez M, Mulliez N, Nap M. The fetoacinar pancreatic protein in the developing human pancreas. Differentiation 1987;34:210.

53. Albers GHR, Escribano MJ. Tissue and serum detection of the 110K fetoacinar pancreatic protein in patients with pancreatic adenocarcinoma. Tumor Biology 1986;7:252.

54. Arai M, Sakamoto K, Otsuka H, Yokoyama Y, Agaki M. Detection of tumor associated antigen, PA8-15, in sera from pancreatic and gastrointestinal carcinoma patients. Jpn J Clin Oncol 1990;20:145.

55. Burtin B, Gold P. Carcinoembryonic antigen. Scand J Immunol 1978;8, Suppl.8:27.

56. Ward MA. Tumor markers. In: Hancock BW, Ward MA, eds. Immunological aspects of cancer. Boston: Martinus Nijhoff, 1985:91.

57. Lindholm L, Holmgren J, Svennerholm L, et al. Monoclonal antibodies against gastrointestinal tumor-associated antigens isolated as monosialogangliosides. Int Arch Allergy Appl Immunol 1983;71:178.

58. Koprowski H, Steplewski Z, Mitchell K, Herlyn M, Herlyn D, Fuhrer P. Colorectal carcinoma antigens detected by hybridoma antibodies. Somat Cell Genet 1979;5:957.

59. Haglund C, Lindgren J, Roberts PJ, Kuusela P, Nordling S. Tissue expression of the tumor associated antigen CA242 in benign and malignant pancreatic lesions. A comparison with CA 50 and CA 19-9. Br J Cancer 1989;60:845.

60. Prat M, Medico E, Rossino P, Garrino C, Comoglio PM. Biochemical and immunological properties of the human carcinoma-associated CAR-3 epitope defined by the monoclonal antibody AR-3. Cancer Res 1989;49:1415.

61. Lan MS, Khorami A, Kaufman B, Metzgar RS. Molecular characterization of a mucin-type antigen associated with human pancreatic cancer. J Biol Chem 1987;262:12863.

62. Yvan S, Ho JJL, Yvan M, Kim YS. Human pancreatic cancer-associated antigens detected by murine monoclonal antibodies. Cancer Res 1985;45:6179.

63. Bosslet K, Kern HF, Kanzy EJ, et al. A monoclonal antibody with binding and inhibiting activity towards human pancreatic carcinoma cells. I. Immunohistological and immunochemical characterization of a murine monoclonal antibody selecting for well-differentiated adenocarcinomas of the pancreas. Cancer Immunol Immunother 1986;23:185.

64. Schmiegel W. Tumor markers in pancreatic cancer-current concepts. Hepato-gastroenterol 1989;36:446.

65. Benini L, Cavallini G, Zordan D, et al. A clinical evaluation of monoclonal (CA19-9, CA50, CA12-5) and polyclonal (CEA, TPA) antibody-defined antigens for the diagnosis of pancreatic cancer. Pancreas 1988;3:61.

66. Kiriyama S, Hayakawa T, Kondo T, et al. Usefulness of a new tumor marker, Span-1, for the diagnosis of pancreatic cancer. Cancer 1990;65:1557.

67. Steinberg W. The clinical utility of the CA 19-9 tumor-associated antigen. Amer J Gastroenterol 1990;85:350.

68. Dietel M, Arps H, Klapdor R, Muller-Hagen S, Sieck M, Hoffman L. Antigen detection by the monoclonal antibodies CA 19-9 and CA 125 in normal and tumor tissue and patients' sera. Cancer Res Clin Oncol 1986;111:257.

69. Ban T, Imai K, Yachi A. Immunohistological and immunochemical characterization of a novel pancreatic cancer-associated antigen MUSE11. Cancer Res 1989;49:7141.

70. Bishop JM. Science 1987;235:305.

71. Schechter AL, Stern DF, Vaidyanathan L, et al. The neu oncogene: an erbB-related gene encoding a 185000 M_r tumor antigen. Nature 1984;312:513.

72. Gullick WJ, Berger MS, Bennet PL, Rothbard JB, Waterfield MD. Expression of the c-erbB-2 protein in normal and transformed cells. Int J Cancer 1987;40:246.

73. Yokota J, Yamamoto T, Toyoshima Y, et al. Amplification of c-erbB-2 oncogene in human adenocarcinomas in vivo. Lancet 1986;i:765.

74. Gullick WJ, Venter DJ. The c-erbB-2 gene and its expression in human tumors. In: Waxman J, Sicora C, eds. The molecular basis of cancer, Oxford: Blackwell, 1989:38.

75. Maguire HC, Greene MI. The neu(c-erbB) oncogene. Seminars in Oncology 1989;16:148.

76. Bargman CI, Hung M-C, Weinberg RA. Multiple independent activations of the neu oncogene by a point mutation altering the transmembrane domain of p 185. Cell 1986;45:649.

77. Yokota J, Yamamoto, T. Miyajima N, et al. Genetic alterations of the c-erbB-2 oncogene occur frequently in tubular adenocarcinoma of the stomach and are often accompanied by amplification of the v-erbA homologue. Oncogene 1988;2:283.

78. Drebin JA, Link VC, Weinberg RA. Inhibition of tumor growth by a monoclonal antibody reactive with an oncogen-encoded tumor antigen. Proc Natl Acad Sci USA 1986;83:9129.

79. Drebin JA, Link VC, Green MI. Monoclonal antibodies reactive with distinct domains of the neu oncogene-encoded p185 molecule exert synergistic antitumor effects. Oncogene 1988;2:273.

80. Drebin JA, Link VC, Greene MI. Monoclonal antibodies specific for the neu oncogene product directly mediate antitumor effects *in vivo*. Oncogene 1988;2:387.

81. Bernards R, Destree A, McKenzie S, Gordon E, Weinberg RA, Panicali D. Effective tumor immunotherapy directed against an oncogene-encoded product using a vaccinia virus vector. Proc Natl Acad Sci USA 1987; 84:6854.

82. Barbacid M. ras genes. Annu Rev Biochem 1987;56: 779.

83. Bos JL. ras oncogenes in human cancer: a review. Cancer Res 1989;49:4682.

84. Almoguera C, Shibata D, Forrester K, Martin J, Arnheim N, Perucho M. Most human carcinomas of the exocrine pancreas contain mutant c-K-ras genes. Cell 1988;53:549.

85. Tada M, Omata M, Ohto M. Clinical application of ras gene mutation for diagnosis of pancreatic adenocarcinoma. Gastroenterology 1991;100:233.

86. Tada M, Yokosuka O, Omata M, Ohto M, Isono K. Analysis of ras gene mutations in biliary and pancreatic tumors by polymerase chain reaction and direct sequencing. Cancer 1990;66:930.

87. Grunewald K, Lyons J, Frohlich A, et al. High frequency of Ki-ras codon 12 mutations in pancreatic adenocarcinomas. Int J Cancer 1989;43:1037.

88. Shibata D, Almoguera C, Forrester K, et al. Detection of c-K-ras mutations in fine needle aspirates from human pancreatic adenocarcinomas. Cancer Res 1990; 50:1279.

89. Smit VT, Boot AJ, Smits AM, Fleuren GJ, Cornelisse CJ, Bos JL. KRAS codon 12 mutations occur very frequently in pancreatic adenocarcinomas. Nucleic Acids Res 1988;16:7773.

90. Nagata Y, Abe M, Motoshima K, Nakayama E, Shiku H. Frequent glycine-to-aspartic acid mutations at codon 12 of c-Ki-ras gene in human pancreatic cancer in Japanese. Jpn J Cancer Res 1990;81:135.

91. Boon T, Van Pel A, De Plaen E, et al. Genetic analysis of tumor antigens. Implications for T-cell mediated immune surveillance. In: Lotze M, Finn OJ, eds. Cellular immunity and the immunotherapy of cancer. Weley-Liss, 1990:287.

92. Peace DJ, Chen W, Nelson H, Cheever MA. T-cell recognition of transforming proteins encoded by a mutated ras proto-oncogene. J Immunol 1991;146:2059.

93. Wahab ZA, Metzgar RS. Human cytotoxic lymphocytes reactive with pancreatic adenocarcinoma cells. Pancreas 1991;6:307.

94. Hilkens J, Buijs F, Ligtenberg M. Complexity of MAM-6, an epithelial sialomucin associated with carcinomas. Cancer Res 1989;49:786.

95. Burchell J, Gendler S, Taylor-Papadimitriou J, et al.

Development and characterization of breast cancer reactive monoclonal antibodies directed to the core protein of the human milk mucin. Cancer Res 1987; 47:5476.

96. Xing PX, Reynolds K, Tjandra JJ, Tang XL, Purcell DFJ, McKenzie IFC. Synthetic peptides reactive with anti-human milk fat globule membrane monoclonal antibodies. Cancer Res 1990;50:89.

97. Girling A, Bartkova J, Burchell J, Gendler S, Gillett C, Taylor-Papadimitriou J. A core protein epitope of the polymorphic epithelial mucin detected by the monoclonal antibody SM-3 is selectively exposed in a range of primary carcinomas. Int J Cancer 1989;43:1072.

98. Gendler SJ, Burchell JM, Duhig T, et al. Cloning of a partial cDNA encoding differentiation and tumor-associated mucin glycoproteins expressed by human mammary epithelium. Proc Natl Acad Sci USA 1987;84: 6060.

99. Gendler SJ, Lancaster CA, Taylor-Papadimitriou J, et al. Molecular cloning and expression of human tumor-associated polymorphic epithelial mucin. J Biol Chem 1990;265:15286.

100. Siddiqui J, Abe M, Hayes E, Shani E, Yunis E, Kufe D. Isolation and sequencing of a cDNA coding for the human DF3 breast carcinoma-associated antigen. Proc Natl Acad Sci USA 1988;85:2320.

101. Ligtenberg MJL, Vos HL, Gennissen AMC, Hilkens J. Episialin, a carcinoma-associated mucin, is generated by a polymorphic gene encoding splice variants with alternative amino termini. J Biol Chem 1990;265:5573.

102. Wreshner D, Harueveni M, Tsarfaty I, et al. Human epithelial tumor antigen cDNA sequences. Differential splicing may generate multiple protein forms. Eur J Biochem 1990;189:463.

103. Lan MS, Batra SK, Qi W-N, Metzgar RS, Hollinsworth MA. Cloning and sequencing of a human pancreatic tumor mucin cDNA. J Biol Chem 1990;265: 15294.

104. Gum JR, Byrd JC, Hicks JW, Toribara NW, Lamport DTA, Kim YS. Molecular cloning of human intestinal mucin cDNAs. Sequence analysis and evidence for genetic polymorphism. J Biol Chem 1989;264:6480.

105. Gum JR, Hicks JW, Swallow DM, et al. Molecular cloning of cDNAs derived from a novel human intestinal mucin gene. Biochem Biophys Res Commun 1990; 171:407.

106. Hanisch F-G, Uhlenbruck G, Peter-Katlinic J, Egge H, Dabrowski J, Dabrowski U. Structures of neutral O-linked polylactosaminoglycans on human skim milk mucins. J Biol Chem 1989;264:872.

107. Finn OJ. Antigen specific, MHC-unrestricted T-cells. Biotherapy, in press.

108. Jerome KR, Barnd DA, Bendt KM, et al. Cytotoxic T-lymphocytes derived from patients with breast adenocarcinoma recognize an epitope present on the protein core of a mucin molecule preferentially expressed by malignant cells. Cancer Res 1991;51:2908.

109. Margalit H, Spouge J, Cornette J, Cease K, Delisi C, Berzofsky J. Prediction of immunodominant T-cell antigenic sites from the primary sequence. J Immunol 1987;138:2213.

110. Yan P-S, Ho SB, Itzkowitz SH, Byrd JC, Siddiqui B, Kim YS. Expression of native and deglycosylated colon cancer mucin antigens in normal and malignant epithelial tissues. Laboratory Investigation 1990;62:698.

111. Moore MW, Carbone FR, Bevan MJ. Introduction of

soluble protein into the class I pathway of antigen processing and presentation. Cell 1988;54:777.

112. Kast WM, Roux L, Curren J, et al. Protection against lethal Sendai virus infection by *in vivo* priming of virus-specific cytotoxic T-lymphocytes with a free synthetic peptide. Proc Natl Acad Sci USA 1991;88:2283.

113. Sugden B, Marsh K, Yates J. A vector that replicates as a plasmid and can be efficiently selected in B-lymph-oblasts transformed by Epstein-Barr virus. Mol Cell Biol 1985;5:410.

114. Kuan S-F, Byrd JC, Basbaum C, Kim YS. Inhibition of mucin glycosylation by aryl-N-acetyl-α-galactosaminides in human colon cancer cells. J Biol Chem 1989; 264:19271.

115. Rigby PWJ. Cloning vectors derived from animal viruses. J Gen Virol 1983;64:255.

Leroy F. Liu
Peter D'Arpa

Topoisomerase-Targeting Antitumor Drugs: Mechanisms of Cytotoxicity and Resistance

5

It has recently been established that many structurally diverse antitumor drugs exert their antitumor activity through their interaction with DNA topoisomerases (Figs. 5-1 and 5-2). Several topoisomerase II drugs are already being widely used in the clinic and others are undergoing development. The only known class of topoisomerase I-targeting drugs, the camptothecins, have shown unprecedented activity against human solid tumors in animal models and are currently undergoing clinical trials. Over the past several years, significant progress has been made on the elucidation of the mechanism of action of these drugs.

Molecular Mechanisms of Drug Action ■

The DNA topoisomerases resolve topological problems in DNA that arise during DNA replication, transcription, mitosis, and possibly other processes.[1] Two types of topoisomerases which are represented by their archetypes, topoisomerase I (type I) and topoisomerase II (type II), have been identified in mammalian cells. Topoisomerases catalyze the interconversion of various topological isomers of DNA by transiently breaking one (type I) or both (type II) DNA strands. Topoisomerase I functions as a monomer and does not require an energy co-factor for catalysis. It relaxes DNA supercoils by transiently cleaving a single strand of duplex DNA and allows the intact complementary strand to pass through the enzyme-bridged cleavage prior to resealing. The energy required for relegation is apparently derived at least in part from the covalent tyrosylphosphate bond formed between the enzyme and $3'$-phosphoryl end of the transiently broken DNA strand.

Topoisomerase II functions as a homodimer and requires ATP hydrolysis for catalysis. Each subunit transiently cleaves one strand of duplex DNA to produce a double-strand break that is bridged by the enzyme. Another duplex DNA, either a portion of the same molecule or a different DNA molecule, can then pass through the enzyme-bridged DNA break prior to resealing. Like DNA topoisomerase I, topoisomerase II can relax DNA supercoils using the strand passing mechanism. In addition, topoisomerase II can catalyze catenation/decatenation and knotting/unknotting of duplex DNA. The importance of a topoisomerase activity in DNA replication and transcription has been well documented.[2]

The topoisomerase-targeting drugs have a similar mechanism of action. They trap the enzymes in putative reaction intermediates; the enzymes

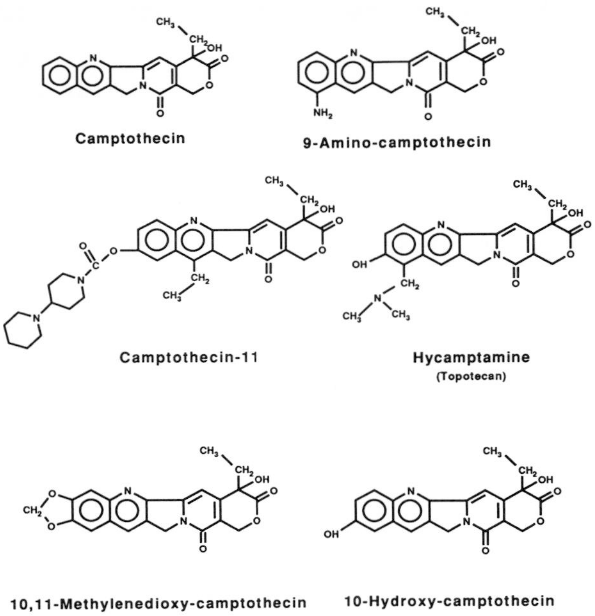

Camptothecin

9-Amino-camptothecin

Camptothecin-11

Hycamptamine
(Topotecan)

10,11-Methylenedioxy-camptothecin

10-Hydroxy-camptothecin

FIG. 5–1 The chemical structures of topoisomerase I drugs.

apparently cleave DNA, but fail to rejoin the cleaved strands in the presence of the drugs. The trapped reaction intermediates are presumably reversible drug-enzyme-DNA ternary complexes, which upon exposure to a strong denaturant, such as SDS or strong alkali, are "cleaved" into topoisomerase-linked DNA fragments. Therefore, they have been termed "cleavable complexes" (Figs. 5-3 and 5-4) (review [2,3]). Models have been proposed to explain how the drugs may interface with DNA and the topoisomerases in putative ternary complexes,[3,4] (see below). In cells, drug-trapped topoisomerase cleavable complexes can be revealed as protein-linked DNA breaks by lysing cells with a strong protein denaturant. Presumably, a small fraction of these reversible cleavable complexes are converted into more lethal DNA lesions in cells.

Topoisomerase I Drugs ■

Only one class of topoisomerase I drug, the camptothecins (Fig. 5-1), has been identified and characterized to date. Camptothecin was originally isolated from the bark of a tree, *Camptotheca acuminata,* which is indigenous to China.[5] It exhibits broad spectrum activity against a number of tumors

in experimental animals[6–8] and has antiviral activity.[9] The sodium salt of camptothecin underwent clinical trials in the early 1970s, but toxic side effects limited further development.[10] Recent studies have suggested that the intact lactone ring is important for camptothecin's activity. Hydrolysis of the lactone form of camptothecin to its sodium salt substantially reduces activity against topoisomerase I.[11] Low activity of the sodium salt may partially explain its failure in early clinical trials.

Studies using a photolinkable camptothecin derivative have demonstrated that camptothecin forms a ternary complex with DNA and topoisomerase I, but does not significantly bind to either DNA or topoisomerase I alone.[4] Many derivatives of camptothecin with varying degrees of antitumor activity have been synthesized.[12] Structure-activity relationships have indicated that the 20S stereoisomer of camptothecin, but not the 20R form, displays both antitumor and anti-topoisomerase activity.[13] In general, modification on the lactone ring abolishes the drug's ability to trap topoisomerase I cleavable complexes.[13,22] On the other hand, modification of the A-ring can sometimes increase the potency of the drug; 10, 11-methylenedioxy-camptothecin is one of the most potent derivatives. Two charged water soluble derivatives, hycamptamine (topotecan) and CPT-11, are currently undergoing clinical trials.[14]

Topoisomerase II Drugs ■

A surprisingly large and structurally diverse group of drugs has been shown to target topoisomerase II (Fig. 5-2). For several classes of these drugs, including the anthracyclines,[16] acridines, and ellipticines,[17] intercalative binding strength has been shown to correlate well with potency in trapping topoisomerase II in the cleavable complex. A model, termed misalignment model, has been proposed that describes the binding of topoisomerase II drugs in the ternary enzyme-drug-DNA complex. It explains why almost all topoisomerase II drugs are intercalators and why such a diverse group of molecular structures can have a common molecular mode of action.[3] In this model, intercalation of the drug within the DNA domain bound by the enzyme causes the transiently cleaved strands to misalign, thereby preventing their rejoining. In addition to an intercalative domain, the drugs have one or two bulky side chains that may interact with topoisomerase II.[18] The structural di-

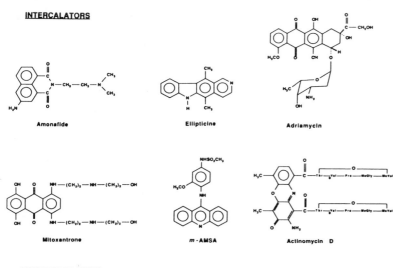

INTERCALATORS

Amonafide   Ellipticine   Adriamycin

Mitoxantrone   m - AMSA   Actinomycin D

NONINTERCALATORS

Etoposide (VP-16)   Teniposide (VM-26)   Genistein

FIG. 5–2 The chemical structures of topoisomerase II drugs.

versity of the side chain domains may indicate a loose drug binding site on the enzyme. This model explains why many topoisomerase II drugs are DNA intercalators, but it fails to explain the action of the nonintercalative epipodopyllotoxins, VM-26 (teniposide), and VP-16 (etoposide). This inconsistency may be resolved by the recent finding that VP-16 and VM-26 do indeed bind to DNA, albeit weakly.[19]

Cytotoxic Mechanisms ■

Many lines of evidence have established that the cleavable complex is the principal mediator of the cytotoxic action of topoisomerase drugs. The clearest example comes from studies in yeast in which the topoisomerase I drug camptothecin is devoid of significant cytotoxic potency in mutants lacking topoisomerase I.[20,21] In addition, topo-

isomerase I and topoisomerase II isolated from topoisomerase drug-resistant mammalian cells are often resistant to drug-induced cleavable complex formation *in vitro* (see below). Furthermore, potency in producing cleavable complexes correlates well with potency in producing lethality for the topoisomerase I drugs[13,22] and for several structural classes of topoisomerase II drugs.[23–25]

Although cleavable complex formation appears to be the necessary first event, subsequent events in the action of the topoisomerase drugs have only recently come into sharper focus. The transient nature of the cleavable complex—that is, their rapid dissociation into free drug, intact DNA, and enzyme—has raised the question, why are short-duration drug exposures lethal? Are a small number of cleavable complexes not reversible, or do cellular processes transform the otherwise reversible cleavable complexes into permanent lesions that are lethal?

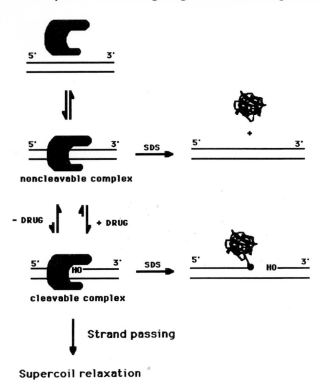

FIG. 5–3 A model for the mechanism of action of topoisomerase I drugs. Topoisomerase I is shown to bind to DNA forming two types of complexes; the cleavable and noncleavable complexes. SDS treatment of the cleavable complex results in a single-strand DNA break and the concurrent covalent linking of the denatured enzyme to the 3′-phosphoryl end of the broken strand. The cleavable complex is presumably a reaction intermediate in the strand-passing reaction.

stant, but significant lethality occurred only when cells were in S-phase during treatment. Therefore, a cell killing mechanism that involves DNA synthesis was indicated.

More recently, the involvement of DNA synthesis in the cell killing mechanism of topoisomerase I-targeting drugs has been studied using the DNA polymerase α and δ inhibitor, aphidicolin, to block DNA synthesis during exposures to camptothecin. Brief treatment with camptothecin (e.g., 30 minutes) that is highly lethal was virtually noncytotoxic when DNA synthesis was inhibited by aphidicolin.[28]

The involvement of DNA synthesis in the cytotoxic mechanism of camptothecin has also been studied at the molecular level in a cell-free SV40 replication system. When DNA synthesis was ongoing and both topoisomerase I and camptothecin were present, strand breakage occurred at replication forks and was associated with replication fork arrest.[28] Breakage was shown to occur particularly on the parental DNA strand complementary to the leading strand of DNA synthesis (Y. P. Tsao and L. F. Liu, unpublished results). Double-strand breakage on replicating SV40 DNA has also been observed in virus-infected cells that were treated with camptothecin.[29–32] These results suggest that the replication fork may collide with the drug-trapped topoisomerase I cleavable complex and transform the otherwise reversible complex into a lethal lesion (Fig. 5-5). DNA breakage at the replication fork, which may be the equivalent of a double-strand break, is expected to be highly lethal. The sensitivity to camptothecin of yeast mutants deficient in double-strand break repair *(rad52)* is consistent with the "collision" model.[20]

Topoisomerase I Drugs ■

Early studies on camptothecin revealed an extreme S-phase sensitivity to cell killing. In CHO cells, S-phase cells were approximately 1000-fold more sensitive to the cytotoxic effect of the drug than cells in other phases of the cell cycle.[26] However, following a 30-minute camptothecin exposure, DNA fragmentation (due to cleavable complex formation) occurred to a similar extent in G1-, S-, and G2- phase cells, and was also equally reversible in the various cell cycle phases within minutes after the drug was washed out.[27] This result showed that the amount of "reversible damage" produced throughout the cell cycle was con-

Topoisomerase II Drugs ■

The topoisomerase II-targeting drugs have often been referred to as inhibitors, which may connote that their primary cell killing mechanism involves inhibition of catalytic activity. While the enzyme cannot catalyze the strand-passing reaction when trapped in the cleavable complex, a cell killing mechanism other than inhibition of catalysis seems more likely. First, studies in yeast have shown the only essential function of topoisomerase II to be the separation of intertwined duplex daughter molecules prior to mitosis. If the mechanism of action of the drugs was inhibition of this

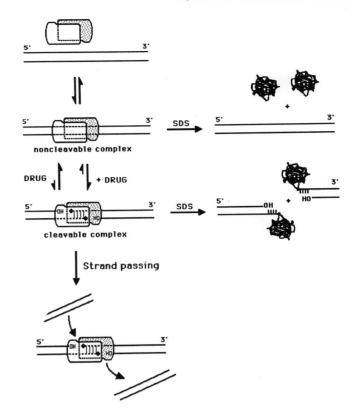

FIG. 5–4 A model for the mechanism of action of topoisomerase II drugs. Topoisomerase II is shown to bind to DNA forming two types of complexes—cleavable and noncleavable. SDS treatment of the cleavable complex results in breakage of duplex DNA and the concomitant covalent linking of each subunit of the homodimeric enzyme to each 5′-phosphoryl end of the broken DNA strand. The cleavable complex is presumably a reaction intermediate in the strand-passing reaction.

activity, G2/M phase cells would be expected to be uniquely sensitive to topoisomerase II-targeting drugs, but this is not the case. More evidence comes from studies of hybrids of drug-resistant cells with their drug-sensitive parental cells.[33] The topoisomerase II from the resistant cells is resistant to drug-induced cleavable complex formation, but its catalytic activity is not inhibited by the drug. The hybrid cell displays the drug-sensitive phenotype, apparently due to the presence of the drug-sensitive enzyme, even though the drug-resistant topoisomerase II is significantly catalytically active in the presence of the drug.

Rather than inhibiting catalytic activity, topoisomerase II drugs appear to kill cells through DNA damage that is mediated by cleavable complexes. However, drug-trapped topoisomerase II-cleavable complexes, like their topoisomerase I counterparts, dissociate rapidly, yet are highly lethal even following brief exposures. As discussed above, DNA synthesis is involved in a mechanism that transforms the transient camptothecin-trapped topoisomerase I cleavable complexes into permanent damage. Topoisomerase II cleavable

complexes similarly appear to be processed by the DNA synthesis machinery into permanent damage, as evidenced by the heightened sensitivity of S-phase cells to topoisomerase II drugs, and the ability of DNA synthesis inhibitors to partially abolish this sensitivity.[34–37]

An additional mechanism of cell killing by topoisomerase II-targeting drugs appears to involve the RNA synthesis machinery.[36,38,39] In the presence of RNA synthesis inhibitors, the slope of the m-AMSA survival curve is significantly reduced.[36] In contrast, DNA synthesis inhibitors have been shown to protect cells from m-AMSA, but only at lower doses of the drug.[36]

Similar to camptothecin-trapped topoisomerase I cleavable complexes, the replication and transcription machineries may transform the topoisomerase II cleavable complex into lethal damage, perhaps a double-strand break, either directly, or indirectly through other enzymatic activities. Consistent with this hypothesis, protein-free double-strand breaks have been shown to arise and persist following m-AMSA or etoposide treatment in a cell line deficient in double-strand

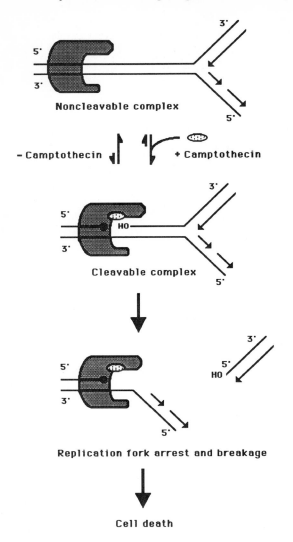

FIG. 5–5 A model for the interaction between the replication fork and the camptothecin-trapped topoisomerase I cleavable complex. The advancing replication fork is shown to "collide" with the topoisomerase I cleavable complex resulting in fork breakage and arrest.

break repair.[40] These breaks were associated with hypersensitivity to cell killing by the drugs.[40]

Cellular Regulation of Topoisomerases ∎

Topoisomerase activity levels may significantly influence cellular sensitivity to topoisomerase drugs. In contrast to other antitumor enzyme inhibitors (e.g., methotrexate) whose cytotoxicity is reduced when the target enzyme is overexpressed, the activity of topoisomerase drugs is expected to be greater in cells that express higher levels of the target topoisomerase.[41]

Studies on the cellular regulation of topoisomerases have shown that topoisomerase I and topoisomerase II are regulated very differently under a variety of conditions of growth and differentiation. In general, topoisomerase II protein levels change dramatically with the proliferative state of cells.[42–49] In contrast, topoisomerase I protein levels differ much less with growth state, although mRNA levels have been shown to be stimulated by serum, the protein kinase C activator PMA (phorbol 12-myristate-13-acetate), and epidermal growth factor.[42,47,50–52] Such changes in topoisomerase I mRNA levels may be due to transcriptional regulation. Recent studies of the human topoisomerase I promoter region show the presence of consensus sequence binding site motifs for the transcription factors Oct1, Sp1 and AP2, as well as a cAMP-responsive element.[53]

Posttranslational modifications may also be involved in the cellular regulation of topoisomerases. Both topoisomerase I and II are phosphorylated *in vivo,* and phosphorylation has been shown to affect their activities *in vitro.*[54–59] Phosphorylation and other posttranslational modifications[60] may also play a role in drug sensitivity.

Topoisomerase levels in human tumor samples and in human tumor xenografts have been measured.[8,61,62] In general, topoisomerase II levels are high in tumor cells. Surprisingly, topoisomerase I levels were elevated in human colon adenocarcinoma and correlated with stage of malignancy.[8] A recent study has also indicated that the adenovirus E1A oncoprotein can cause elevated topoisomerase I levels.[63] It seems plausible that activated oncogenes in tumor cells may lead to elevated levels of topoisomerase expression.

Mechanisms of Resistance ∎

Resistance to the cytotoxic effects of topoisomerase drugs has generally been studied in cells selected for their ability to survive continuous exposure to incremental concentrations of drug. Compared to the parental cells, high-level resistance often appears to be due to multiple alterations, which probably arise from the combination of drug-induced mutagenesis and continuous selection for mutants that survive drug exposure.[64-66]

Resistance to the cytotoxic effects of the topoisomerase drugs may potentially be due to alterations that affect (1) the intracellular concentration of drug; (2) the catalytic activity of the target topoisomerase; (3) the sensitivity of the target topoisomerase to drug; (4) the processing of drug-trapped cleavable complexes into lethal damage; (5) subsequent steps along the cell killing pathway. Recent studies of drug resistant cells have provided evidence for some of these mechanisms.

Reductions in Topoisomerase Levels ■

Reduced levels of topoisomerases have been found to occur frequently in tumor cells continuously selected in the presence of topoisomerase I or II drugs.[15,66-69] It has been suggested that resistance may more frequently occur due to a reduction in topoisomerase levels than to the creation of a drug-resistant enzyme.[69] Presumably, mutations in any of several genes affecting topoisomerase levels may down-regulate the enzyme, and even a mutation within the topoisomerase coding region is more likely to disrupt the gene[67] than to create an enzyme resistant to drug-induced cleavable complex formation.

In most cases, the mutations that lead to reduced topoisomerase levels have not been identified. In two cases, rearrangement of one of the topoisomerase alleles has been associated with reduced topoisomerase I[69] or topoisomerase II activity[67] in camptothecin- and adriamycin-resistant cells, respectively.

Intrinsic resistance, as opposed to drug-induced or acquired resistance, has also been demonstrated to result from down-regulation of topoisomerase II in differentiated or nutrient deprived cells, and in some cancers that have low proliferative index.[37,50,61,70-72]

Resistance Due to Altered Topoisomerases ■

Many drug-resistant cells have also been shown to contain approximately wild-type cellular levels of topoisomerases; however, these enzymes are resistant to cleavable complex formation in cells, in extracts, or in purified form.[73-78] In some cases, topoisomerase II from drug-resistant mutant cells displays cross-resistance to other topoisomerase II drugs,[79-81] but not always.[81,82] In addition, catalytic activity of drug-resistant enzyme has been shown to be either relatively unaffected,[82] or noticeably impaired.[76] This type of resistance could be due to a mutation that alters the drug-binding site on the enzyme, or some other characteristic of the enzyme that prevents cleavable complex formation.[83,84] One cell line selected under continuous exposure to camptothecin has been shown to contain topoisomerase I having a single amino acid change that confers camptothecin resistance.[84-86] Another VM-26-resistant cell line may contain an altered topoisomerase II with a possible change in the ATP binding domain.[76]

Studies of resistant cell lines have also provided important information about the possible mechanism of drug-induced topoisomerase II cleavable complex formation. As suggested previously, all topoisomerase II drugs have a common bipartite structure comprised of a planar fused ring system and one or two bulky side chains. The planar ring system is important for DNA intercalation, which is crucial for the action of topoisomerase II drugs, while the bulky side chain is important for stabilizing the intercalated drugs in the ternary complex by interacting with the enzyme.[3] The structural diversity of the bulky side chains suggests that they interact only loosely with topoisomerase II. Based on this model, drug-resistant topoisomerase II may be altered with respect to its drug sensitivity due to structural changes within the enzyme's drug-binding domain. Studies of m-AMSA resistant topoisomerase II in the T4 model system are consistent with such a model.[81,83,87] Interestingly, one of the m-ASMA resistant T4 topoisomerases was found to be hypersensitive to VP-16.[81] Other studies have shown that m-AMSA derivatives can overcome resistance due to altered topoisomerase II in a cell line selected with m-AMSA.[18]

Lengthened Cell Cycle Time ■

Some cells resistant to topoisomerase I or topoisomerase II drugs have significantly longer cell cycle times.[65,73] Presumably, the sensitivity of cells to camptothecin would be lessened if the total cell cycle time increased, but the duration of S-phase remained constant. Indeed, cell cycle time has been shown to correlate with resistance to camptothecin in cells in which cell cycle time was varied by growth in different concentrations of fetal bovine serum.[88] Lengthening of the cell cycle may also be a mechanism of resistance in certain tumors that contain a large fraction of non-S-phase cells.

Multidrug Resistance ■

Overexpression of MDR-1 has been found in many tumor types.[89] Whether the expression of MDR-1 is responsible for the intrinsic resistance of these tumors to topoisomerase II drugs or other drugs is not known. Studies have shown that MDR-1 overexpressing cells are not equally cross-resistant to topoisomerase II drugs. Analysis of the structure-activity relationship for aminoacridines in inhibiting cell growth has suggested that certain synthetic modifications can overcome MDR-1-mediated resistance.[18]

In contrast, the topoisomerase I drugs, camptothecin, 9-amino-camptothecin, 10,11-methylenedioxy-camptothecin, or CPT-11 (a prodrug of SN38), have been shown not to be susceptible to the MDR-1-mediated resistance mechanism (A. Chen and L. F. Liu, unpublished results).[90] Interestingly, some of these camptothecin derivatives have shown unprecedented effectiveness in the human colon tumor xenograft model in nude mice.[9] Whether this effectiveness is related to their ability to overcome MDR-1-mediated resistance remains unknown.

The drug selectivity of MDR-1 has been a mystery. Studies of both topoisomerase I and II drugs have indicated that MDR-1 overexpressing cells display more resistance to positively charged derivatives than their noncharged counterparts (A. Chen and L. F. Liu, unpublished results). For example, MDR-1 overexpressing KB-V1 cells are more resistant to the positively charged camptothecin derivative hycamptamine (topotecan) than to camptothecin. These studies may indicate that the membrane permeability of these drugs may be an important factor in their susceptibility to the MDR-1-mediated resistance mechanism.

Other Mechanisms ■

It has been reported that m-AMSA can be activated by microsomes to a form that is more potent in trapping topoisomerase II.[91] If such activation normally increases the sensitivity to m-AMSA, then inactivation of such a pathway may be a resistance mechanism.

In some instances, the magnitude of the resistance cannot be explained by any of the mechanisms discussed above. For example, reduced levels of topoisomerase II in a doxorubicin-resistant human fibroblast cell line could not account for the full resistance. This line had no evidence of p-glycoprotein expression, but the activity of several enzymes was shown to be altered (glucose-6-phosphate dehydrogenase, glutathione-S-transferase, glutathione reductase, glutathione peroxidase, catalase).[73] Whether these altered enzyme activities can account for some of the unexplained resistance remains to be determined.

Summary and Perspectives ■

Topoisomerase drugs have a unique mechanism of action; they convert essential cellular enzymes into DNA "cleaving" agents. Unlike other DNA damaging agents, topoisomerase drugs produce an initial reversible DNA lesion, the cleavable complex, which is then transformed into lethal DNA damage upon interaction with cellular factors. Recent studies have identified both DNA and RNA synthesis to be involved in the processing of a fraction of these reversible cleavable complexes into lethal DNA damage. Further studies are needed to dissect the pathway that leads to cell death.

Because cell killing by this class of drugs is mediated by topoisomerases, knowledge concerning the regulation of topoisomerases in tumor and normal tissues may lead to pharmacological means for sensitizing tumor cells. Recent studies have also revealed the presence of additional topoisomerases in cells; however, their involvement in drug-induced cytotoxicity and resistance has yet to be investigated.

Structure-activity studies of topoisomerase drugs have revealed that certain structural modifications can overcome MDR-1-mediated resistance as well as resistance due to drug-resistant topoisomerases. These modified drugs may be important not only for their possible utility in treating some MDR-1 overexpressing tumors, but also in investigating the molecular mechanism of drug selectivity of MDR-1. Knowledge of the drug selectivity of MDR-1-mediated resistance may direct drug design in the future.

Investigation of the mechanisms of action of topoisomerase-targeting antitumor drugs may also lead to new concepts for antimicrobial, antiparasitic, and antiviral therapies.

Acknowledgment. We are grateful to Drs. Erasmus Schneider, Annette Bodley, Carolyn Hendricks, and Gilbert Nyamuswa for their critical reading of the manuscript. This work was supported by NIH grant CA39662.

References ■

1. Wang JC. Recent studies of DNA topoisomerases. Biochim Biophys Acta 1987;909:1.
2. Liu LF. DNA topoisomerase poisons as antitumor drugs. Ann Rev Biochem 1989;58:351.
3. D'Arpa P, Liu LF. Topoisomerase-targeting antitumor drugs. Biochem Biophys Acta 1989;989:163.
4. Hertzberg RP, Busby RW, Caranfa MJ, et al. Irreversible trapping of the DNA-topoisomerase I covalent complex. Affinity labeling of the camptothecin binding site. J Biol Chem 1990;265:19287.
5. Wall ME, Wani MC, Cooke CE, et al. Plant antitumor agents. I. The isolation and structure of camptothecin, a novel alkaloidal leukemia and tumor inhibitor from *Camptotheca acuminata*. J Am Chem Soc 1966;88:3888.
6. Gallo RC, Whang-Peng J, Adamson RH. Studies on the antitumor activity, mechanism of action, and cell cycle effects of camptothecin. J Nat Cancer Inst 1971;46:789.
7. Suffness M, Cordell GA. Antitumor alkaloids. In: Brossi, A, ed. Chemistry and pharmacology, 1985, Orlando, Academic Press: 3.
8. Giovanella BC, JS, Stehlin WE, Wall MC, et al. DNA topoisomerase I-targeted chemotherapy of human colon cancer in xenografts. Science 1989;246:1046.
9. Horwitz SB, Chang C-K, and Grollman AP. Antiviral action of camptothecin. Antimicro Agents and Chemo 1972;2:395.
10. Muggia FM, Creaven PJ, Hansen HH, Cohen MH, and Selawry OS. Phase I clinical trial of weekly and daily treatment with camptothecin (NSC-100880): Correlation with preclinical studies. Cancer Chemother Rep Prt I 1972;56:515.
11. Hertzberg RP, Caranfa MJ, Holdern KG, et al. Modification of the hydroxy lactone ring of camptothecin: inhibition of mammalian topoisomerase I and biological activity. J Med Chem 1989;32:715.
12. Wani MC, Nicholas AW, Wall ME. Synthesis and antitumor activity of camptothecin analogues. J Med Chem 1986;29:1553.
13. Jaxel C, Kohn KW, Wani MC, Wall ME, Pommier Y. Structure-activity study of the actions of camptothecin derivatives on mammalian topoisomerase I: Evidence for a specific receptor site and a relation to antitumor activity. Cancer Res 1989;49:1465.
14. Kuhn J, Wall J, Burris S, Rodriguez M, Marshall M, Smith B, Johnson R, Von Hoff D. Phase I clinical and pharmacokinetic trial of the topoisomerase I inhibitor, topotecan. Abs. 49. Third Conference on DNA Topoisomerases in Therapy. 1990;35.
15. Sugimoto Y, Tsukahara S, Oh HT, Isoe T, Tsuruo T. Decreased expression of DNA topoisomerase I in camptothecin-resistant tumor cell lines as determined by a monoclonal antibody. Cancer Res 1990;50:6925.
16. Bodley AL, Liu LF, Israel M, et al. DNA topoisomerase II-mediated interaction of doxorubicin and daunomycin congeners with DNA. Cancer Res 1989;49:5969.
17. Tewey KM, Chen GL, Nelson EM, Liu LF. Intercalative antitumor drugs interfere with the breakage-reunion reaction of mammalian DNA topoisomerase II. J Biol Chem 1984;259:9182.
18. Baguley BC, Holdaway KM, Fray LM. Design of DNA intercalators to overcome topoisomerase II-mediated multidrug resistance. J Natl Cancer Inst 1990;82:398.
19. Chow K-C, MacDonald TL, Ross WE. DNA binding by epipodophyllotoxins and N-acyl anthracyclines: implications for mechanism of topoisomerase II inhibition. Mol Pharm 1988;34:467.
20. Nitiss J, Wang JC. DNA topoisomerase-targeting antitumor drugs can be studied in yeast. Proc Natl Acad Sci USA 1988;85:7501.
21. Eng W-K, Faucette L, Johnson RK, Sternglanz R. Evidence that DNA topoisomerase I is necessary for the cytotoxic effects of camptothecin. Mol Pharm 1989;34:755.
22. Hsiang Y-H, Liu LF, Wall ME, et al. DNA topoisomerase I mediated DNA cleavage and cytotoxicity of camptothecin analogs. Cancer Res. 1989;49:4385.
23. Rowe TC, Chen GL, Hsiang Y-H, Liu LF. DNA damage by antitumor acridines mediated by mammalian DNA topoisomerase II. Cancer Res 1986;46:2021.
24. Monnot M, Mauffret O, Simon V, et al. DNA-drug recognition and effects on topoisomerase II-mediated cytotoxicity. J Biol Chem 1991;266:1820.
25. Rowe T, Kupfer G, Ross W. Inhibition of epipodophyllotoxin cytotoxicity by interference with topoisomerase-mediated DNA cleavage. Biochem Pharm 1985;34:2483.
26. Li LH, Fraser TJ, Olin EJ, Bhuyan BK. Action of camptothecin on mammalian cells in culture. Cancer Res 1972;32:2643.
27. Horwitz SB, Horwitz MS. Effects of camptothecin on the breakage and repair of DNA during the cell cycle. Cancer Res 1973;33:2834.
28. Hsiang YH, Lihou MG, Liu LF. Arrest of replication forks by drug-stabilized topoisomerase I-DNA cleavable complexes as a mechanism of cell killing by camptothecin. Cancer Res 1989;49:5077.
29. Horwitz MS, Brayton C. Camptothecin: mechanism of inhibition of adenovirus formation. Virol 1972;48:690.
30. Avemann K, Knippers R, Koller T, Sogo JM. Camptothecin, a specific inhibitor of type I DNA topoisomerase, induces DNA breakage at replication forks. Mol & Cell Biol 1988;8:3026.
31. Snapka RM. Topoisomerase inhibitors can selectively interfere with different stages of simian virus 40 DNA replication. Mol & Cell Biol 1986;6:4221.
32. Champoux JJ. Topoisomerase I is preferentially associated with isolated replicating simian virus 40 molecules after treatment of infected cells with camptothecin. J Virol 1988;62:3675.
33. Glisson B, Gupta R, Smallwood-Kentro S, Ross W. Characterization of acquired epipodophyllotoxin resistance in a Chinese hamster ovary cell line: loss of drug-stimulated DNA cleavage activity. Cancer Res 1986;46:1934.
34. Wilson WR, Whitmore GF. Cell-cycle-stage specificity of 4'-(9-acridinylamino)methanesulfon-m-anisidide(m-AMSA) and interaction with ionizing radiation in mammalian cell cultures. Radiation Res 1981;87:121.
35. Estey E, Adlakha RC, Hittelman WN, Zwelling LA. Cell cycle stage dependent variations in drug-induced topo-

isomerase II mediated DNA cleavage and cytotoxicity. Biochem 1987;26:4338.

36. D'Arpa P, Beardmore C, Liu LF. Involvement of nucleic acid synthesis in cell killing mechanisms of topoisomerase poisons. Cancer Res 1990;50:6919.

37. Markovits J, Pommier Y, Kerrigan D, Covey JM, Tilchen EJ, Kohn KW. Topoisomerase II-mediated DNA breaks and cytotoxicity in relation to cell proliferation and the cell cycle in NIH 3T3 fibroblasts and L1210 leukemia cells. Cancer Res 1987;47:2050.

38. Schneider E, Lawson PA, Ralph RK. Inhibition of protein synthesis reduces the cytotoxicity of 4'-(9-acridinylamino)methanesulfon-m-anisidide without affecting DNA breakage and DNA topoisomerase II in a murine mastocytoma cell line. Biochem Pharm 1989;38:263.

39. Kaufmann SH. Antagonism between camptothecin and topoisomerase II-directed chemotherapeutic agents in a human leukemia cell line. Cancer Res 1991;51:1129.

40. Caldecott K, Banks G, Jeggo P. DNA double-strand break repair pathways and cellular tolerance to inhibitors of topoisomerase II. Cancer Res 1990;50:5778.

41. Smith PJ, Makinson TA. Cellular consequences of overproduction of DNA topoisomerase II in an ataxia-telangiectasia cell line. Cancer Res 1989;49:1118.

42. Duguet M, Lavenot C, Harper H, Mirambeau G, De Recondo AM. DNA topoisomerases from rat liver: physiological variations. Nucleic Acids Res 1983;11:1059.

43. Miskimins R, Miskimins WK, Bernstein H, Shimizu N. Epidermal growth factor-induced topoisomerase(s). Intracellular translocation and relation to DNA synthesis. Exper Cell Res 1983;146:53.

44. Taudou G, Mirambeau G, Lavenot C, Garabedian A, Vermeersch J, Duguet M. DNA topoisomerase activities in Concanavalin A stimulated lymphocytes. FEBS letts 1984;176:431.

45. Heck MMS, Earnshaw WC. Topoisomerase II: a specific marker for cell proliferation. J Cell Biol 1987;103:2569.

46. Earnshaw WC, Heck MMS. Cell biology of topoisomerase II. Cancer Cells 1988;6:279.

47. Heck MMS, Hittelman WN, Earnshaw WC. Differential expression of DNA topoisomerase I and II during the eukaryotic cell cycle. Proc Natl Acad Sci USA 1988; 85:1086.

48. Woessner RD, Chung TDY, Hofmann GA, et al. Differences between normal and ras-transformed NIH-3T3 cells in expression of the 170kD and 180kD forms of topoisomerase II. Cancer Res 1990;50:2901.

49. Zwelling LA, Hinds M, Chan D, Altschler E, Mayes J, Zipf TF. Phorbol ester effects on topoisomerase II activity and gene expression in HL-60 human leukemia cells with different proclivities toward monocytoid differentiation. Cancer Res 1990;50:7116.

50. Hsiang Y-H, Wu H-Y, Liu LF. Proliferation-dependent regulation of DNA topoisomerase II in cultured human cells. Cancer Res 1988;48:3230.

51. Romig H, Richter A. Expression of the topoisomerase-I gene in serum stimulated human fibroblasts. Biochim Biophys Acta 1990;1048:274.

52. Champoux JJ, Young LS, Been MD. Studies on the regulation and specificity of the DNA-untwisting enzyme. Cold Spring Harbor Symp Quant Biol 1978;43:53.

53. Kunze N, Klein M, Richter A, Knippers R. Structural characterization of the human DNA topoisomerase-I gene promoter. Eur J Biochem 1990;194:323.

54. Durban E, Goodenough M, Mills J, Busch H. Topoisomerase I phosphorylation in vitro and in rapidly growing Novikoff hepatoma cells. EMBO J 1985;4:2921.

55. Pommier Y, Kerrigan D, Hartman KD, Glazer RI. Phosphorylation of mammalian DNA topoisomerase I and activation by protein kinase C. J Biol Chem 1990;265:9418.

56. Coderoni S, Paparelli M, Gianfranceschi GL. Role of calf thymus DNA topoisomerase I phosphorylation on relaxation activity expression and on DNA-protein interaction: role of DNA topoisomerase I phosphorylation. Mol Biol Rep 1990;14:35.

57. Heck MMS, Hittelman WN, Earnshaw WC. In vivo phosphorylation of the 170-KDA form of eukaryotic DNA topoisomerase. J Biol Chem 1989;264:15161.

58. Ackerman P, Glover CVC, Osheroff N. Phosphorylation of DNA topoisomerase II in vivo and in total homogenates of Drosophila Kc cells. J Biol Chem 1988; 263:12653.

59. Ackerman P, Glover CVC, Osheroff N. Phosphorylation of DNA topoisomerase II by casein kinase II: modulation of eukaryotic topoisomerase II activity in vitro. Proc Natl Acad Sci USA 1985;82:3164.

60. Kasid UN, Halligan B, Liu LF, Dritschilo A, Smulson M. Poly (ADP-ribose) -mediated postranslational modification of chromatin-associated human topoisomerase I. Inhibitory effects on catalytic activity. J Biol Chem 1989;264:18687.

61. Potmesil M, Hsiang Y-H, Liu LF, et al. Resistance of human leukemic and normal lymphocytes to drug-induced DNA cleavage and low levels of DNA topoisomerase II. Cancer Res 1988;48:3537.

62. Priel E, Aboud M, Feigelman J, Segal S. Topoisomerase II activity in human leukemic and lymphoblastoid cells. Biochem Biophys Res Comm 1985;130:325.

63. Romig H, Richter A. Expression of the type-I DNA topoisomerase gene in adenovirus-5 infected human cells. Nucleic Acids Res 1990;18:801.

64. Singh B, Gupta S. Mutagenic responses of thirteen anti-cancer drugs on mutation induction at multiple genetic loci and on sister chromatid exchanges in Chinese hamster ovary cells. Cancer Res 1983;43:577.

65. Matsuo K, Kohno K, Takano H, Sato S, Kiue A, Kuwano M. Reduction of drug accumulation and DNA topoisomerase II activity in acquired teniposide-resistant human cancer KB cell lines. Cancer Res 1990; 50:5819.

66. Ferguson PJ, Fisher MH, Stephenson J, Li D, Zhou B, Cheng Y. Combined modalities of resistance in etoposide-resistant human KB cell lines. Cancer Res 1988; 48:5956.

67. Deffie AM, Bosman DJ, Goldenberg GJ. Evidence for a mutant allele of the gene for DNA topoisomerase II in adriamycin-resistant P388 murine leukemia cells. Cancer Res 1989;49:6879.

68. Deffie AM, Batra JK, Goldenberg GJ. Direct correlation between DNA topoisomerase-II activity and cytotoxicity in adriamycin-sensitive and adriamycin-resistant P388 leukemia cell lines. Cancer Res 1989;49:58.

69. Eng WK, McCabe FL, Tan KB, et al. Development of a stable camptothecin-resistant subline of P388 leukemia with reduced topoisomerase I content. Molec Pharm 1990;38:471.

70. Sullivan DM, Glisson BS, Hodges PK, Smallwood-Kentro S, Ross WE. Proliferation dependence of topoisomerase II mediated drug action. Biochem 1986;25:2248.

71. Sullivan DM, Latham MD, Ross WE. Proliferation-dependent topoisomerase II content as a determinant of antineoplastic drug action in human mouse and Chinese hamster ovary cells. Cancer Res 1987;47:3973.

72. Zwelling LA, Estey E, Silberman L, Doyle S, Hittelman

W. Effect of cell proliferation and chromatin conformation on intercalator-induced protein-associated DNA cleavage in human brain tumor cells and human fibroblasts. Cancer Res 1987;47:251.

73. Zwelling LA, Slovak ML, Doroshow JH, et al. Ht1080/DR4: A p-glycoprotein-negative human fibrosarcoma cell line exhibiting resistance to topoisomerase-II-reactive drugs despite the presence of a drug-sensitive topoisomerase II. J Natl Can Inst 1990;82:1553.

74. Zwelling LA, Hinds M, Chan D, et al. Characterization of an amsacrine-resistant line of human leukemia cells: evidence for a drug-resistant form of topoisomerase-II. J Biol Chem 1989;264:16411.

75. Drake FH, Zimmerman JP, McCabe FL, et al. Purification of topoisomerase II from amsacrine-resistant P388 leukemia cells. J Biol Chem 1987;262:16739.

76. Danks MK, Schmidt CA, Cirtain MC, Suttle DP, Beck WT. Altered catalytic activity of and DNA cleavage by DNA topoisomerase II from human leukemic cells selected for resistance to VM-26. Biochem 1988;27:8861.

77. Sullivan DM, Latham MD, Rowe TC, Ross WE. Purification and characterization of an altered topoisomerase II from a drug-resistant Chinese ovary cell line. Biochem 1989;28:5680.

78. Gupta RS, Gupta R, Eng B, et al. Camptothecin-resistant mutants of Chinese hamster ovary cells containing a resistant form of topoisomerase I. Cancer Res 1988;48:6404.

79. Charcosset J-Y, Saucier J-M, Jacquemin-Sablon A. Reduced DNA topoisomerase II activity and drug-stimulated DNA cleavage in 9-Hydroxyellipticine resistant cells. Biochem Pharm 1988;37:2145.

80. Robson CN, Hoban PR, Harris AL, Hickson ID. Cross-sensitivity to topoisomerase II inhibitors in cytotoxic drug-hypersensitive Chinese hamster ovary cell lines. Cancer Res 1987;47:1560.

81. Huff AC, Kreuzer KN. Evidence for a common mechanism of action for antitumor and antibacterial agents that inhibit type-II DNA topoisomerase. J Biol Chem 1990;265:20496.

82. Estey EH, Silberman L, Beran M, Anderson BS, Zwelling LA. The interaction between nuclear topoisomerase II activity from human leukemia cells, exogenous DNA, and 4′-(9-acridinylamino) ethanesulfon-m-anisidide (m-AMSA) or 4-6-0-ethylidene-β-D-glucopyranoside) (VP-16) indicates the sensitivity of the cells to the drugs. Biochem Biophys Res Comm 1987;144:787.

83. Huff AC, Ward RE IV, Kreuzer KN. Mutational alteration of the breakage resealing subunit of bacteriophage T4 DNA topoisomerase confers resistance to antitumor agent m-AMSA. Mol & Gen Genet 1990;221:27.

84. Tamura H, Kohchi C, Yamada R, et al. Molecular cloning of a cDNA of a camptothecin-resistant human DNA topoisomerase I and identification of mutation sites. Nucleic Acids Res 1991;19:69.

85. Andoh T, Ishii K, Suzuki Y, et al. Characterization of a mammalian mutant with a camptothecin resistant DNA topoisomerase I. Proc Natl Acad Sci USA 1987;84:5565.

86. Kjeldsen E, Bonven BJ, Andoh T, et al. Characterization of a camptothecin-resistant human DNA topoisomerase I. J Biol Chem 1988;263:3912.

87. Huff AC, Leatherwood JK, Kreuzer KN. Bacteriophage-T4 DNA topoisomerase is the target of antitumor agent 4′-(9-acridinylamino)methanesulfon-meta-anisidide(m-AMSA) in T4-infected *Escherichia coli*. Proc Natl Acad Sci USA 1989;86:1307.

88. Kaufmann S. Inhibition of topoisomerase II-mediated cytotoxicity in a human leukemia cell line by camptothecin and other inhibitor of RNA synthesis. Third conf. on DNA topoisomerases in therapy. 1990. p37 (abs. #62)

89. Noonan KE, Beck C, Holzmayer TA, et al. Quantitative analysis of MDR1 (multidrug resistance) gene expression in human tumors by polymerase chain reaction. Proc Natl Acad Sci USA 1990;87:7160.

90. Tsuruo T, Matsuzaki T, Matsushita M, Saito H, Yokokura T. Antitumor effect of CPT-11, a new derivative of camptothecin, against pleiotropic drug-resistant tumors *in vitro* and *in vivo*. Cancer Chemother Pharma 1988;21:71.

91. Gorsky LD, Morin MJ. Microsomal activation and increased production of 4′-(9-acridinylamino)-3-methanesulfon-m-anisidide (m-AMSA) -dependent, topoisomerase-associated DNA lesions in nuclei from human HL-60 leukemia cells. Biochem Pharm 1990;39:1481.

Part Two

Clinical Progress

Scott M. Lippman
Waun Ki Hong

Retinoid Chemoprevention of Upper Aerodigestive Tract Carcinogenesis

6

Introduction ■

Epithelial cancers of the upper aerodigestive tract (UADT) along with those of the esophagus and lung (lower aerodigestive tract) are a devastating group. In 1991, they will cause 160,000 deaths in the United States alone, fully one-third of all U.S. cancer deaths in that year.[1]

Cancers of this group also are profoundly heterogeneous.[2] Striking variations in their patterns of sites and incidences occur among different regions, cultures and demographic groups.[3] These variations are the result of different patterns of the use of one causative agent—tobacco. Tobacco, through a process known as "field" carcinogenesis, is the underlying link connecting diverse cancers of the aerodigestive tract.

Worldwide, tobacco is smoked by one billion people. Smoking rates are rising by 2% per year in developing countries. Although smoking rates in industrialized nations are decreasing by 1.5% per year, the surgeon general reported that, in 1989, 50 million people smoked habitually in the United States.

Tobacco is chewed by 600 million people around the world, and the rate of smokeless tobacco use is growing. In Asia, the Philippines, and islands of the South Pacific, 450 million people chew betel quids consisting of areca nut, betel leaf, tobacco, and spice. In India and Africa, 100 million people use a tobacco-lime mixture placed in the gingival groove. In the Soviet Union, Iran, and Afghanistan, 20 million people use a mixture of tobacco, lime, ash, and oil placed under the tongue.[4] More than 30 million people in North America and Europe use smokeless tobacco.

These data indicate that, despite intensified programs to achieve tobacco cessation, tobacco use remains a major health problem and the number-one cause of head and neck and other aerodigestive tract cancers. Also, rates of survival for patients with aerodigestive tract cancers have not improved significantly despite treatment advances. Even among patients "cured" of UADT cancers, a significant percentage go on to develop second primary tumors, usually in the head and neck, esophagus, or lung.[5] Unless new approaches can be found, tobacco will continue to cause aerodigestive tract cancers that will kill hundreds of thousands of people throughout the world every year. For these reasons, research into the management and control of this devastating cancer group has begun to focus on the promising new field of chemoprevention.

In 1976 Sporn coined the term "cancer chemoprevention" and defined it as the reversal of carcinogenesis in the premalignant phase.[6] This concept forms the rationale for clinical chemoprevention trials. A body of preclinical and epidemiologic data support the premise that carcinogenesis in preinvasive stages is reversible. Chemoprevention trials can be designed for a broad spectrum of subjects: (a) for general populations at low risk of a broad spectrum of cancer types; (b) for specific populations with either high- or low-risk premalignant lesions; and (c) for subjects at extremely high risks of second primary tumors.

The focus of this chapter will be on chemoprevention study of retinoids in the region of the UADT, also called the head and neck. The term *retinoids,* also coined by Sporn in 1976,[7] refers to the class of agents including vitamin A, or retinol and its more than 3000 natural derivatives and synthetic analogues.[8-10] The retinoid 13-*cis*-retinoic acid (13-cRA), or isotretinoin, is the most studied chemopreventive agent in the UADT region. Three landmark developments within the last five years have raised unprecedented interest in retinoids as cancer preventive and therapeutic agents. These include (1) preclinical work that identified the retinoic acid nuclear receptors and may ultimately resolve retinoids' primary mechanism of action,[11-14] (2) spectacular clinical results with the retinoid all-*trans*-retinoic acid in acute promyelocytic leukemia,[15] and (3) chemopreventive trials of the retinoid 13-cRA, which significantly reduced incidences of *de novo* tumors in patients "cured" of skin cancer[16] and reduced incidences of second primary tumors in patients "cured" of head and neck squamous cell carcinoma.[17] The third retinoid achievement marks the first time that any agent has been shown to prevent the development of invasive cancer in humans.

The UADT region, which includes the oral cavity, pharynx, and larynx, provides an ideal *in vivo* model system for studying carcinogenesis within the epithelia of the entire aerodigestive tract (Fig. 6-1).[2,4] UADT carcinogenesis can be easily and relatively noninvasively monitored, and it shares features of biology and etiology (tobacco) with premalignancy of the esophagus and lung. Short-term chemoprevention trials of retinoids in UADT subjects have focused on suppression of carcinogen-

Aerodigestive Tract Epithelia

FIG. 6–1 This diagram illustrates the shared epithelium between the upper aerodigestive tract and esophagus and that between the larynx and lung.

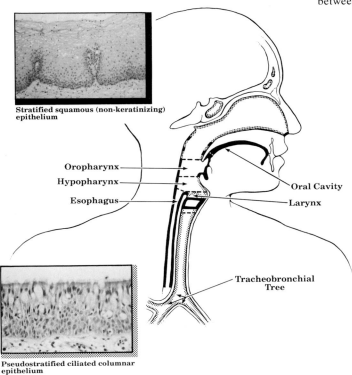

Stratified squamous (non-keratinizing) epithelium

Oropharynx
Hypopharynx
Esophagus

Oral Cavity
Larynx

Tracheobronchial Tree

Pseudostratified ciliated columnar epithelium

esis in the progression phase, that is, the phase between the appearance of a premalignant lesion and the onset of invasive cancer.

This chapter will review the following major areas: the multistep biology of UADT carcinogenesis, mechanism(s) of retinoid action, preclinical retinoid research, clinical retinoid trials, chemoprevention safety issues, and future directions of this research.

Biology of UADT Carcinogenesis ■

Field Carcinogenesis ■

In 1953 Slaughter and associates[18] published a classic report describing the novel concept they called "field cancerization." This term referred to

the basic pathogenic process that linked their oral cancer patients' originally diagnosed tumors with multiple other primary tumors in the oropharynx, esophagus, and lung. Slaughter realized that in subjects at risk the entire aerodigestive epithelial surface, or "field," is exposed to repeated carcinogenic insults, usually from tobacco use (Fig. 6-2). The exposed epithelial field encompasses a group of multiple synchronous independent premalignant foci which develop and progress at variable rates.[5] This concept of multistep field carcinogenesis opened the door for modern chemopreventive research in the aerodigestive tract region.

Today, field carcinogenesis refers to the clinical and biologic (that is, cellular, biochemical, and molecular) alterations that occur in multiple epithelial sites within the aerodigestive tract of a high-risk individual. This process provides a tremendous challenge for clinicians. Local therapy of

FIG. 6–2   This diagram illustrates carcinogenesis within an early stage laryngeal cancer patient. Premalignant lesions were present in the oral cavity and lung. The histologically "normal" bronchial epithelium was shown to be "premalignant" by more sensitive biomarker studies. "Field" carcinogenesis refers to this pattern of diffuse exposure of the epithelia of the upper aerodigestive tract, lung, and esophagus to carcinogens (commonly, cigarette smoke).

"Field" Carcinogenesis in Aerodigestive Tract Epithelia

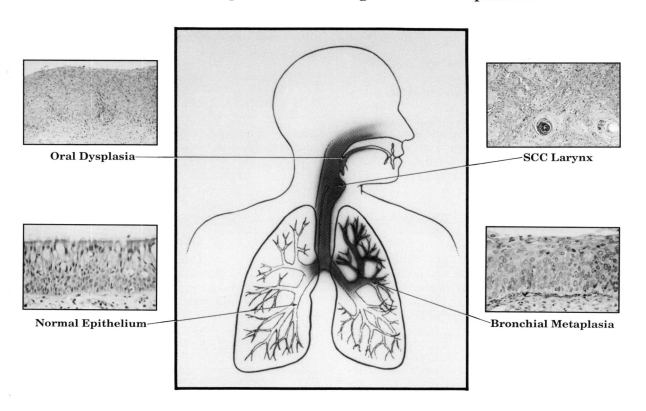

Oral Dysplasia

SCC Larynx

Normal Epithelium

Bronchial Metaplasia

malignant tumors and premalignant lesions is inadequate in the face of the following field-wide developments: high incidence of second primary tumors in head and neck squamous cell carcinoma; *de novo* appearances of oral premalignancy in over one-third of locally treated oral premalignancy patients; and the frequent presentation of a patient's premalignant lesions at multiple aerodigestive tract sites. Clinicians require chemopreventive approaches in addition to standard therapies if they are to suppress the multistep progression of dysplastic sites of preinvasive disease.

Intermediate Endpoints of Carcinogenesis ■

Aerodigestive tract epithelial carcinogenesis is an extremely complex multistep process. Rather late, gross markers of this process are observable histologic and clinical stages that are incapable of detecting the subtle cellular, molecular, and biochemical changes occurring in the earliest preneoplastic phases. Basic science advances in the biology of carcinogenesis are leading to the development of exciting new markers of subtle intermediate stages, or endpoints, of the multistep process. Called intermediate endpoint biomarkers, these markers may provide far earlier and more specific indicators of cancer risk and drug efficacy in prevention trials than currently are possible with standard clinical and histologic evaluations.[19]

The multistep carcinogenic process begins with genetic alterations and proceeds to altered expressions of regulatory gene products and dysregulated tissue growth, or proliferation, and differentiation. Biomarkers of intermediate endpoints therefore fall into four main classes—genetic alterations, differentiation, proliferation, and gene regulatory processes.

Currently, investigators are studying most intensively markers in the class of proliferation, such as proliferating cell nuclear antigen, or PCNA. New preliminary data indicate that in the future certain markers in the class of genetic alterations (for example, the oncogene product markers c-erb B1, INT-2, and HST-1) and in the class of differentiation (*e.g.,* carbohydrate antigens such as blood group antigens) will be the most hotly pursued.[2]

Although preliminary data indicate promise for several markers, no marker has yet been established as a valid biomarker of intermediate endpoints of carcinogenesis; in other words, no one-to-one correlation exists between any marker

Table 6–1
Biologic Markers As Intermediate Endpoints For Chemoprevention Trials

Criteria
- Differential expression in normal and high-risk sites
- Degree or pattern correlate with stage of carcinogenesis
- Ability to analyze in small tissue specimens
- Modulatable by chemopreventive agent

Utility
- Identify high-risk subject/site (enhance statistical power).
- Trial monitor—early indicator of response/relapse
- Short-term *in-vivo* estimate of biologic activity.
- Study mechanism(s) of drug activity/resistance.
- Provide rationale for long-term phase III trial.

expression and long-term clinical outcome. Listed in Table 6-1 are elements of two important facets of biomarker study—the criteria upon which potential biomarkers are selected for study, and the potential uses biomarkers will have in chemoprevention trials.

UADT carcinogenesis is an excellent model for conducting biomarker studies. It has extremely reliable preclinical study models, easy accessibility for the surveillance and tissue acquisition necessary for studying the carcinogenic process and its pharmacologic reversal, and an agent, 13-cRA, with established activity against it.

Mechanism of Retinoid Action ■

Vitamin A and other retinoids have been studied in carcinogenesis for over 60 years.[20] Established retinoid effects—that is, inducing differentiation and suppressing proliferation of malignant cells—occur primarily in the post-initiation phase (promotion and progression phases). Until very recently, only modest gains had been made in understanding these agents' mechanism for achieving these results. We knew that potential anticarcinogenic mechanisms of retinoids include modulations of growth factor receptors, apoptosis, protein kinase-C and gap-junction protein synthesis.[10] The specific nature of the molecular mechanism of action, however, remained unclear.

Then, in 1987, researchers studying nuclear steroid receptors in two independent labs simultaneously stumbled onto something that retinoid researchers had not been able to find in 60 years of investigation—a nuclear receptor for retinoic acid.[11,12] They called it "RAR-α." This discovery has revolutionized basic science research in the retinoid field. For the first time, the primary mechanism of retinoic acid began to emerge into the light.

Nuclear receptors are the protein products of certain genes. Four human retinoic acid receptors (RARs), along with most of their chromosomal origins, now have been identified. These are RAR-α (chromosome 17q21), RAR-β (chromosome 3p24), RAR-γ (chromosome 12), and the structurally unique RXR-α. RAR-α, -β and -γ and their multiple isoforms have different biologic properties, tissue distributions, and expression patterns. The RAR series is strongly homologous (especially in the DNA binding, or zinc-finger, domain) to steroid and thyroid hormone receptors.[11-14]

The gene family responsible for RARs has been highly conserved throughout the evolution of humans and many other animals. These genes did not appear suddenly in response to pharmacologically introduced retinoic acid. Therefore, they must play a critical role in the regulation of normal cell growth and function by producing the receptors that bind to the extremely low endogenous levels of *trans*- and *cis*-retinoic acids found in normal cells.[21] (It is a recent discovery that *cis*-retinoic acid also is found naturally in human cells and serum.)

Because RARs are part of the well-studied and -understood steroid receptor family, researchers have a tremendous advantage in understanding the nuclear RARs. The α, β, and γ receptors consist of proteins of approximately 50,000 daltons that combine with the free carboxyl groups on retinoic acid molecules. Recent data indicate that the α and β receptors have similar affinity for binding retinoic acid.[22] All RARs have a much higher affinity for binding retinoic acid than for binding retinol. After binding with retinoic acid, the receptors undergo conformational changes that allow them to bind to DNA sequences (retinoic acid response elements) that, through transactivation, directly modulate gene transcription.

Whether or not RAR-mediated retinoid effect on DNA transcription directly influences carcinogenesis is the focus of intensive current research. Two pieces of recent data suggest that RAR alterations do influence carcinogenesis. Study in UADT and lung carcinogenesis shows that loss of the gene that produces RAR-β is associated with progression. Study in promyelocytic leukemia shows that the 15;17 translocation transects the RAR-α gene on chromosome 17 and fuses it to a chromosome 15-specific locus (PML).[23]

Preclinical Retinoid Study ■

Vast data from epidemiologic, *in vitro,* and animal studies strongly support the role of retinoids in suppressing epithelial carcinogenesis.[2,4,7-10,16,17,19,20,24] One of vitamin A's major physiologic functions is to prevent squamous differentiation of epithelial cells in nonkeratinizing tissues. Retinoids can modulate the growth and differentiation of normal, premalignant, and malignant epithelial cells in culture and can suppress carcinogenesis *in vivo* in a variety of human and animal epithelial tissues, including mucosa of the skin, trachea, lungs, and UADT.[10]

In vivo models of UADT carcinogenesis are critical for identifying new single agents and agent combinations, establishing dose-response relationships, and conducting intermediate biomarker studies. The most utilized model system is that of DMBA-induced carcinogenesis in the Syrian golden hamster buccal pouch.[25] Work in this model is supplemented by work in lingual and palatal carcinogenesis systems.[4] Several different retinoids, including 13-cRA, are active in all UADT carcinogenesis study systems.[25-29]

A number of other chemopreventive agents— crude extracts of onion, soybean-derived Bowman-Birk protease inhibitor, vitamin E (dietary and topical), β-carotene (topical only), and extracts of *Spirulina-Dunaliella* algae (rich in β-carotene, other carotenoids, and vitamin E)—inhibit cancer development to varying degrees in the hamster buccal pouch model.[4,25,30,31] Although active in the hamster buccal pouch,[32] β-carotene was ineffective in the hamster lingual model, even at doses that turned the hamster's tongue yellow.[28]

Up to the present, clinical UADT data are limited to retinoids (natural and synthetic), β-carotene, and selenium. Of these agents, only the retinoids have a record of established clinical effect.

Retinoid Chemoprevention Trials ■

Oral Premalignancy ■

Overview. Most clinical chemoprevention trials in head and neck squamous cell carcinoma (HNSCC) to date have used pharmacologic doses of the synthetic retinoids and the natural agent β-carotene (a carotenoid) in reversing oral premalignant lesions.

The premalignant oral lesion is called oral leukoplakia and is defined clinically as a white patch or plaque on the oral mucosa that will not rub off and cannot be removed by scraping, reversed by elimination of obvious local irritants such as dentures, or classified clinically or histologically as any other specific disease.[33] Its histologic pattern ranges from hyperkeratosis with hyperplasia to severe dysplasia and carcinoma *in situ*. In clinical trials, we use the term *oral premalignancy* to refer to the clinical spectrum from whitish low-risk lesions to red or speckled high-risk lesions, with further classification and stratification based on histologic differences.

Leukoplakia is classified as a premalignant lesion in part because of its epidemiologic, geographic, and etiologic similarities to oral squamous cell carcinoma (SCC). More important are leukoplakia's frequent occurrence adjacent to oral SCC in over 30% (range 10%–100%) of cancers[34] and the relationship between its malignant transformation rates and the presence and degree of dysplasia. Red (erythroplasia) or speckled sites within lesions are associated highly with dysplastic epithelium, and therefore are useful indicators of biopsy sites.

A broader definition of oral premalignancy includes normal-appearing mucosa at risk of malignant transformation as a result of field carcinogenesis. Oral leukoplakia's etiology, pathogenesis, and demographic characteristics are similar to those for HNSCC, especially in regard to its strong relationship with tobacco use.[2–5] The strongest risk factor for developing oral premalignancy is prolonged exposure to smokeless tobacco. This disorder afflicts millions of people in Asia, where highly carcinogenic betel quid mixtures are endemic. "Inverse" smoking—placing the lit end in the mouth—is associated highly with palatal lesions. Cigarette smoking is a weaker risk factor for oral lesion development, and smoking cessation has only a marginal influence on this lesion's natural history.[33] Recent laboratory work suggests that human papilloma viruses (HPVs) contribute to the progression of oral premalignancy.[2]

Many characteristics of oral premalignancy make it an ideal system in the human body for the study of chemopreventive agents with potential for preventing other tobacco-related epithelial neoplastic disorders. First is its well-described role as a precursor of oral cancer. Silverman, of the University of California, San Francisco, conducted the most comprehensive long-term study of oral leukoplakia in this country.[33] Silverman observed an overall malignant transformation rate of

18%, which rose to 36% in the subset of patients with dysplastic leukoplakia lesions. Hyperplastic oral lesions can undergo spontaneous partial improvement. The spontaneous improvement rate of dysplastic lesions is not well studied, although in Silverman's study dysplastic lesions rarely resolved. These data indicate the variable natural history of this disorder and the importance of histologic monitoring and randomized trial designs to distinguish drug effects from naturally occurring changes. Oral premalignancy's second advantage as a model system is that the oral cavity is easily and noninvasively monitored. This system contrasts with other tobacco-related high-risk sites where premalignant lesions have not been identified (such as the esophagus) or require invasive procedures for monitoring (*e.g.*, lung). The third and perhaps the major attribute of this model system is its implications for other epithelial cancers. Oral premalignancy chemoprevention studies already have contributed to the design of a retinoid trial, discussed later, that achieved a significant suppression of second primary tumors in head-and-neck cancer patients.

Although high-risk dysplastic lesions account for fewer than 10% of all oral lesions, this percentage represents hundreds of thousands of people worldwide. In a significant percentage of cases, advanced premalignant, or dysplastic, lesions are not amenable to such local control as surgery because of the diffuse field carcinogenic process with multiple precancerous foci. Therefore, a systemic approach, or chemoprevention, is necessary for control of high-risk lesions. No effective systemic approach currently exists.

NATURAL-AGENT TRIALS □

The first intervention studies in oral premalignancy began in the mid-1950s and used high doses of topical and systemic vitamin A (Table 6-2). These early studies reported clinical and/or histologic activity and response, relapse, and toxicity patterns that are still relevant today. One dramatic trial produced a response rate of 90% with systemic vitamin A.[35] Despite early promising results and insights, however, further work in this area was suspended for over two decades. Stich then conducted a small randomized trial of single-agent systemic vitamin A and reported a 57% clinical complete remission rate with histologic documentation that confirmed the earlier trial.[40]

Single-agent β-carotene has been evaluated in five nonrandomized trials that included a total of

Table 6–2
Natural Agent Chemoprevention Trials in Oral Premalignancy

Investigators	Agent(s)	N	Clinical Response
Wulf (1957)[35]	Vitamin A	20	90%
Silverman (1965)[36,37]	Vitamin A[a]	503[b]	57%
Stich (1985)[38]	β-carotene	23	0%
Stich (1988)[39]	β-carotene	27	15%[c,d]
	β-carotene plus vitamin A	51	28%[c,d]
Stich (1988)[40]	Vitamin A	21	57%[c]
Toma (1990)[41,42]	β-carotene	24	8%(27%)[e]
Garewal (1990)[43]	β-carotene	24	71%
Toma (1990)[42]	Selenium	25	33%
Malaker (1991)[44]	β-carotene	18	22%(44%)[e]

[a]Topical only

[b]Total from this report and literature review

[c]Only complete resolution reported

[d]Lesion resolution and *new* lesion development rates vs placebo: β-carotene (p = .16); β-carotene plus vitamin A (p = .004).

[e]3-month (6-month) response rates

over 100 subjects. These trials' clinical response rates varied widely, from 0%–71%. In the mid-1980s, Stich and colleagues reported the first series of β-carotene trials in Asian betel nut chewers with oral premalignant lesions. No clinical activity was detected in the initial trial of a ten-week course of β-carotene.[38] This study was expanded to include canthaxanthine, a synthetic carotenoid not converted to retinol *in vivo,* and again produced no clinical response. The next series of trials compared a six-month intervention of β-carotene to β-carotene plus vitamin A.[39] In the single-agent β-carotene group, lesion response (15%) was countered equally by new lesion development (15%). The vitamin A/β-carotene combination produced a complete response rate of 28%, two times higher than that of β-carotene alone and nine times greater than placebo. Recent data from this group suggest that low-dose vitamin A (and, to a lesser degree, β-carotene) partially can maintain remission of micronuclei, a biomarker of genetic damage, after combined vitamin A/β-carotene induction.[4,19] Stich's high-risk trial subjects were unique by virtue of intense localized carcinogen exposure, uniform lifestyle, and a diet that was often deficient in vitamin A and carotenoids. The applicability of Stich's results, from subjects in underdeveloped countries, to populations at risk in more industrialized nations is not clear. For example, the micronuclei frequencies of Stich's groups are far higher than those indicated by the data from all other aerodigestive tract studies.[4]

In a pilot trial, Garewal[43] reported a remarkable response rate of 71% in 24 patients with oral leu-

koplakia treated with β-carotene at 30 mg/day for three months. Fewer than half of these subjects had dysplastic lesions, none severe. In contrast, Toma[41,42] and Malaker[44] recently reported lower response rates in patients with oral leukoplakia who were treated with 3–4 fold higher doses of β-carotene (Table 6-2).

Besides being nonrandomized, none of the β-carotene studies included systematic histologic assessments. Nontoxic β-carotene's clinical value therefore remains unproved.

The only other agent with published clinical results in oral premalignancy is selenium, an agent with proven activity in the lingual model.[28] The one reported trial of this agent included 25 subjects and produced a 33% response rate at 3 months.[42] No toxicity has been reported in this or any of the natural-agent trials.

SYNTHETIC-AGENT TRIALS □

Limited to retinoids, nine synthetic-agent trials at daily doses of 1 mg/kg/day or greater have consistently produced objective response rates in leukoplakia of 60%–90%, with a median response rate of over 75% (Table 6-3). In contrast to the limited and recent data with nontoxic natural agents, synthetic retinoid trials began over two decades ago and include more than 250 treated patients. In the first of his two comparative trials, Koch treated 75 patients for two months with 70 mg/day of 13-cRA, all-*trans*-retinoic acid, or etretinate.[48] Response rates were 87%, 59%, and 92%, respectively. On the basis of these results (etretinate was

Table 6–3
Synthetic Agent Chemoprevention Trials in Oral Premalignancy

Investigator(s)	Agent(s)	N	Clinical Response
Ryssel (1971)[45]	β-all *Trans*-Retinoic Acid	10	70%
Stuttgen (1975)[46]	β-all *Trans*-Retinoic Acid	8	100%
Raque (1975)[47]	β-all *Trans*-Retinoic Acid	5	100%
Koch (1978)[48]	β-all *Trans*-Retinoic Acid	27	59%
	13-*cis*-Retinoic Acid	24	87%
	Etretinate	24	92%
Koch (1981)[49]	Etretinate[a]	24	83%
	Etretinate	21	71%
Cordero (1981)[50]	Etretinate	3	100%
Shah (1983)[51]	13-*cis*-Retinoic Acid[b]	11	100%
Hong (1986)[52]	13-*cis*-Retinoic Acid	24	67%[c]
Han (1990)[53]	N-4-(Hydroxy-carbophenyl) Retinamide	31	87%[c]
Lippman (1990)[54]	13-*cis*-Retinoic Acid	56	62%

[a]Oral and Topical

[b]Topical

[c]Randomized placebo-controlled trials

not only the most active but also the least toxic), Koch designed a second study to compare oral etretinate alone with oral etretinate plus topical etretinate paste.[49] Response rates were high and roughly equivalent between the two study arms.

The variable natural history of oral premalignancy and lack of histologic confirmation of retinoid results led to the most recently reported final data from a randomized, placebo-controlled trial of 13-cRA (1–2 mg/kg/day for 3 months) conducted by Hong and associates.[52] The clinical objective response rate was 67% in the treated group, compared to only 10% in the placebo group (p = .0002). This was the first study to assess histologically all patients before and after therapy. Pretreatment biopsies of 63% of the retinoid-treated group and 40% of the placebo group had varying degrees of dysplasia. Reversal of dysplasia occurred in 54% of the retinoid group (including all severely dysplastic lesions), and only a 10% reversal occurred in the placebo group (p = .01).

Toxicity was significant in those receiving 2 mg/kg/day—cheilitis, facial erythema, and skin dryness and peeling occurring in 88% and conjunctivitis in 76%. Forty-seven percent in this group required dose reduction (to 1 mg/kg/d). With 1 mg/kg/d, only 57% experienced mild skin toxicity and 29% had conjunctivitis. All subjects at this lower dose completed the three-month therapy.

Response rates were not significantly different between patients receiving the lowest (1 mg/kg/day) or highest (2 mg/kg/day) doses. The study was prematurely terminated, after only 44 patients, because of highly significant response differences between treated and placebo subjects.

Although this randomized trial established the efficacy of 13-cRA in premalignant oral lesions, two serious problems were encountered—significant toxicity with high-dose 13-cRA and a relapse rate of over 50% within three months after stopping the drug. This relapse finding is a consistent finding in all oral premalignancy trials reported to date. Hong therefore designed a second study to prolong remission with less toxic maintenance therapy.[54] After 3 months' induction with high-dose 13-cRA (1.5 mg/kg/day), responding (or stable) patients were randomized to a nine-month maintenance program with either low-dose 13-cRA (0.5 mg/kg/d) or β-carotene (30 mg/d). Clinical, histologic and biomarker endpoints were analyzed before therapy and after the induction and maintenance phases. Two-thirds of subjects had dysplastic lesions, which were severe in over 20%.

This trial's high-dose induction phase produced a response rate consistent with the overall response rate of over 60% established in our earlier definitive trial. Preliminary data from the ongoing randomized maintenance phase indicate that low-dose 13-cRA is significantly more effective than β-carotene in maintaining clinicopathologic remission. Relapse rates after the nine-month maintenance phase were 10% in the 13-cRA group and 54% in the β-carotene group (2-sided p < .01).[54]

This trial included laboratory analyses of the genomic biomarker micronuclei. Micronuclei results correlated in general with the clinical data—that is, lowered counts present in the clinically active retinoid arm, increased counts present in the clinically less active β-carotene arm. The data, however, did not establish a significant one-to-one correlation between micronuclei changes and clinical results. Low-dose 13-cRA not only effectively maintained remission but also further improved lesion and micronuclei response.

Other than skin yellowing, no toxic effects occurred in the β-carotene arm. Low dose 13-cRA also was well tolerated, although grade 2 or greater skin or lip dryness occurred more frequently in this arm. No patient dropped off study during maintenance because of toxicity in either arm. Low-dose 13-cRA was associated with mild and reversible toxicities. These data indicate that low-dose 13-cRA is effective and well-tolerated maintenance therapy for oral premalignancy.

ADJUVANT RETINOID TRIAL IN HNSCC □

During the past twenty to thirty years, only marginal improvement in overall survival has occurred for patients with early and locally advanced HNSCC.[2] This is true even though the standard therapies of surgery and/or radiotherapy and, more recently, primary chemotherapy are effective for the control of primary tumors.[55]

Treatment advances have been undermined by the significant percentage of patients initially "cured" of HNSCC who go on to develop second primary tumors—usually in the head and neck, lung, or upper two-thirds of the esophagus and usually of squamous histology.[5] Second primary tumors (SPTs) are the major threat to long-term survival after successful therapy of early-stage HNSCC. Data from tumor registries, multicenter oncology groups, and cancer centers indicate that second primaries, either synchronous or metachronous, develop conservatively at a constant yearly rate of 3%–6% in previously treated patients and contribute to a 6%–9% excess annual mortality rate for these patients.[5,56–58] These rates are higher in prospective studies. SPTs probably result from the field-wide effects of the same carcinogenic exposure responsible for the initial primary. Local curative therapy for early stage disease does not ameliorate the multifocal mucosal field effect. SPTs presumably evolve from premalignant foci that continue to progress throughout the exposed field at risk. This pathogenesis differs from *de-novo* malignancies in other disorders, such as ovarian cancer and Hodgkin's disease, which are clearly treatment-related and include a diverse group of hematologic disorders and solid tumors.[5] It is conceptually difficult, therefore, to develop a chemopreventive strategy for all these diverse cancers. The clinical significance of SPTs is that a patient who presents with HNSCC, even in its earliest stage, is a patient for life.

Multistep field carcinogenesis involving multiple independent sites within the aerodigestive tract,[5] significant activity of 13-cRA in reversing oral premalignancy,[52] and the high rate of SPTs in HNSCC led to the design of an adjuvant trial of 13-cRA in HNSCC.[5,56–59] All patients selected for this study were clinically disease free after surgery and/or radiation therapy for SCC of the head and neck. All patients had histologically confirmed primary SCC in the oral cavity, oropharynx, hypopharynx, or larynx. (Salivary gland and nasopharyngeal carcinoma were excluded from these studies since these sites are outside the field at risk of tobacco-related carcinogenesis.)

Patients were stratified by site (oral cavity, oropharynx, hypopharynx, or larynx) and treatment (surgery, radiation, or both) and randomized in a double-blind fashion to receive for 12 months either 13-cRA (50–100 mg/m^2 of body weight per day) or placebo. The treatment was initiated no later than 10 weeks after primary surgery or 16 weeks after primary radiation therapy in patients who had received radiation therapy alone or radiation combined with surgery.

The primary endpoint of this adjuvant study was the emergence of new disease and its development into either of two major pattern types—progression (local recurrence and regional or distant metastasis), and SPTs. Emergence of any form of new histologically confirmed disease was considered treatment failure. The criteria for second primary tumors that follow were based on a modification of those given by Warren and Gates:[60]

A new cancer with different histology
Any cancer, regardless of site, occurring after three or more years
In the head and neck, a distinct lesion separated from the primary site by more than 2 cm of normal epithelum
In the lung, if histology is squamous cell cancer (within three years), lesion must present as a solitary mass; must be free of local–regional recurrence of original tumor; and have histologic findings of dysplasia or carcinoma-*in-situ* in bronchial epithelium

A total of 103 patients was registered into this study, and patient characteristics were approximately equivalent between the two groups (Table 6-4). Table 6-5 shows the pattern of treatment failures within the retinoid and placebo groups at a median follow-up of all patients of 42 months. The differences between local, regional, and distant failure proportions (ignoring time) in the 13-cRA group (8%, 16%, and 16%) and those in the placebo group (14%, 14%, and 10%) were not statistically significant. But the difference between the percentage of patients developing SPTs in the two patient groups was highly significant—6% (3/49) in

Table 6–4
Adjuvant Trial Patient Characteristics

Characteristics	13-cis-Retinoic Acid Group	Placebo Group
Total Registered Patients	51	52
Inevaluable Patients	2	1
Evaluable Patients	49 (100%)	51 (100%)
Primary site		
Larynx	17 (35%)	19 (37%)
Pharynx	13 (27%)	7 (14%)
Oral cavity	19 (39%)	25 (49%)
Stage		
I, II	20 (41%)	29 (57%)
III, IV	29 (59%)	22 (43%)
Prior therapy		
Surgery alone	20 (41%)	26 (51%)
Radiotherapy alone	10 (20%)	10 (20%)
Surgery and radiotherapy	19 (39%)	15 (29%)
Smoking history		
Active	17 (35%)	16 (31%)
Former	27 (55%)	30 (59%)
Never	5 (10%)	5 (10%)
Alcohol drinker	29 (59%)	26 (51%)

the 13-cRA group compared with 28% (14/51) in the placebo group; p = .005. None of the three SPT failures in the 13-cRA group had multiple SPTs, whereas four of the placebo failures had SPTs in multiple sites. One of these multiple-site failures developed three second primaries and severe dysplasia at two other sites. Figure 6-3 shows the time-adjusted SPT failure rates in the placebo and retinoid-treatment groups.

Follow-up at 3 1/2 years strengthened the trends

Table 6–5
Primary Treatment Failures by Study Group.*

Type of Failure	13-cis-Retinoic Acid Group (N = 49)	Placebo Group (N = 51)	P Value[a]
No. Relapse	15 (31%)[b]	17 (33%)[b]	0.77
Local	4 (8%)	7 (14%)	0.37
Regional	8 (16%)	7 (14%)	0.72
Distant	8 (16%)	5 (10%)	0.33
No. SPTs	3 (6%)	14 (28%)[c]	0.005
Total	18 (37%)	31 (61%)	0.016

*Median follow-up 42 months

[a]By chi-square test without Yates correction. All p-values represent two-sided tests.

[b]Some patients had disease relapse in more than one site category.

[c]Four patients developed more than one second primary tumor.

reported after 32 months;[17] the overall failure rate in the 13-cRA group was significantly smaller than that of the placebo group (Table 6-5).

No patient developed an SPT while on the retinoid intervention. The SPT rate in the placebo arm of this prospective study (10% per year) was higher than the 3%–6% per year reported from retrospective studies and tumor registries.

A total of 17 patients developed SPTs (14 in the placebo, 3 in the retinoid group after therapy). Sites of the SPTs were the UADT, esophagus, or lung in 14 (82%) of the 17 patients (Table 6-6, Fig. 6-4). Nine patients developed SPTs at different sites in the head and neck region; three in the esophagus; and three in the lung. One SPT occurred in the bladder, which, although not strictly within the aerodigestive tract, clearly is within the broader field of tobacco-related epithelial carcinogenesis. One patient in the placebo group developed acute myelogenous leukemia. This pattern is consistent with the site-dispersal patterns of second primary disease reported in other head and neck cancer series and is predicted by tobacco-related field cancerization. Patterns and rates of SPTs indicate that field cancerization is not homogeneous. SPTs are not predicted by exposed surface area but are related to the primary cancer site. Patients with oral cancer have a relatively higher rate of UADT and esophageal SPTs whereas larynx cancer patients seem to have a greater rate of lung SPTs. These patterns may relate to a "ripple" effect, with the most intensive tissue damage close to the primary. These patterns also may be related to shared epithelial types—columnar for larynx and lung cancers, stratified squamous for UADT and esophageal cancers (Fig. 6-1). In analyses of three subsets of SPTs—(a) one that excludes those occurring within 6 months of the primary tumor (synchronous), (b) one that excludes all SPTs not within the carcinogenic field (UADT, lung, esophagus), and (c) one that excludes both—the differences between the placebo and retinoid-treatment groups remain statistically significant (Table 6-7).

Although smoking indisputably is a major risk factor for the development of primary cancers of the UADT and lung, the influence of smoking cessation on the rate of SPT occurrences in patients after developing their first primary is controversial.[4,5] Most reports suggest that, in the long-term, smoking cessation reduces the incidence of second cancers. These reports, however, have experienced difficulties in collecting accurate smoking-related data and have lacked biochemical con-

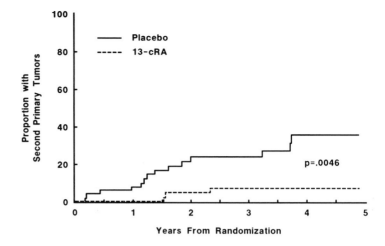

FIG. 6–3 This graph clearly depicts the earlier and significantly greater rate of second primary tumor failures that occurred in the placebo group.

firmation of smoking behavior such as cotinine levels and therefore do not render a clear quantitative assessment of smoking's impact on SPT development. Some investigators have gone so far as to question the unconfirmed association between smoking and SPT risk.

In our study, SPTs developed in only four active smokers; 12 (71%) of the patients who developed SPTs were ex-smokers (Table 6-6). Smoking cessation may have a greater beneficial effect at earlier stages of the multistep carcinogenic process,

or stages that precede premalignant or malignant primary lesions. Other genetic and environmental factors such as viruses and alcohol may have influences on SPT development equal to or even greater than that of smoking.

These variations on the etiologic effects of smoking indicate that an effective chemopreventive approach is needed for the prevention of SPTs in head and neck cancer patients as an adjunct to the important primary preventive measure of smoking cessation. Although the data are limited,

Table 6–6
Characteristics of Patients Who Developed Second Primary Tumors (SPTs)*

Patient No.	Study Group	Age Yr	Sex	Primary Site	Initial Stage	Primary Therapy	Time to SPT	SPT Site(s)	Smoking Status
1	Placebo	53	M	Floor of mouth	II	Surgery	45	Esophagus	Active
2	Placebo	52	M	Palatine arch	II	Surgery	6	False cord, Pyriform sinus, Pharyngeal wall	Active
3	Placebo	57	M	Larynx	II	Surgery + XRT	45	Lung	Active
4	Placebo	71	M	Floor of mouth	II	Surgery	16	Pyriform sinus	Never
5	Placebo	58	F	Pharyngeal wall	II	XRT	13	Lateral tongue	Former
6	Placebo	60	F	Larynx	IV	Surgery	22	Pharyngeal wall	Former
7	Placebo	57	M	Buccal mucosa	IV	Surgery + XRT	2	Ventral tongue	Former
8	Placebo	41	F	Tongue	II	Surgery	2	Pyriform sinus	Former
							27	Lung	
9	Placebo	73	F	Lateral tongue	II	Surgery	14	Floor of mouth, Retromolar trigone	Former
10	Placebo	50	M	Larynx	III	Surgery + XRT	23	AML	Former
11	Placebo	56	F	Soft palate	II	Surgery + XRT	19	Lung, Trachea	Former
12	Placebo	63	M	Soft palate	III	XRT	38	Esophagus	Former
13	Placebo	61	M	Tongue	I	Surgery + XRT	11	Tongue	Former
14	Placebo	48	M	Oropharynx	II	XRT	14	SCC Skin	Former
15	13-cRA	62	M	Floor of mouth	II	Surgery	18	Pharynx	Former
16	13-cRA	66	M	Larynx	IV	Surgery + XRT	18	Esophagus	Active
17	13-cRA	60	M	Oropharynx	II	XRT	28	Bladder	Former

*13-cRA denotes 13-*cis*-retinoic acid; XRT, external x-irradiation; AML, Acute myelogenous leukemia

Site Patterns of Second Primary Tumor Patients

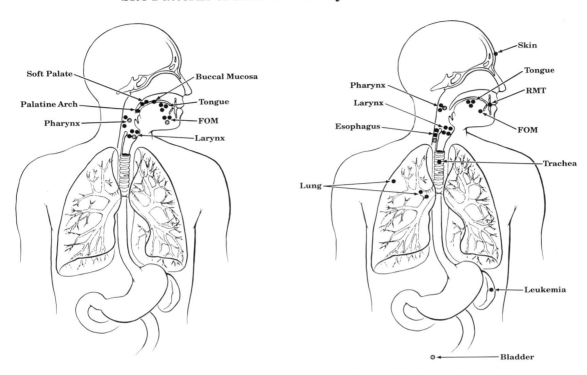

Primary Tumor Sites   **Second Primary Tumor Sites**

...ant trial (which involved patients "cured" of UADT cancer) patients developed
...ese patients' primary tumor sites appear in diagram at left; SPT sites appear at
...group tumors; speckled circles represent retinoid-group tumors. The right dia-
...PTs occurred in the placebo group (black circles) and that a predominance of all
...act, as predicted by "field" carcinogenesis. (FOM) floor of mouth; (RMT) ret-

onchial metaplasia
(a smoking-related premalignant lung lesion) suggest that the chemopreventive activity of retinoids
is enhanced by smoking cessation.[4]

Mucocutaneous toxicities were significant in the
high-dose 13-cRA group (Table 6-8). Only 47%
of the retinoid group completed the one-year
therapy. Thirty-four percent of the patients in the
retinoid group dropped out before completing the
12-month course of therapy because of toxicity-
related issues. This comparatively high dropout
rate enhances the significance of SPT reduction
among retinoid-treated patients, the failure analysis of which included patients who dropped out.

Although this significant adjuvant retinoid trial
is an important first step, the study must be expanded and elaborated through a large-scale phase

III trial. If proven effective in HNSCC alone, this
retinoid strategy would translate into a 10%–20%
improvement in overall survival.[4,5,56] This survival
benefit with adjuvant 13-cRA in early-stage head-
and-neck cancer patients falls within the range of
the survival benefit from standard adjuvant therapy with tamoxifen in breast cancer. HNSCC currently accounts for more than 12,000 deaths per
year in the United States. Worldwide, HNSCC
mortality figures are much higher, and adjuvant
retinoid therapy could save many lives each
year.

We believe that these survival data may provide
the basis for designing primary and adjuvant
chemoprevention studies of retinoids and related
agents in all tobacco-related cancers of the UADT
and lung. This group of deadly cancers constitute

Table 6–7
Subset Analyses of Second Primary Tumor (SPT) Development

	13-cRA (n = 49)	Placebo (n = 51)	p Value
Total SPT	3 (6%)	14 (28%)	p = .005
Excluding Synchronous SPT	3 (6%)	11 (22%)	p = .026
Excluding Out-of-Field SPT	2 (4%)	12 (24%)	p = .005
Excluding Synchronous Plus Out-of-Field SPT	2 (4%)	9 (18%)	p = .03

a major and increasing national and worldwide health problem that has yet to come under control through tobacco cessation programs alone.

The toxicity data and the need for long-term therapy suggest the need for continued investigation of new strategies. To extend the positive adjuvant study in HNSCC, we are planning a new study of low-dose 13-cRA to treat patients with early-stage HNSCC who have been rendered disease-free by local therapy. This multicenter study will include over 1000 patients and is aimed at preventing the major cause of death in patients with early-stage disease—epithelial SPTs within the aerodigestive tract with no relationship to primary treatment.

Safety Issues of Chemoprevention

The safety issue is a chemopreventive age in chemoprevention healthy. As with tamo

oprevention, agents for the chemoprevention of UADT cancers will have to be taken for a long time. Potential chronic side-effects, whether subjective or objective, must therefore be studied carefully. Acceptable toxicity for a chemopreventive agent will vary with the degree of risk—for example, moderate toxicity of effective agents may be acceptable for subjects with dysplastic premalignant lesions or "cured" cancer patients at risk of SPTs.

The major classes of retinoid toxicity are mucocutaneous, visual, skeletal, lipid, liver, and teratogenic side-effects.[10] Although no randomized comparisons have been reported, toxicities appear to vary in incidence and intensity with regard to specific retinoids, doses, durations of administration, and methods of toxicity assessment. The mechanism(s) of toxicity is likely different among the different classes and is largely dose-related and reversible. The clear exception to this view of the mechanism is teratogenicity, the most serious side-effect, which is not reversible and can occur at low doses of synthetic retinoids. Teratogenicity is not a major exclusion factor for aerodigestive cancers, which occur mostly in men and post-menopausal women.

Adjuvant Trial Mucocutaneous Toxicity

Toxicity	13-cis-Retinoic Acid Group (N = 49)*	Placebo Group (N = 50)*	P Value
Skin dryness			<0.001
Mild	14 (29%)	30 (60%)	
Mod/Severe	31 (63%)	4 (8%)	
Cheilitis			0.001
Mild	20 (41%)	17 (34%)	
Mod/Severe	12 (24%)	1 (2%)	
Conjunctivitis			0.184
Mild	6 (12%)	5 (10%)	
Mod/Severe	9 (18%)	4 (8%)	

*Three patients (one in 13-cis-retinoic acid group, two in placebo) who never started adjuvant therapy (i.e., never took pills) were not evaluated for toxicity.

The mechanism of visual toxic effects from synthetic retinoids has been studied most with fenretinide (4HPR). This retinoid can produce reversible night blindness, although asymptomatic electroretinogram abnormalities are more common.[61] This side-effect may result from the synthetic retinoid-lowering serum retinol levels and competing with the endogenous (physiologic) vitamin A metabolite retinal for the retinal receptor, which creates a deficiency of necessary retinol (vitamin A) in the ocular tissue. In this case, 4HPR curiously can produce ocular vitamin A deficiency simultaneously with symptoms of hypervitaminosis A such as skin toxicity. Besides this mechanism causing reversible night blindness and that of teratogenicity, apparently regulated by RARs, precise mechanisms of other retinoid toxicities have not been worked out.

The most troublesome toxicity is mucocutaneous toxicity, which limits long-term use for chemoprevention. It should be noted, however, that it is difficult to determine the true frequency of this effect since it is common in the general population and is reported in more than 50% of placebo recipients in retinoid trials (Table 6-8). Moderate or grade-2 skin toxicity, clearly drug related, is far less common. Toxicities are clearly dose-related. Only 14% of patients who received high dose ($\geq$ 2 mg/kg/d) 13-cRA therapy were able to complete one year without dose reduction. In contrast, 80% who received low-dose (0.5 mg/kg/d) retinoid therapy completed treatment without dose reduction.

In contrast to clinical studies using high-dose synthetic retinoids, no drug-related toxicities occurred in any natural-agent trials. The most attractive agent in this context is β-carotene, which has no side-effects except a dose-dependent yellowing of the skin.[4] The conversion of β-carotene to retinaldehyde is tightly regulated, which prevents hypervitaminosis A, even with extremely high β-carotene doses. Doses of more than 300 mg/d are known to be safe. Trial doses are empiric and range from <30 to 120 mg/d with no attempt to standardize doses by body weight or surface area calculations.

Natural vitamin A is generally well tolerated, and recent data refute early reports of great toxicity with natural vitamin A. Retinyl esters (retinyl palmitate) appear especially tolerable. Doses of 200,000 IU/week of retinol were associated with no clinical toxicities,[40] and the extremely high doses of 200,000 IU/m²/day (approximately 350–400,000 IU/day) were associated with non-specific, generally mild side-effects in only a third of the subjects.[4,10]

Although it is clear that in general retinoid toxicities are less severe than those of cytokine or cytotoxic antitumor agents, the identification of nontoxic (and effective) agents is a high priority for the chemoprevention effort. There is great interest in the retinol/β-carotene combination for long-term use. Preclinical and clinical studies have shown it to be active in oral and lung preneoplasia, and it is well tolerated. Two large trials—one in Tyler, Texas, and the other in Seattle, Washington—are studying the short- and long-term toxicities of the combination. These two long-term trials (>15,000 subjects) have thus far demonstrated that moderate doses of β-carotene and retinol substantially increase serum β-carotene and serum retinyl palmitate levels without producing significant clinical or laboratory toxicity.

Summary and Future Directions ∎

UADT carcinogenesis is a worldwide problem of great magnitude. Despite increased smoking cessation programs and advances in the primary therapies of surgery, irradiation, and chemotherapy, survival rates for patients with these tobacco-related neoplasias have improved only marginally over the past 30 years.[1] Clinicians have therefore begun to focus on chemopreventive approaches to improve the ability to control cancers of the UADT and lung.

Although many agents, including β-carotene, have demonstrated promise as chemopreventives in this region, only the retinoid 13-cRA has a record of established activity against the development of UADT neoplasia.[62,63] In trials in human oral premalignancy, or leukoplakia, 13-cRA has achieved a significant objective response rate of 67%.[52] In an adjuvant trial to prevent second primary tumors in patients initially "cured" of HNSCC, 13-cRA significantly reduced the statistically high incidence of these usually fatal second malignancies.[17]

Not only do these retinoid trials in the UADT have important implications for saving lives directly, they also may have important implications for chemoprevention of other aerodigestive tract cancers. UADT carcinogenesis is a model human system for chemoprevention study. Its tobacco-related etiology and the process of field cancerization link carcinogenesis in this region to that in other areas of the aerodigestive tract. The UADT is easily and relatively noninvasively monitored. This is especially important in chemoprevention study, which involves relatively healthy subjects for whom invasive procedures are not appropriate. Agents with clinical, histologic, and biologic activity in the oral cavity can reasonably be expected to have potential in the lung, which is difficult to monitor.

Many high-risk subjects will need long-term, perhaps even lifelong, chemoprevention therapy to prevent UADT cancers. Toxicity with established retinoid doses, although largely reversible, can be unacceptable for many subjects. Therefore, an important direction of retinoid chemoprevention study is toward establishing effective lowest doses of the agent 13-cRA for toxicity-free long-term maintenance therapy. Other promising synthetic retinoids under study include all *trans*-retinoic acid and 4HPR. Also planned are trials of toxicity mitigating agents[64] and natural-agent combinations, such as retinol plus β-carotene, for nontoxic chemoprevention. These toxicity issues do not apply to the problem of teratogenecity. The vast majority of subjects at high risk of UADT and lung neoplasia, however, are women beyond the age of child-bearing potential and men.

Recent laboratory research has identified the retinoic acid receptor family of genes, which may lead to understanding the precise mechanism of retinoid action. Investigators now are intensively attempting to establish the role of nuclear (and cytoplasmic) retinoic acid receptors in mediating retinoid effects on carcinogenesis. This work should contribute greatly to the future design of retinoid trials and to understanding the role of intermediate endpoint biomarkers in monitoring retinoid anticarcinogenic effects.

Recent retinoid chemoprevention trials in the UADT have incorporated laboratory analyses of biomarkers of intermediate endpoints of carcinogenesis. Preliminary results show many positive correlations between clinical/histologic changes and modulations of certain biomarkers of genetic damage, differentiation, and proliferation. The genomic marker micronuclei has been studied the most. Increased micronuclei frequencies have occurred in cells of nonresponding oral premalignancy subjects; decreased frequencies have occurred in cells of subjects who respond to retinoids and carotenoids.[4,38,39,54] No biomarker, however, has demonstrated a statistically significant correlation between its modulation by retinoid and a positive clinical/histologic response.[19]

The most critical long-term issue facing investigators in the very new field of intermediate endpoint biomarker research is the establishment of biomarkers, probably interrelated in panels, as valid measures of carcinogenesis and chemoprevention. The difficult issue of validation is extremely complicated. All early markers, even premalignant lesions, are variable. These lesions can progress but not result in cancer, or can regress in advance of cancer. General correlations in oral premalignancy trials between micronuclei and lesion results did not reach significance. Over time, discrepancies between micronuclei frequencies and lesion responses may disappear. We anticipate that long-term relationships between biomarkers of various stages of carcinogenesis and its modulation by agents will form the basis of valid panels of intermediate endpoint biomarkers. For example, an earlier micronuclei change may be established as having a significant correlation with a lesion response (or cancer) occurring years later.

Ideal markers will be those with early patterns of expression and modulation by chemopreventive agents that correlate directly with later stages of invasive cancer. The immediate task for cancer chemoprevention is to continue to pursue positive data from the most promising intermediate endpoint markers we now have so as to provide the best candidates for future validation studies.

The continuing resolution of the associations between molecular and cellular events and specific stages of carcinogenic transformation will play an increasingly important role in the design and evaluation of clinical chemoprevention trials. All full-scale phase III chemoprevention trials should include biomarker assessments. Although no marker has yet been validated by this new research, it is currently reasonable and feasible to design new large-scale, long-term phase III chemoprevention trials in high-risk populations based in part on supportive data from intermediate endpoint analyses of short-term trials. These short-term marker data can be extremely helpful in selecting drugs (single agents or combinations), doses, and schedules.

Validated panels of intermediate endpoint biomarkers may one day replace the endpoint of invasive cancer in phase III chemoprevention trials of retinoids and other promising agents. This would cut down enormously on the tremendous expense these trials now incur because they involve following thousands of subjects for many years.

References ∎

1. Boring CC, Squires TS, Tong T. Cancer statistics. 1991; CA 1991;41:19–36.

2. Wolf G, Lippman SM, Laramore G, Hong WK. Head and Neck Cancer. In: Holland JF, Frei E, Bast RC Jr, Kufe DW, Morton DL, Weichselbaum R eds. Cancer Medicine, 3rd edn. Philadelphia: Lea & Febiger, 1991, in press.

3. Decker J, Goldstein JC. Risk factors in head and neck cancer. N Engl J Med 1982;306:1151–1155.

4. Lippman SM, Hong WK. Differentiation therapy for head and neck cancer. In: Snow G, Clark JR, eds. Multimodality therapy for head and neck cancer. Leipzig: Verlag, in press.

5. Lippman SM, Hong WK. Second malignant tumors in head and neck squamous cell carcinoma: the overshadowing threat for patients with early-stage disease. Int J Radiat Oncol Biol Phys 1989;17:691–694.

6. Sporn M. Approaches to prevention of epithelial cancer during the preneoplastic period. Cancer Res 1976; 36:2699–2702.

7. Sporn M, Dunlop N, Newton D, Smith J. Prevention of chemical carcinogenesis by vitamin A and its synthetic analogs (retinoids). Federation Proc 1976;35:1332–1338.

8. Lotan R. Effects of vitamin A and its analogs (retinoids) on normal and neoplastic cells. Biochim Biophys Acta 1980;605:33–91.

9. Bollag W. Vitamin A and retinoids: from nutrition to pharmacotherapy in dermatology and oncology. Lancet 1983;1:860–863.

10. Lippman SM, Kessler JF, Meyskens FL Jr. Retinoids as preventive and therapeutic anticancer agents. Cancer Treat Rep 1987;71:391–405, 493–515.

11. Blomhoff R, Green MH, Berg T, Norum KR. Transport and storage of vitamin A. Science 1990;250:399–404.

12. Evans RM. The steroid and thyroid hormone receptor superfamily. Science 1988;240:889–895.

13. Krust A, Kastner P, Petkovich M, Zelent A, Chambon P. A third human retinoic acid receptor, hRAR-gama. Proc Natl Acad Sci USA 1989;886:5310–5314.

14. Mangelsdorf D, Ong E, Dyck J, Evans R. Nuclear receptor that identifies a novel retinoic acid response pathway. Nature 1990;345:224–229.

15. Warrell P, Frankel S, Miller W, Scheinberg D, et al. Differentiation therapy of acute promyelocytic leukemia with tretinoin (all-transretinoic acid). N Engl J Med 1991;324:1385–1393.

16. Kraemer KH, DiGiovanna JJ, Moshell AN, Tarone RE, Peck GL. Prevention of skin cancer in xeroderma pigmentosum with the use of oral isotretinoin. N Engl J Med 1988;318:1633–1637.

17. Hong WK, Lippman SM, Itri LM, Karp DD, Lee JS, Byers RM, Schantz SP, Kramer AM, Lotan R, Peters LJ, Dimery IW, Brown BW, Goepfert H. Prevention of second primary tumors with isotretinoin in squamous cell carcinoma of the head and neck. N Engl J Med 1990; 323:795–801.

18. Slaughter DP, Southwick HW, Smejkal W. "Field cancerization" in oral stratification squamous epithelium: Clinical implications of multicentric origin. Cancer 1953; 6:963–968.

19. Lippman SM, Lee JS, Lotan R, Hittelman W, Wargovich MJ, Hong WK. Biomarkers as intermediate endpoints in chemoprevention trials. JNCI 1990;82:555–560.

20. Wolbach SB, Howe PR. Tissue changes following deprivation of fat soluble A vitamin. J Exp Med 1925;42:753–777.

21. Tang G, Russell RM. 13-*cis*-Retinoic acid is an endogenous compound in human serum. J Lipid Res 1990;31: 175–182.

22. Crettaz M, Baron A, Siegenthaler G, Hunziker W. Ligand specifities of recombinant retinoic acid receptors RAR alpha and RAR beta. Biochem J 1990;272:391–397.

23. de The H, Lavau C, Marchio A, Chomienne C, Degos L, Dejean A. The PML-RARα fusion mRNA generated by the t(15:17) translocation in acute promyelocytic leukemia encodes a functionally altered RAR. Cell 1991; 66:675–684.

24. Lippman SM, Meyskens FL. Treatment of advanced squamous cell carcinoma of the skin with isotretinoin. Ann Intern Med 1987;107:499–501.

25. Shklar G. Oral leukoplakia. N Engl J Med 1986; 315:1544–1546.

26. Burge-Bottenbley A, Shklar G. Retardation of experimental oral cancer development by retinyl acetate. Nutr Cancer 1983;5:121–129.

27. Shklar G, Schwartz J, Grau D, Trickler D, Wallace H. Inhibition of hamster buccal pouch carcinogenesis by 13-*cis*-retinoic acid. Oral Med Oral Pathol 1980;50:45–52.

28. Goodwin WJ, Bordash GD, Huijing F, Altman N. Inhibition of hamster tongue carcinogenesis by selenium and retinoic acid. Ann Otol Rhinol Laryngol 1986;95:162–166.

29. Shklar G, Marefat P, Korhauser A, Trickler D, Wallace H. Retinoid inhibition of lingual carcinogenesis. Oral Surg Oral Med Oral Pathol 1980;49:325–332.

30. Schwartz J, Shklar G, Reid S, Trickler D. Prevention of experimental oral cancer by extracts of Spirulina-Dunaliella algae. Nutr Cancer 1988;11:127–134.

31. Trickler D, Shklar G. Prevention by vitamin E of experimental oral carcinogenesis. JNCI 1987;78:165–169.

32. Suda D, Schwartz J, Shklar G. Inhibition of experimental oral carcinogenesis by topical beta-carotene. Carcinogenesis 1986;7:711–715.

33. Silverman S, Gorsky M, Lozada F. Oral leukoplakia and malignant transformation: A follow-up study of 257 patients. Cancer 1984;53:563–568.

34. Bouquot JE, Weiland LH, Kurland LT. Leukoplakia and carcinoma *in situ* synchronously associated with invasive oral/oropharyngeal carcinoma in Rochester, Minn., 1935–1984. Oral Surg Oral Med Oral Pathol 1988;65: 199–207.

35. Wulf K. Zur vitamin A behandlung der leukoplakien. Arch Klin exp Derm 1957;206:495–498.

36. Silverman S, Renstrup G, Pindborg JJ. Studies in oral leukoplakias: III. Effects of vitamin A comparing clinical, histopathologic, cytologic and hematologic responses. Acta Odont Scandinav 1963;21:271–292.

37. Silverman S, Eisenberg E, Renstrup G. A study of the effects of high doses of vitamin A on oral leukoplakia (hyperkeratosis), including toxicity, liver function and skeletal metabolism. J Oral Therapeutics and Pharm 1965;2:9–23.

38. Stich HF, Hornby AP, Dunn BP. A pilot beta-carotene intervention trial with Inuits using smokeless tobacco. Int J Cancer 1985;36:321–327.

39. Stich HF, Rosin MP, Hornby AP, Mathew B, Sankaranarayanan R, Nair MK. Remission of oral leukoplakias and micronuclei in tobacco/betel quid chewers treated

with beta-carotene and with beta-carotene plus vitamin A. Int J Cancer 1988;42:195–199.

40. Stich HF, Hornby AP, Mathew B, Sankaranarayanan R, Nair MK. Response of oral leukoplakias to the administration of vitamin A. Cancer Lett 1988;40:93–101.

41. Toma S, Albanese E, De Lorenzi M, Nicolo G, Mangiante P, Galli A, Cancedda R. Beta-carotene in the treatment of oral leukoplakia. ASCO 1990;9:695.

42. Toma S, Coialbu T, Collecchi P, Cavallari M, Bacigalupo A, Michelotti A, Albanese E, Giacchero A, Cantoni E, Merlano M. Aspetti biologici e prospettive applicative della chemioprevenzione nel cancro delle vie aerodigestive superiori. Acta Otohinol ital 1990;10:41–54.

43. Garewal HS, Meyskens FL, Killen D, Reeves D, Kiersch TA, Elletson H, Strosberg A, King D, Steinbronn K. Response of oral leukoplakia to beta-carotene. J Clin Oncol 1990;8:1715–1720.

44. Malaker K, Anderson BJ, Beecroft WA, Hodson DI. Management of oral mucosal dysplasia with β-carotene retinoic acid: A pilot cross-over study. Cancer Detect Prev 1991;15:335–340.

45. Ryssel HJ, Brunner KW, Bollag W. Die perorale Anwendung von Vitamin-A-Saure bei Leukoplakien, Hyperkeratosen und Plattenepithelkarzinomen: Ergebnisse und Vertraglichkeit. Schweiz Med Wschr 1971;101:1027–1030.

46. Stuttgen G. Oral vitamin A acid therapy. Acta Derm Venereol Suppl 1975;74:174–179.

47. Raque CJ, Biondo RV, Keeran MG, Honeycutt WM, Jansen GT. Snuff dippers keratosis (snuff-induced leukoplakia). South Med J 1975;68:565–568.

48. Koch HF. Biochemical treatment of precancerous oral lesions: the effectiveness of various analogues of retinoic acid. J Maxillofac Surg 1978;6:59–63.

49. Koch HF. Effect of retinoids on precancerous lesions of oral mucosa. In: Orfanos CE, Braun-Falco O, Farber EM eds. Retinoids, Advances in Basic Research and Therapy. Berlin, Springer-Verlag: 1981;307–312.

50. Cordero AA, Allevato MAJ, Barclay CA, et al. Treatment of lichen planus and leukoplakia with the oral retinoid RO 10-9359. In: Orfanos CE, ed. Retinoids, Advances in Basic Research and Therapy. Berlin: Springer-Verlag, 1981;273–278.

51. Shah JP, Strong EW, DeCosse JJ, Itri L, Sellers P. Effect of retinoids on oral leukoplakia. Am J Surg 1983;146:466–470.

52. Hong WK, Endicott J, Itri LM, Doos W, Batsakis JG, Bell R, Fofonoff S, Byers R, Atkinson EN, Vaughan C. 13-*cis*-retinoic acid in the treatment of oral leukoplakia. N Engl J Med 1986;315:1501–1505.

53. Han J, Jiao L, Lu Y, et al. Evaluation of N-4-(Hydroxycarbophenyl) retinamide as a cancer prevention agent and as a cancer chemotherapeutic agent. In Vivo 1990;4:153–160.

54. Lippman SM, Toth BB, Batsakis JG, Lee JS, Weber RS, McCarthy KS, Martin JW, Hays G, Wargovich MJ, Lotan R, Hong WK. Low-dose 13-*cis*-Retinoic Acid (13cRA) maintains remission in oral premalignancy: more effective than β-carotene in randomized trial. Proc Am Soc Clin Oncol 1990;9:59.

55. Hong WK, Bromer R. Chemotherapy in head and neck cancer. Current concepts. N Engl J Med 1983;308:75–79.

56. Cooper JS, Pajak TF, Rubin P, et al. Second malignancies in patients who have head and neck cancers: Incidence, effect on survival and implications for chemoprevention based on the RTOG experience. Int J Radiat Oncol Biol Phys 1989;17:449–456.

57. Tepperman BS, Fitzpatrick PJ. Second respiratory and upper digestive tract cancers after oral cancer. Lancet 1981;2:547–549.

58. Vikram B. Changing patterns of failure in advanced head and neck cancer. Arch Otolaryngol 1984;110:564–565.

59. Lippman SM, Kessler JF, Al-Sarraf M, et al. Treatment of advanced squamous cell carcinoma of the head and neck with isotretinoin: A phase II randomized trial. Invest New Drugs 1988;6:51–56.

60. Warren S, Gates O. Multiple primary malignant tumors: A survey of the literature and statistical study. Am J Cancer 1932;51:1358–1403.

61. Modiano MR, Dalton WS, Lippman SM, et al. Ocular toxic effects of fenretinide. JNCI 1990;82:1063.

62. Meyskens FL Jr. Coming of Age—the chemoprevention of cancer. N Engl J Med 1990;323:825–827.

63. Greenberg E, Baron J, Stukel T, et al. A clinical trial of beta carotene to prevent basal-cell and squamous-cell cancers of the skin. N Engl J Med 1990;323:789–795.

64. Besa E, Abrahm J, Bartholomew M, Hyzinski M, Nowell P. Treatment with 13-cis-retinoic acid in transfusion-dependent patients with addition of alpha-tocopherol. Am J Med. 1990;89:739–747.

Michael L. Grossbard
Lee M. Nadler

Immunotoxin Therapy of Malignancy

7

Targeted Therapy: General Concepts ■

Despite recent advances in the use of high dose chemoradiotherapy in the treatment of malignancy, the majority of patients still succumb to their disease. While increased dosages of chemotherapeutic agents, combinations of drugs, or even high dose ablative regimens are frequently more effective at tumor cell cytoreduction, progressive dose escalation of these agents is ultimately limited by their nonspecific end organ toxicity. Therefore, the thrust of clinical investigation will continue to explore the role of dose intensity with the goal to enhance cytotoxicity by overcoming tumor cell resistance.

In contrast to the nonspecificity of conventional chemotherapeutic agents, antibodies and natural ligands that can specifically bind to targets on the tumor cell surface represent potential reagents to widen the therapeutic index of cancer treatment. Such serotherapy has the potential advantage of specifically killing the malignant cell. Moreover, serotherapy may circumvent conventional tumor cell resistance by killing cells by means of a different mechanism from standard chemotherapeutic agents.

Although the concept of treating tumors with antibodies and natural ligands has intrigued investigators for several decades, extensive clinical studies were impossible because of the limited supply of appropriate reagents. It is only in the past 10–15 years that monoclonal antibodies have been readily available for testing as therapeutic agents.[1] Moreover, the first reported serotherapy with a monoclonal antibody dates only to 1980.[2] Indeed, the majority of the monoclonal antibodies that have been administered thus far to patients were developed in the first half of the 1980s. During the past five years these antibodies have been conjugated to drugs, toxins, and radionuclides, and are being evaluated as delivery vehicles for these cytotoxic agents.

To bring about optimal tumor cell targeting and resultant cytotoxicity, the first major hurdle was to define the properties of cell surface molecules, (Table 1) which were identified as follows:[3]

Specificity
Heterogeneity of expression
Capacity to internalize
Capacity for shedding
Quantity (density) of target on cell surface
Affinity of ligand for receptor

The single most important characteristics to be considered are the specificity of the selected target molecule and its uniformity of expression on malignant cells. Ideally, the target should be expressed on the surface of malignant cells but not

111

on normal cells. Although few, if any, tumor-specific antigens have thus far been identified, numerous surface molecules have enhanced expression on the surface of malignant cells and therefore are potential targets. Antibodies could be directed against differentiation antigens expressed on the surface of both malignant and normal cells if these antigens were absent from the surface of stem cells that were capable of renewing the population of normal cells. Alternatively, the patient might tolerate the destruction of both normal and malignant cells if the cell death occurred in a tissue or organ that is not critical for the patient's survival. In order to be a potentially effective target, heterogeneity of expression of the surface molecule optimally should be limited. The antigen should be strongly expressed on all targeted tumor cells and weakly expressed on normal cells. Antigen negative cells should be rare. If a native ligand is directed against the malignant cell, it is essential that the cell surface receptor be expressed on all malignant cells in order to obliterate the mature population of malignant cells. Moreover, the putative clonogenic tumor cell should express the antigen. An example of this problem is seen in the case of anti-idiotype therapy (in which an antibody is directed at the variable region of immunoglobulin uniquely present on the surface of the malignant B cell), where the emergence of an idiotype negative clone can blunt the efficacy of the targeting antibody.[4,5] Likewise, the emergence of antigen negative cells due to somatic cell mutation can prove a limiting factor.

The second major consideration addresses the membrane stability of the target molecule. Depending on the type of therapy to be delivered, the ability of the target molecule to be internalized or fixed in the membrane will determine the potential therapeutic effect. For instance, if an antibody alone is used therapeutically, fixation of the target antigen may enhance antibody-mediated cytotoxicity. However, if the ligand is used to deliver a toxin or drug to the cell, the cell surface target should be capable of internalizing, since such toxins often must be delivered to the cytosol to exert their cytotoxic effect. By contrast, the receptor should have minimal capacity to be shed from the cell since an excess of circulating receptor could bind to the ligand and prevent it from reaching its target.

The quantity or density of the antigen or receptor on the cell surface can affect the efficacy of the targeting antibody or ligand. A critical number of molecules of the antibody or ligand may need to bind to the cell for it to be killed by either endogenous mechanisms or toxin delivery. Finally, the affinity of the ligand for the receptor can influence the interaction between ligand and receptor.

The ability of unconjugated monoclonal antibodies to induce cytotoxicity depends on the nature of the antibody and its capacity to mediate endogenous pathways of killing. Figure 7-1 schematically portrays several postulated cytotoxic mechanisms. Monoclonal antibodies binding to antigens on the surface of malignant cells are capable of triggering complement-mediated cytotox-

FIG. 7–1 Antibody-mediated tumor cell cytotoxicity. Antibodies binding to receptors on the cell surface of a tumor cell can trigger endogenous mechanisms of cytotoxicity. Antibody binding can trigger the complement pathway. Natural killer (NK) cells can participate in antibody-dependent cell-mediated cytotoxicity (ADCC). Macrophages (Mac) can release cytokines, including tumor necrosis factor (TNF) and interleukin-1 (IL-1), that can assist in toxicity. Antibodies can also be used to carry toxins and radioisotopes to the target tumor cell.

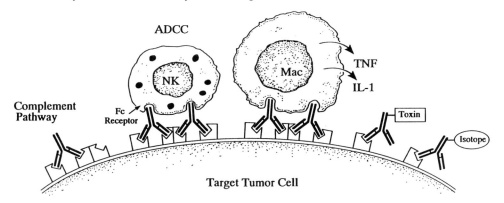

icity. Monoclonal antibodies also might serve a role in antibody-dependent cell-mediated cytotoxicity (ADCC) by Fc binding to malignant cells and promoting the cytotoxic effect of lymphocyte-activated natural killer cells, monocytes, and macrophages. The release of lymphokines such as TNF and IL-1 from activated macrophages can enhance cytotoxicity directly or through other cellular mechanisms. Binding of the ligand alone could lead to direct antiproliferative or cytotoxic effects on the malignant cells. Lastly, antibodies could be used to transport toxins and radioisotopes to the tumor cell surface. Because the preponderance of clinical trials during the past decade has employed murine monoclonal antibodies, clinical responses must be evaluated in the context of the ability of a murine antibody to activate or augment a human effector mechanism.

Numerous investigators have treated both hematologic malignancies and solid tumors with unconjugated monoclonal antibodies.[2,6–25] Tables 7-1 and 7-2 show a number of representative trials completed in a variety of disease types. In general, these trials have enrolled small numbers of patients; the overwhelming majority represent pilot studies in which a selected dose of antibody was administered in a Phase I trial without attempting to determine the maximal tolerated dose. These trials were largely undertaken to determine the safety of administration of monoclonal antibodies, to identify whether the antibody could reach the target cell, and to assess response. Approximately half of the patients treated with unconjugated monoclonal antibodies had solid tumors, whereas the remainder had either a leukemia or a lymphoma. The trials uniformly demonstrated that murine monoclonal antibodies could be safely administered to patients. Just 10–15% of patients demonstrated evidence of allergic reaction to the murine proteins as characterized by rashes, pruritus, dyspnea, and fever. Systemic reversible toxicities including fever, elevation of hepatic transaminases, rigors, diaphoresis, and nausea were observed.[26] Severe organ-specific toxicities, however, have been extremely rare. Despite the fact that many of the monoclonal antibodies tested possess significant cross-reactivity with normal tissues, the low cytotoxicity of these agents has yielded limited nonspecific toxicity.

Although clinical responses occasionally have been seen, responses often occurred only when large quantities (500 mg to more than 1 gram) of antibody were administered,[5,19] and responses were nearly always transient. In the case of leukemias, the observed reductions in malignant cells often lasted merely hours and were attributable to sequestration of antibody-coated malignant cells.[9,27] Occasional long-term responses have been seen in lymphomas, including one complete response lasting six years with anti-idiotype therapy of B-cell non-Hodgkin's lymphoma.[5] In solid tumors, the frequency of reported responses has also been low and durations have been brief.

Nevertheless, these preliminary studies did affirm the safety of murine monoclonal antibody administration. Biopsies of tumor sites after treatment also have frequently demonstrated binding of the antibody to malignant cells.[19,21,25] Moreover, post-therapy biopsies have demonstrated complement deposition, infiltration of T lymphocytes, and increased numbers of mast cells within the tumor, indicating several potential endogenous mechanisms by which malignant cells might be killed.[25]

With over 200 patients treated with unconjugated monoclonal antibodies, the lack of sustained responses has been disappointing; it appears that the majority of these antibodies fail to activate sufficient endogenous cytotoxicity. The encouraging preliminary results with several of these targeted therapies, such as R24 monoclonal antibody therapy of malignant melanoma and CAMPATH-1 and anti-idiotype antibody therapy of lymphoid malignancies, have led to larger on-going trials with

Table 7–1
Clinical Studies with Unconjugated Monoclonal Antibodies in Hematologic Malignancies

Disease	Monoclonal AB	# Pts	Reference
AML	PMN 6, PMN 29, PM-81, AML-2-23	4	6
	M195 (CD33)	10	7
ALL	J5 (CD10)	4	8
	CAMPATH-1G	5	9
CLL	T101 (CD5)	4	10
	T101 (CD5)	13	11
	CAMPATH-1M	1	9
B-NHL	AB89	1	2
	Anti-idiotypic	14	12
	CAMPATH-1H	2	13
	CAMPATH-1M	1	9
	CAMPATH-1G	9	9
	OKB7	18	14
T-NHL	Anti-Leu-1	1	15
CTCL	Anti-Leu-1	6	15
	T101 (CD5)	4	10
ATL	Anti-Tac	9	16

Table 7–2
Clinical Studies with Unconjugated Monoclonal Antibodies in Solid Tumors

Disease	Monoclonal AB	# Pts	Reference
Colorectal	1083-17-1A	20	17
	16.88, 28A32	28	18
	L6	2	19
GI Adenoca	CO17-1A	25	21
Lung Ca	KS1/4	6	20
	L6	3	19
	MoAB 225 (Anti-EGF)	19	22
Melanoma	MAb 96.5, 48.7	5	23
	3F8 (Anti-ganglioside GD2)	9	24
	R24 (Anti-GD3 ganglioside)	24	25
Neuroblastoma	3F8	8	24
Breast Ca	L6	5	19
Ovarian Ca	L6	9	19

these specific antibodies, which may provide answers regarding their utility.[5,9,25]

Through these preliminary investigations, several limitations to the serotherapy of malignancies became apparent. These obstacles to serotherapy are outlined below.

Delivery of carrier to target cells
Presence of free circulating target
Nonspecific binding of carrier
Receptor negative tumor cells
Development of resistance
Development of immune response to carrier

Delivery of the antibody or ligand to tumor cells in bulky, fibrotic tumor masses is frequently difficult if not impossible. The presence of free circulating antigen that is either shed from or secreted by malignant cells may bind to the antibody and prevent it from reaching the tumor. Receptor negative tumor cells, derived from somatic mutations or secondary to antigen heterogeneity, may permit a clone of the malignant cells to escape the effects of the delivered antibody. In the case of anti-idiotype therapy, idiotype negative cells would have the same advantage.[5] Antigenic modulation, by which the antigen disappears from the targeted cell, has been observed clinically[11] and can result in a decrease of the antigen density on the cell surface to a level below which sufficient molecules of the antibody are deposited to exert their cytotoxic effects. As is observed with standard chemotherapy, the malignant cells could develop resistance to one or more of the potential cytotoxic mechanisms. Finally, since the majority of monoclonal antibodies are of murine derivation, the patient's immune system recognizes them as foreign. The production of anti-mouse antibodies can neutralize the delivered antibody or potentially lead to serum sickness.

Immunotoxins: Concepts of Immunotoxin Development ■

The above studies with unconjugated monoclonal antibodies demonstrate that targeted therapy can be delivered safely to the patient and to the malignant cell. Unfortunately, these monoclonal antibodies rely on endogenous mechanisms to mediate cytotoxicity and therefore, in most instances, display relatively low potency. In an effort to enhance cytotoxicity beyond that which could be achieved with unconjugated ligands, monoclonal antibodies and other ligands were evaluated as potential delivery vehicles for cytotoxic agents. These highly cytotoxic antibody-toxin or ligand-toxin conjugates are known as immunotoxins.[28,29] Their cytotoxicity does not rely exclusively on the activation of the host effector system, but rather depends on their ability to deliver a toxin to the malignant cell.[30] This chapter focuses on the concepts of immunotoxin development including preclinical studies, toxicity, potential obstacles to the therapy, clinical trials to date, and future directions in immunotoxin therapy.

Although the concept underlying immunotoxin development is relatively simple, the development of highly cytotoxic and specific immunotoxins has been more difficult. The following three major components are essential for a successful immunotoxin:

I. Ligand with restricted specificity
   a. Monoclonal antibodies
   b. Growth factors
   c. Natural ligands
II. Potent toxin with limited nonspecificity
III. Conjugation procedure with stable linkage which conserves antibody binding and toxin potency

As this summary indicates, the carrying ligand should first have restricted specificity with minimal or no cross-reactivity with normal tissues. This condition can be met by monoclonal antibodies, growth factors, or other natural ligands such as adhesion molecules. Second, the toxin must be potent and should not react with tissues unless bound to the ligand. Third, between the antibody or ligand and the toxin a stable linkage must exist which prevents release of the toxin into the circulation but facilitates efficient release of the toxin at the targeted site. In this review, we will focus on the first two components of an immunotoxin since the issue of linkers has been extensively reviewed elsewhere.[31,32]

Of critical importance in the development of an immunotoxin is the nature of the selected carrier molecule and its receptor. Similar to the issues previously addressed for unconjugated monoclonal antibodies, the targeted antigen must be expressed in a sufficiently high density so that an adequate number of molecules of immunotoxin can be delivered to the cell surface. Moreover, the targeted epitope expressed on the cell surface antigen should be sufficiently close to the cell membrane to permit the toxin to penetrate the membrane.[33] Antibodies that have a more rapid internalization rate have greater cytotoxicity.[34] The routing of the antigen and toxin after internalization is also important. For instance, conjugates that are directed to lysosomes after internalization are often ineffective because the toxic moiety may be rapidly degraded. Hence, immunotoxins that traffic through the Golgi may be more potent.[33]

An intact immunoglobulin molecule is not required to carry the toxin. Figure 7-2 schematically represents an immunoglobulin molecule and its functional domains. The Fab (one arm of the bifunctional antibody) or the F(ab')₂ fragment (both arms of the antibody) alone can confer the specificity of the entire antibody and may be conjugated to a toxin.[35,36] Even more specific is the use of an Fv fragment, which consists of a light and heavy chain variable domain.[37] These smaller molecules may be more effective in penetrating to the periph-

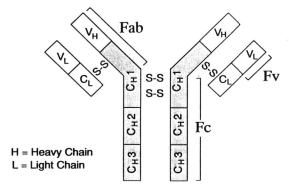

FIG. 7–2 Schematic structure of a murine immunoglobulin molecule. The constant (C) and variable (V) domains of the light chain (L) and the heavy chain (H) can be chemically cleaved to provide suitable domains (Fv and Fab) for binding to toxins and isotopes.

ery of the targeted tumor both because of their reduced size and because their lower avidity for the targeted antigen may make them less likely to be irreversibly bound by the first antigen they contact. Moreover, the fragments may prove less immunogenic than the intact immunoglobulin.

A recently developed alternative is the use of chimeric antibodies consisting of murine variable regions and constant regions. The variable region of the mouse immunoglobulin is retained, preserving the specificity of the antibody. By using the Fc portion of the human immunoglobulin, its interaction with the human effector system may be enhanced in comparison with that of the murine Fc. Again, chimeric antibodies are likely to be less immunogenic than whole murine antibodies.[38,39]

In addition to monoclonal antibodies, other molecules have receptors in the cell membrane and therefore are candidates for immunotoxin therapy. These natural ligands bind to the cell surface and undergo receptor-mediated endocytosis. For example, alpha-melanocyte stimulating hormone, epidermal growth factor, and interleukin-2 have been used as carriers.[40–42] Because circulating levels of these ligands can be elevated in the malignant state, binding of the ligand-toxin complex may be reduced due to competition from unconjugated ligand.

Originally, investigators considered conjugating standard chemotherapeutic agents to the antibodies in the hope that a greater concentration of the chemotherapeutic agent could be delivered to the tumor site with reduced systemic toxicity of the agent. In fact, this enhanced cytotoxicity did not manifest itself and the use of standard chemotherapeutic agents did not circumvent the difficulty of tumor cell resistance. Several candidate toxins with exquisite potency have long been available which are five to seven logs more toxic to cells than are conventional chemotherapeutic agents. If administered directly to patients, however, these compounds are lethal at nanomolar concentrations because of their cytotoxic effects on both normal and malignant cells. These single and multichain plant and bacterial protein toxins operate by inhibiting protein synthesis within the cell. Their extreme potency requires only a few molecules to enter the cytoplasm to be lethal. In fact, fewer than ten molecules of the plant toxin ricin inside a cell are lethal. Furthermore, because these candidate toxins possess a different mechanism of cytotoxicity from that of conventional chemotherapeutic agents such as Cyclophosphamide and Doxorubicin, they have the potential to kill cells that are resistant to chemotherapy.[43] Extensive laboratory studies have been conducted to examine the cytotoxicity of these toxins on a variety of tumor cell lines, both in a native state and when they are conjugated to monoclonal antibodies and other carrying ligands.

Following is a partial list of the candidate toxins that have undergone preclinical and clinical testing when conjugated to carrying ligands.

Single-chain Toxins
  Gelonin
  Pokeweed antiviral protein (PAP)
  Saporin

Two-chain Plant Toxins
  Ricin
  Abrin

Two-chain Bacterial Toxins
  Diphtheria toxin
  Pseudomonas exotoxin A

Fungal Toxin
  α-sarcin

Drugs
  Methotrexate
  Melphalan
  Doxorubicin

The single-chain toxins are ribosomal inactivating proteins (RIP) that consist of single polypeptide chains. Although they are extremely effective at inactivating ribosomes in cell-free systems (50% inhibition of protein synthesis at concentrations ranging from 0.002nM to 0.6nM), they are relatively nontoxic to intact cells because they lack a binding chain.[44] Since they fail to bind to the cell surface, these toxins rely on pinocytosis for internalization.[45] Thus, when combined with antibodies to make immunotoxins, the specificity that they possess is conferred by the specificity of the antibody to which they are bound. Gelonin, a representative RIP whose structure–function relationship is depicted in Figure 7-3, functions by enzymatically attacking the 60S ribosomal subunit.

The other major class of toxins includes plant and bacterial toxins which possess not only an enzymatically active subunit, but also a subunit that binds to targeted cells and aids the toxin in entering the cell. Figure 7-3 demonstrates the functional domains of three representative toxins that have been used most frequently—ricin, diphtheria toxin (DT), and Pseudomonas exotoxin (PE). Ricin is a heterodimer, composed of an A chain (toxic moiety) and a B chain (binding and translocation). The A chain has N-glycosidase activity and inactivates the 60S subunit of the ribosome, disrupting protein synthesis.[46] The B chain binds via two high affinity galactose binding sites to galactose residues present on cell-surface glycoproteins and glycolipids.[47] The B chain also serves a role in transporting the A chain across the cell membrane.[48] The structure of DT is conceptually similar to that of ricin. The A chain (toxic moiety) has adenosine

FIG. 7–3   Natural toxins and their functional domains. The functional toxin domains participate in binding to target cells, translocating the toxin through a membrane, and lead to cytotoxicity via the toxic moiety. RIP indicates ribosomal inactivating protein. Ricin and diphtheria toxin have two chains. Each has a unique A chain and a unique B chain. In contrast, Pseudomonas exotoxin has three domains termed I, II, and III. In this figure, shading has been used to indicate the various functional regions. ▨ indicates the binding region, ||| indicates the translocation region, and ▨ indicates the toxic moiety.

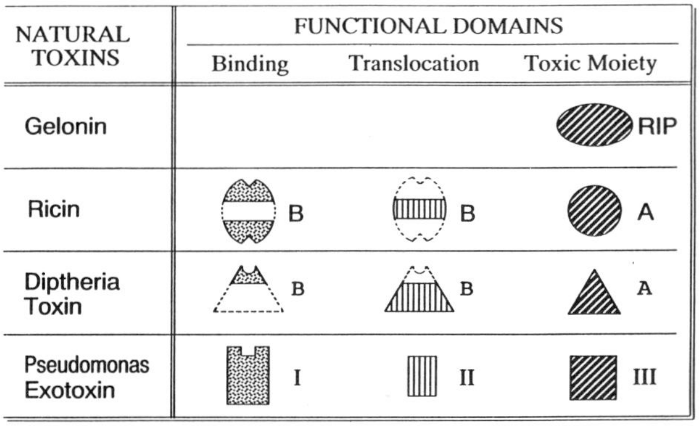

NATURAL TOXINS	FUNCTIONAL DOMAINS		
	Binding	Translocation	Toxic Moiety
Gelonin			⬭ RIP
Ricin	⬭ B	⬭ B	● A
Diptheria Toxin	▲ B	▲ B	▲ A
Pseudomonas Exotoxin	▮ I	▮ II	▮ III

diphosphate ribosylation activity which inhibits protein synthesis by inactivating elongation factor 2 (EF-2), a protein required for the translocation reaction in polypeptide chain elongation on ribosomes.[49] As in the case of ricin, the B chain of DT mediates nonspecific binding to cells and translocation. By contrast, PE is structurally dissimilar to ricin and DT. PE contains three structural domains. Domain 1 of PE mediates binding, domain 2 mediates translocation of the toxin into the cell, and domain 3 (toxic moiety) possesses adenosine diphosphate ribosylation activity that inactivates elongation factor 2.[30,50]

Figure 7-4 depicts the binding, internalization, and cytotoxic mechanism of native ricin. The receptors for ricin binding are galactose residues, which are present on glycolipids and glycoproteins, which are ubiquitous on eucaryotic cell surfaces. The receptors for DT and PE are unknown.

FIG. 7–4 Cytotoxicity of the native toxins—(DT) diphtheria toxin, (PE) Pseudomonas exotoxin, (R) receptor. Ricin is presented as a representative toxin. The binding, internalization, translocation, and toxic steps are described in detail in the text.

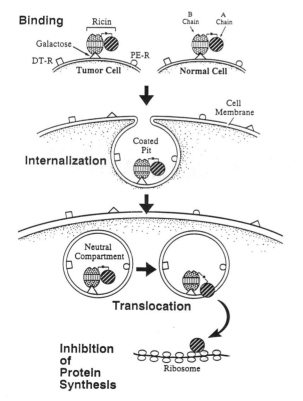

As shown, binding receptors are present on both tumor cells and normal cells, so the binding of the native toxin is not specific for normal cells. After binding, the toxins must be internalized, and it appears that endocytosis is necessary for this transport.[47] Ricin enters cells by both coated vesicles and an alternative pathway, perhaps via the trans-Golgi reticulum.[51] DT and PE enter the cell via coated vesicles. Once inside the cell, the active toxin fragment needs to enter the cytosol. For ricin, the toxin is translocated from the internalized vesicle to the cytosol via a neutral pH dependent process, but the precise mechanism of translocation is poorly understood.[52] For DT, a conformational change is induced by low pH in the endosomes, which results in insertion of the hydrophobic domains into the endosome membrane and subsequent translocation of the active fragment to the cytosol.[53] PE also moves into the cytoplasm in a low pH dependent process, but again the mechanism is less well understood. After the toxic moiety is liberated, the A chain of ricin travels to the ribosome, where it disrupts protein synthesis. Similarly, the toxic moieties of DT and PE are now free to inactivate EF-2.

Obviously, if the native two-chain toxins are conjugated to monoclonal antibodies, the resultant immunotoxins would have significant nonspecific activity via the nonspecific binding of the holotoxin through the B chain in the case of ricin and DT, and through domain 1 in the case of PE. Such whole ricin immunotoxins would only exhibit specificity in the presence of high concentrations of lactose, which can compete with cell surface carbohydrates for nonspecific binding of the B chain. This may be practical *in vitro* where high concentrations of lactose can be achieved, but is not feasible *in vivo*. Thus the native toxins must undergo modification to delete the cell-binding function. Figure 7-5 portrays some of the potential modifications that will be described in following paragraphs. As shown, optimal modifications require the deletion of the binding moiety, but preservation of the translocation and toxin domains.

The simplest solution to this dilemma would be to use the single-chain RIPs and conjugate them to the chosen antibodies. Extensive studies have characterized the cytotoxicity of immunotoxins containing gelonin, PAP, and saporin on a variety of cell lines.[54] The cytotoxicity of these conjugates depends on conjugate binding to the target cell surface, the internalization of the immunotoxin, and the nature of the linkage between the toxin and the antibody. Many of the immunotoxins de-

NATIVE AND ALTERED TOXINS

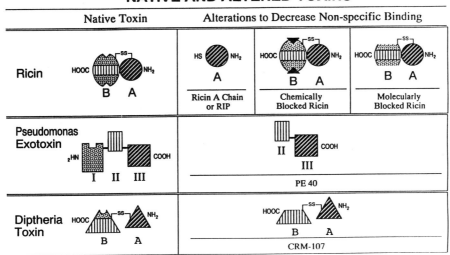

FIG. 7–5 Native and altered toxins. Alterations or deletion in the binding region of ricin, Pseudomonas exotoxin, and diphtheria toxin can decrease or eliminate nonspecific binding to cells. Several altered toxins are depicted as examples.

veloped using RIPs are 1000 times as potent as the single chains themselves. Unfortunately, some of the immunotoxins prepared using the single-chain RIPs possess little more toxicity than the native single chain. For example, when gelonin is conjugated to antibodies that are poorly internalized, the compounds have low cytotoxicity. While RIPs may occasionally be useful in toxin development, they may only be appropriate for conjugation to a limited spectrum of antibodies and ligands. Yet the use of RIPs would seem to have several advantages over the use of the two-chain toxins. Because the RIPs lack a binding chain, they are extremely safe to work with in the laboratory. Also, several immunologically distinct toxins have been characterized, which might permit multiple toxins to be conjugated to the same antibody in an effort to enhance the likelihood of retreatment.

An understanding of the structure–function relationship of toxins permits the development of novel immunotoxins which are selectively toxic for cells with a particular target on their surface. Hence, another possible modification of the toxin would be to remove its binding chain and link the toxic moiety to the appropriate monoclonal antibody. For example, immunotoxins can be constructed using the ricin A chain alone. Vitetta has defined these as "first generation immunotoxin-As."[33] A chains can be made available by chemical separation of the A and B chains or by recombinant DNA technology. Both types of ricin A chain immunotoxins have been developed and are undergoing clinical testing.[55,56] Unfortunately, ri-

cin A chains may suffer from a similar drawback to the RIPs in that they only are potent cytotoxic agents when conjugated to a limited spectrum of antibodies. Indeed, conjugates made with ricin A chain alone lack the domain of the toxin that is instrumental in translocation of the toxin to the cytosol. An alternative possibility is therefore to construct toxins in which both the A and B chains are used but in which nonspecific binding is blocked either by attaching ligands to the galactose binding sites or by molecular reconstruction of the B chain. Such blocked ricin conjugates have been developed and appear to have enhanced cytotoxicity when compared with toxins composed of ricin A chain alone.

Other approaches involve manipulation of the toxin to alter nonspecific binding (Fig. 7-5). An amino acid located near the C-terminus of DT mediates this binding; if that amino acid is changed from serine to phenylalanine, a DT mutant (CRM107) is produced which has little nonspecific binding.[57] Similarly, chemical modification of key amino acids in the binding domain of PE results in a toxin with altered nonspecific binding.[58] A more elegant approach involves the development of a recombinant form of PE, known as PE40, in which the DNA that codes for the binding domain is deleted. PE40 contains domains II and III of PE, but not domain I. When conjugated to a carrying ligand, as has been accomplished in the case of the anti-Tac antibody, the toxin can kill specifically.[59,60]

The selection of the ligand and toxin can be influenced by the availability of a suitable linker. The optimal linker should be one which is poorly cleaved in the blood, but readily cleaved in the target tissue.[31] If the linkage is broken prior to the IT reaching the target cell, not only would the amount of IT reaching the target cell be diminished, but free antibody would also compete with the IT for binding to the target. The production of antibody-toxin conjugates has usually involved the placement of a reducible disulfide bond between the antibody and the enzymatic portion of the toxin. Within the target cell, reduction of the disulfide bond by thiol-containing compounds such as glutathione liberates the toxic chain. In contrast to chemical linkers, recombinant DNA technology can be used to construct fusion genes in which the portion of the toxin gene that encodes the binding domain is replaced with the DNA encoding the ligand of choice. Fusion toxins have been developed between IL-2 and DT (Fig. 7-6).[42]

Ultimately, it should be possible to construct immunotoxins entirely through recombinant DNA technology. The A and B chains of ricin toxin have been cloned, and both recombinant chains have been expressed.[33] Likewise, it is possible to clone the various targeting antibodies. Such "designer immunotoxins" could circumvent many of the difficulties inherent in immunotoxin therapy by providing a human antibody, a selective toxin and a molecular linkage.

By applying the previously discussed features of toxin development, numerous groups have constructed immunotoxins that have undergone clinical testing (see Fig. 7-6 for examples). In these immunotoxins the various functional domains mediating binding, translocation, and cytotoxicity have been deleted, modified, or replaced. Thus, in anti-T101-RTA, the binding domain is replaced with the T101 antibody, the translocation domain is deleted, and the toxic domain is conserved in ricin A chain.[61] In anti-B4 (CD19)-blocked ricin (anti-B4-bR), the anti-B4 (CD19) antibody serves the binding role, the blocked B chain no longer participates in binding but still contributes its translocation function, and the ricin A chain constitutes the toxic moiety. In transforming growth factor alpha (TGFα)-PE40, TGFα replaces domain I of PE and provides the binding function to cells bearing the receptor for epidermal growth factor. The translocation and toxin functions are contributed by domains II and III of PE40.[62] Finally, DAB486IL-2 is a recombinant fusion protein that combines the toxin and translocation functions of DT with the binding function of IL-2.[63]

Figure 7-7 displays the mechanism of action of anti-B4-blocked ricin, a representative immunotoxin. With CD19(B4) providing the binding function, and with the natural binding sites of the B chain blocked, this molecule binds to cell surfaces through antibody binding to the CD19 antigen. As noted, CD19 is present on both normal and malignant B lymphocytes, so the immunotoxin will bind to both types of cells. However, all other normal cells lack the CD19 antigen and will not bind the immunotoxin. After binding, anti-B4-blocked ricin is internalized via a coated pit. The blocked B chain still functions in translocation, assisting the A chain in crossing the cell membrane to the cytosol. After reaching the cytosol, the A chain travels to the ribosome and inhibits protein synthesis.

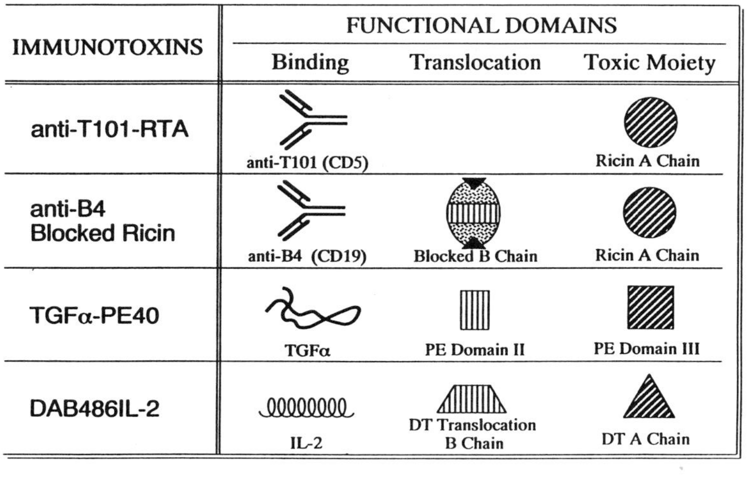

FIG. 7–6 Representative immunotoxins. Altered toxins can be conjugated to either antibodies or ligands. This provides a binding domain for the altered toxins and permits them to bind specifically to targeted cells. (PE = Pseudomonas exotoxin, DT = diphtheria toxin, IL-2 = Interleukin 2.)

IMMUNOTOXINS	FUNCTIONAL DOMAINS		
	Binding	Translocation	Toxic Moiety
anti-T101-RTA	anti-T101 (CD5)		Ricin A Chain
anti-B4 Blocked Ricin	anti-B4 (CD19)	Blocked B Chain	Ricin A Chain
TGFα-PE40	TGFα	PE Domain II	PE Domain III
DAB486IL-2	IL-2	DT Translocation B Chain	DT A Chain

IMMUNOTOXINS: CYTOTOXICITY

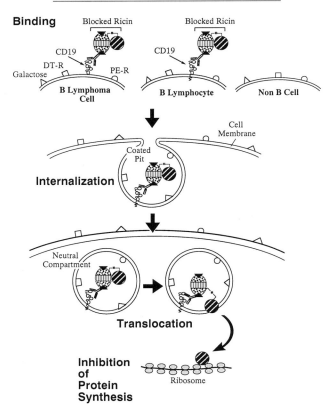

FIG. 7–7 The mechanism of action of anti-CD19-blocked ricin is depicted. In contrast to native ricin, the binding regions of the B chain are chemically blocked. The immunotoxin can only bind to B-lymphoma cells and normal B cells that bear the CD19 antigen. Immunotoxin binding, internalization, translocation, and inhibition of protein synthesis are described in the text.

Clinical Trials ■

In Vitro and Preclinical Evaluation of Immunotoxins ■

Many investigators have developed immunotoxins using both single-chain and multiple-chain toxin molecules. *In vitro* and *in vivo* preclinical studies performed with these agents have demonstrated the three essential functional properties of immunotoxins—specificity for the targeted surface molecule, selectivity for a specific population of cells, and exceptional potency of killing.

In vitro studies with immunotoxins have been undertaken to determine the specific and nonspecific cytotoxicity of the agents. To determine the cytotoxicity of the conjugate, the fraction of targeted cells that survive after exposure to the immunotoxin can be measured. Alternatively, the reduction in protein synthesis after cells are exposed to immunotoxin may be ascertained. By testing the immunotoxin against cell lines that contain or

lack the targeted antigen, its specificity can be defined.

Extensive *in vitro* studies using the immunotoxin anti-B4-bR are presented in Figure 7-8 to illustrate the principals of cytotoxicity, antigen specificity, and immunotoxin selectivity. Figure 7-8 (upper left) demonstrates the cytotoxicity of anti-B4-bR on Namalwa B cells, a B4 positive lymphoma cell line. At concentrations of anti-B4-bR less than 10^{-11}M, more than three logs of cells can be killed. When Namalwa cells are treated with blocked ricin alone, however, less than one log of cells is killed at concentrations of anti-B4-bR 1000 times higher. This emphasizes the importance of antibody-mediated binding and translocation of the toxin moiety. Without the presence of the B4 antigen, the toxin only enters the cell slowly, likely via pinocytosis, and the efficiency of killing is markedly reduced.

Figure 7-8 (lower left) also depicts the selectivity of anti-B4-bR for B4 antigen negative cell lines. The two curves represent the cytotoxicity of anti-B4-bR and native ricin for MOLT-4, a

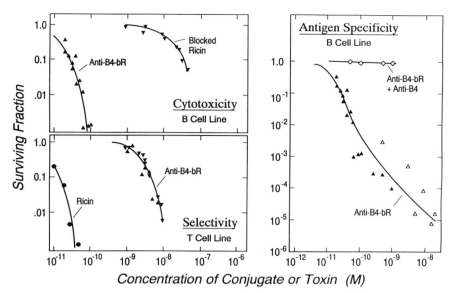

FIG. 7–8 *In Vitro* Immunotoxin Cytotoxicity. The cytotoxicity (upper left), selectivity (lower left), and antigen specificity (right) of anti-B4-bR is depicted. Cell killing was assessed by determining the fraction of cells surviving after a 24-hour incubation with the immunotoxin.

T-cell leukemia cell line that does not bear the target antigen. Less than one log of cells is killed at 10^{-9}M concentrations of the immunotoxin. Such concentrations have been achieved *in vivo* in patients with B-cell leukemias and lymphomas during treatment with anti-B4-bR. Because MOLT-4 cells lack the B4 antigen, the limited toxicity secondary to immunotoxin treatment must be secondary to nonspecific uptake of the immunotoxin. When whole ricin is used to treat MOLT-4 cells, the B chain binds through cell membrane galactose residues and ricin proves a potent toxin.

Lastly, Figure 7-8 (right) shows the specificity with which anti-B4-bR binds to Namalwa B cells via the B4 antigen. As previously seen, the curve for treatment with anti-B4-bR alone demonstrates potent cytotoxicity. When unconjugated Anti-B4 is added to the incubation mixture, however, it competes with the immunotoxin for binding to the surface receptor and the cytotoxicity of the immunotoxin is markedly reduced. If the binding of anti-B4-bR were through galactose residues, then unconjugated B4 antigen would not compete and reduce cytotoxicity.

Similar *in vitro* cytotoxicity studies have demonstrated that the time the malignant cells are exposed to the immunotoxin appears to be critical in determining cytotoxicity. For any given concentration of immunotoxin, increased time of incubation with the target cells will lead to enhanced cytotoxicity. This time dependence may reflect the time required for the ligand-receptor interaction to occur and for toxin internalization.

Comparable evidence of cytotoxicity and antigen specificity has been accumulated for many immunotoxins. With a particular target cell selected and minimal nonspecific toxicity, the immunotoxins can be moved to preclinical animal toxicity trials and then to the clinic for potential clinical trials.

Clinical Studies with Immunotoxins ■

A number of clinical trials have been undertaken using immunotoxins. These studies can be grouped into two major categories. The first group employs immunotoxins to kill malignant cells *in vitro*, in a direct application of the preclinical studies. When the immunotoxins are not administered directly to the patient, concerns regarding nonspecific toxicity may be reduced. Such studies permit a determination of the selectivity and specificity of immunotoxins without concern for systemic toxicity for the patient. The second large group of trials involves administration of the immunotoxin directly to the patient in an effort to determine specific and nonspecific toxicities, the maximal tolerated dose that can be delivered, and efficacy.

In Vitro Purging ■

Immunotoxins may have a role in the *in vitro* manipulation of marrow cells used for reinfusion in both autologous and allogeneic bone marrow transplantation (BMT). A major concern in autologous BMT is the potential for reinfusion of malignant cells that may be harbored within the patient's marrow. In allogeneic BMT, a significant factor leading to morbidity and mortality is graft versus host disease (GVHD), which is mediated by donor T cells. Immunotoxins have also been used *in vitro* to deplete malignant cells and T cells from harvested bone marrow prior to its reinfusion. In autologous BMT, immunotoxins can be used to purge malignant cells from the marrow. In the case of allogeneic BMT, immunotoxins directed against T cells may eliminate these cells and ameliorate graft versus host disease in the marrow recipient. Previous studies have reported the effective use of monoclonal antibodies and complement for the depletion of malignant cells and T cells, but this procedure is technically difficult and can be dependent on the activity of the lot of complement.[64–66]

Several clinical trials have been conducted that use immunotoxins for purging (Table 7-3). Preijers and associates purged autologous bone marrow obtained from 13 patients with T-cell acute lymphoblastic leukemia or T-cell lymphoblastic lymphoma with an anti-CD7-ricin A chain immunotoxin.[67] CD7 is a T-cell antigen expressed on most T-cell malignancies. *In vitro* studies showed that concentrations of immunotoxin ranging from 7×10^{-12} to 1×10^{-9} mol/liter could inhibit protein synthesis 50% in the malignant cells obtained from patients. Moreover, the anti-CD7-ricin A chain could induce more than six logs cell kill on a malignant T-cell line.[68] Nonspecific killing of hematopoietic progenitor cells was relatively insignificant since neutrophil engraftment was not delayed, occurring at a median of 17 days. However, in three patients, platelet engraftment was delayed. Studies of immunologic reconstitution after reinfusion indicated that normal numbers of T cells were achieved within one month. Seven patients remained in complete remission from 6 to 44 months after BMT. Four patients relapsed within six months of BMT and two of the four had the lowest expression of CD7 on their tumor cells. Thus, the immunotoxin was cytotoxic and selective for T-lineage cells.

Uckun and colleagues have reported their results on the use of a cocktail of two immunotoxins directed against the T-lineage differentiation antigens CD5 and CD7 in combination with 4-hydroperoxycyclophosphamide to purge marrow obtained from patients with T-cell ALL undergoing autologous BMT.[69,70] The immunotoxins were conjugates of CD5 and CD7 with whole ricin. The immunotoxins were incubated with malignant cells in the presence of lactose to avoid nonspecific binding via the B chain. In this instance, the binding function of the B chain was conserved, but its po-

Table 7–3
Immunotoxins in Bone Marrow Purging

Immunotoxin	Marrow Source	Disease	# Patients	Purging Outcome *in vitro*
Anti-CD7-RTA	AUTOLOGOUS	T-Leukemia	7	Not Available
		T-Lymphoma	6	
Cocktail of: Anti-CD5-ricin + Anti-CD7-ricin + 4-HC	AUTOLOGOUS	T-ALL	14	0.8 to 3.4 log kill
T101Fab-RTA	ALLOGENEIC	CML	19	2 to 3 log kill
		AML	9	
		ALL	6	
		NHL	2	
		MDS	2	
Anti-CD3-RTA	ALLOGENEIC	CML	5	2.9 to 3.3 log kill
		ALL	2	
		NHL	2	
Cocktail of: Anti-CD3-ricin + Anti-CD5-ricin + Anti-TA-1-ricin	ALLOGENEIC	CML	5	1 to 2 log kill
		ALL	5	
		AML	7	

tential to bind to galactose residues was overwhelmed by the addition of lactose to the incubation mixture. Fourteen patients were treated and 13 engrafted at a median of 23 days post-BMT. Residual leukemic cells were effectively depleted in the marrow with 0.8 to > 3.4 logs killed in 10 of 11 evaluable patients. In assessing log depletion of residual leukemic cells, it is important to recognize that all patients were in complete morphologic remission at the time of purging and the accuracy of the log depletion calculation is hampered by the sensitivity of the assay. Despite this effective purging, 9 of the 14 patients relapsed at a median of 2.2 months post-BMT. Relapse may have been due to an ineffective conditioning regimen or inadequate purging of leukemic progenitor cells.

Immunotoxins have also been used to deplete T cells from allogeneic marrow. Previously, numerous groups have used anti-T-cell monoclonal antibodies together with complement or magnetic beads to deplete T cells from bone marrow prior to reinfusion and decrease the incidence and severity of GVHD. There is less experience with the use of immunotoxins in T-cell depletion. Laurent and associates used a T101 Fab fragment-ricin A chain immunotoxin to deplete T cells from the marrows of 38 histocompatible donors prior to reinfusion.[71] A previous study by this group had attempted to use a whole immunoglobulin ricin A chain immunotoxin for T-cell depletion, but found poor T-cell cytoreduction and a high incidence of acute and chronic GVHD.[36] This condition was partly attributable to a critical dependence on the *pH* of the medium. Despite the lower affinity of the Fab fragment immunotoxin, there was improved cytoreduction with a lesser dependence on *pH*. A median cytoreduction of 99.5% of T101 positive cells was achieved and in 32 of the cases T-cell depletion was greater than 99%. Thirty-seven of the patients engrafted, but six patients demonstrated marrow rejection. Only three patients developed grade II acute GVHD, and no patients developed chronic GVHD with a median follow-up of 300 days. However, the magnitude of the effect of T-cell depletion remains undetermined since all patients received post-transplant immunosuppression with methotrexate, cyclosporin A, or both. Only one patient failed to engraft, but, of greater concern, six patients developed a documented bone marrow rejection after initial engraftment.

Martin and associates used an anti-CD3-ricin A chain immunotoxin for purging of HLA identical marrow prior to reinfusion in allogeneic BMT patients.[72] Marrows from eight donors were treated, and 2.9 to 3.3 log depletion of T cells was achieved. Seven of the 8 patients engrafted promptly with a median of 22 days to the achievement of 1000 granulocytes. Two patients had graft failure, one after having had evidence of initial engraftment. Two patients developed Grade II GVHD and one developed Grade I GVHD. Notably, only one patient received prophylactic post-transplant immunosuppression. The clinical outcome of three relapses in this patient population was similar to that seen in a comparable group of patients previously transplanted by the Seattle group.

Another trial used a combination of three T-cell targeting immunotoxins to deplete T lymphocytes from the marrow of HLA identical donors prior to reinfusion.[73] Three antibodies, anti-CD3, anti-CD5, and anti-TA-1 were conjugated to whole ricin and the marrows from 17 donors were treated. Again, to avoid nonspecific binding of the immunotoxin through the ricin B chain, bone marrow cells were incubated in the presence of high concentrations of lactose. No routine post-transplant GVHD prophylaxis was given, and 5 patients developed skin GVHD without evidence of liver or gastrointestinal involvement. Unfortunately, as was observed in the Laurent trial, episodes of early rejection were observed in four patients. Eight of 13 evaluable patients had post-transplant relapse of disease.

These small trials have demonstrated the feasibility of purging with immunotoxins. The advantage of immunotoxins for purging is their relative ease of use when compared with monoclonal antibodies and complement. Immunotoxins can potentially provide a simple, reproducible depletion of T cells and malignant cells from marrows. A difficulty inherent in the use of monoclonal antibodies and complement for purging is the lot-to-lot variability of the complement. This situation should not prove to be a problem with immunotoxin purging. The selection of a carrying antibody may prove less important when the whole ricin molecule can be used *in vitro,* allowing the B chain to function in its translocation role. *In vitro* immunotoxins have repeatedly shown depletion of more than three logs of malignant cells from the marrow, and combinations of immunotoxins directed against different cell surface molecules and used simultaneously may prove even more effective at purging. The encouraging preliminary evidence indicates the need for larger follow-up trials.

Serotherapy with Immunotoxins ■

As the previous studies were on-going, several groups of investigators began clinical trials with immunotoxins administered directly to patients with leukemias, lymphomas, and solid tumors. Also, in a direct correlate to *in vitro* T-cell depletion for the prevention of GVHD, a trial was conducted to deplete T cells *in vivo* in patients with established GVHD. These trials used a spectrum of immunotoxins based upon the previously discussed concepts of immunotoxin development. Trials of single-chain immunotoxins all used the ricin A chain, either after chemical separation from the B chain or as recombinant ricin A chain. Ricin has been tested in patients with the B chain binding sites chemically blocked. Pseudomonas exotoxin has been directly conjugated to an antibody and tested clinically. Finally, a fusion protein between IL-2 and diphtheria toxin has been used clinically. The features of these clinical trials are outlined in Tables 7-4 and 7-7. The vast majority of the published reports are Phase I/II trials which treat patients with escalating doses of immunotoxins to determine toxicity, safety, and the maximum tolerated dose that can be administered to patients.

Several objectives were critical in developing these trials. Because immunotoxins had not previously been administered *in vivo*, it was necessary to determine whether blood levels of the immunotoxin could be achieved that were comparable to those that had proved cytotoxic in *in vitro* systems. The systemic and organ-specific toxicity at therapeutic blood levels required evaluation. Specifically, the dose limiting toxicities and the toxicities at the maximal tolerated dose needed definition. These toxicities are listed in Tables 7-5 and 7-6. Finally, responses to therapy needed to be assessed.

Hematologic Malignancies ■

E. S. Vitetta and colleagues (written communication, 1991) have used an anti-CD22 ricin A chain immunotoxin to treat patients with refractory B-cell lymphomas (Table 7-4). In this immunotoxin, the ricin A chain has been deglycosylated, which prolongs the serum half-life by removing mannose and fucose residues in the A chain.[74-77] These residues lead to uptake of A chain by Kupffer cells in the liver. Also tested was an immunotoxin between deglycosylated ricin A chain and the Fab' fragments of the anti-CD22 antibody (RFB4). The Fab' immunotoxin has an IC50 (dose of immunotoxin at which protein synthesis is inhibited 50%) of 10^{-11}M on Daudi cells, an RFB4 positive cell

Table 7–4
Immunotoxins: Clinical Trials in Leukemias and Lymphomas

Immunotoxin	Disease	Phase	# Pts	Schedule	MTD	HAMA	HARA
Anti-B4-BR	B-NHL B-CLL B-ALL	I/II	25	BOLUS	250 ug/kg	9/25	9/25
Anti-B4-BR	B-NHL B-CLL B-ALL	I/II	43	C.I.	350 ug/kg	25/43	25/43
T101-RTA	CLL T-ALL	I	11	BOLUS	112,000 ug/m²	0/11	1/11
Fab'-RFB4-dgA	NHL	I	15	BOLUS	75,000 ug/m²	1/14	4/14
Anti-CD22-dgA	NHL	I	22	BOLUS	52,000 ug/m²	3/18	4/18
DAB486IL-2	B-NHL B-CLL CTCL Hodgkin's Disease Kaposi's Sarcoma	I	47	BOLUS and INFUSION	2000 ug/kg	60%	

MTD = Maximum tolerated dose

C.I. = Continuous Infusion

HAMA and HARA = # of positive patients / total # of patients line, and an IC50 of 10,000 fold greater on an RFB4 negative cell line.[78] Twenty-two patients with refractory B cell malignancies have been treated in a Phase I trial. The dose-related toxicities have been vascular leak syndrome, myalgias, and low-grade fevers, and the dose-limiting toxicities were aphasia, pulmonary edema, and rhabdomyolysis (Tables 7-5 and 7-6). A partial response was reported in 40% of the patients at one month, and a partial response was seen in 55% of the patients whose tumor cells were more than 50% CD22 positive. Vitetta also described in detail the 15 patients who received the immunotoxin composed of glycosylated RTA and the Fab fragments of the antibody. The mean serum half-life of the smaller conjugate was just 1.5 hours, so therapeutic blood concentrations were poorly maintained. Although the doses limiting toxicities were identical, the MTD of the conjugate made of Fab fragments was higher at 75 mg/m^2 than at 52 mg/m^2. Antibody formation was reduced, with only three patients making antibody against just A chain and a fourth producing antibody against both A chain and murine immunoglobulin. Forty-three percent of patients showed greater than a 50% reduction in tumor within a week after completion of the therapy, but these responses were often not maintained at one month.

At the Dana-Farber Cancer Institute we have conducted two Phase I trials using anti-B4-blocked ricin (anti-B4-bR), a conjugate between the anti-B4 monoclonal antibody and blocked ricin, a derivative of ricin in which the nonspecific binding of the B chain has been chemically blocked by conjugating ligands to the binding sites (Table 7-4). Preclinical data on this immunotoxin is presented in Figure 7-8. An initial Phase I trial administered daily bolus injections of the drug to patients with relapsed B-cell leukemias and lymphomas. Of the 25 patients treated, 23 had non-Hodgkin's lymphoma, 1 had non-T ALL, and one had CLL. All patients had disease that relapsed after previous chemotherapy, and seven patients had failed BMT. The majority of patients failed to exhibit any clinically significant side-effects after therapy with anti-B4-bR. The toxicity was limited, consisting of transient elevations of hepatic transaminases, two cases of transient thrombocytopenia, low-grade fevers, and hypoalbuminemia without edema (Tables 7-5 and 7-6). One complete response lasted 21 months and two partial responses were of a shorter duration. Eight patients

Table 7–5
Frequency of Systemic Toxicity

Immunotoxin	Fever	Fatigue/ Malaise	Arthralgias Myalgias	Edema/ Weight Gain
Hematologic Malignancies				
Anti-B4-bR (Bolus)	+	+		
Anti-B4-bR (C.I.)	+ + +	+ +	+	+ +
T101-RTA	+ + + +			
Fab-RFB4-dgA	+ + +		+ +	+ + + +
Anti-CD22-dgA				
DAB486IL-2	+			
Solid Tumors				
Xomazyme-Mel RTA	+ + +	+ + +		+ +
Xmme-001-RTA	+	+ + + +	+ +	+
Cyclophosphamide				
79IT/36-RTA	+ +	+ +		+ +
OVB3-PE (I.P.)	+			
260F9-RTA (Bolus)	+ +	+ +		+ + +
260F9-RTA (C.I.)	+ + + +	+ + + +	+ + + +	+ + + +
Anti-CD5-RTA	+ + +	+ +	+	+ + +

Frequency of Specific Toxicity

+	1–25% of patients
+ +	26–50% of patients
+ + +	51–75% of patients
+ + + +	76–100% of patients

Table 7–6
Frequency of Organ-Specific Toxicity

Immunotoxin	Hematological	Hepatic	Albumin	Renal	Neuro	Cardiac	GI
Hematologic Malignancies							
Anti-B4-bR (Bolus)	+ +	+ + + +	+ + + +				+
Anti-B4-bR (C.I.)	+ +	+ + + +	+ + +				+
T101-RTA							
Fab¹-RFB4-dgA			+ + + +			+ +	+ +
Anti-CD22-dgA							
DAB486IL-2	+	+ +	+	+			+
Solid Tumors							
Xomazyme-Mel RTA	+ +		+ + + +	+		+ + +	+ + +
Xmme-001-RTA	+ + +		+ + +		+		+ + + +
Cyclophosphamide							
79IT/36-RTA		+	+ + + +	+ + + +	+ +		+
OVB3-PE (I.P.)		+ +			+		+ + +
260F9-RTA (Bolus)	+ + + +		+ + + +		+ +		
260F9-RTA (C.I.)							
Anti-CD5-RTA			+ +	+	+ +		

Frequency of Specific Toxicity

+	1–25% of patients
+ +	26–50% of patients
+ + +	51–75% of patients
+ + + +	76–100% of patients

experienced transient reductions in adenopathy but they did not persist for four weeks. Human anti-mouse antibodies (HAMA) and human anti-ricin antibodies (HARA) were observed in 13 of the patients. Blood levels in the therapeutic range of 200 nM were maintained for only transient periods of time.

Because preclinical studies of anti-B4-bR demonstrated that increased dosages of the immunotoxin could be administered with lower toxicity by prolonged continuous infusion than by bolus injection, a second Phase I trial was undertaken using a seven-day continuous infusion (Table 7-4). Forty-three patients were treated. Thirty-three patients had NHL, five had CLL, and five had non-T-ALL. All patients had relapsed from or were refractory to prior chemotherapy and 19 had failed prior BMT. Transient elevations of SGOT and SGPT lasting 7 to 14 days were observed in all patients and represented the dose limiting toxicity (Tables 7-5 and 7-6). Twenty-three patients developed transient hypoalbuminemia with a 20% or greater reduction in serum albumin and 11 patients developed peripheral edema. Thirty patients had fevers greater than 101°. Although many patients developed transient 20–30% reductions in platelet counts, only two patients developed platelet counts below 20,000 which required transfusion support. Most patients receiving anti-B4-bR at the

MTD obtained therapeutic blood levels within 48 hours of initiating the infusion, and sustained those levels until the infusion was discontinued. Twenty-six patients developed HAMA or HARA, which limited retreatment. There were two complete responses, five partial responses, and 12 transient responses to the continuous infusion. Nearly 50% of the treated patients with low and intermediate grade NHL or CLL demonstrated significant responses, while similar responses were less frequent in patients with high grade NHL and ALL. In contrast to Vitetta's trial with a ricin A chain based immunotoxin, hepatotoxicity was dose limiting and capillary leak syndrome was less prominent.

A third trial with a ricin derived immunotoxin was undertaken in patients with CLL and T-ALL (Table 7-4).[61,79] This immunotoxin was composed of the T101 monoclonal antibody and recombinant ricin A chain. A total of 11 patients received the immunotoxin, with three patients receiving the highest dose of 14,000 ug/m². Fever, nausea, and a transient rash were all observed as side-effects, but in contrast to other immunotoxins, hypoalbuminemia and edema were not seen (Tables 7-5 and 7-6). Clinical effects were limited to transient reductions in the peripheral white blood count, but no intact immunotoxin was detected in bone marrow or lymph node aspirates. Moreover, pharmacokinetic studies revealed that the serum half-life was 43 minutes. The brief half-life and associated reduction in drug levels may be attributable to the presence of accessible circulating antigen. These same factors may account for the comparatively low toxicity in this trial.

Clinical trials have also been undertaken using a recombinant fusion protein produced by expression in *E. coli* of a hybrid gene in which the receptor binding domain of diphtheria toxin has been replaced with DNA sequences for IL-2 (Table 7-4).[42,80] The resultant toxin (DAB486IL-2) binds to IL-2 receptors expressed on the surface of a variety of lymphoid, epidermoid, and sarcomatoid malignancies. This fusion protein has undergone testing in 70 patients with IL-2 expressing malignancies, 47 of whom are evaluable for response (JC Nichols, Seragen Inc., written communication, 1991). Side-effects at the maximum tolerated dose have included transient hepatic transaminase elevations in 30% of patients, hypoalbuminemia in 10% of patients, hypersensitivity-like syndromes (consisting of fever, chest tightness, rash) in 20% of patients, occasional transient creatinine elevations, and occasional thrombocytopenia (Tables 7-5 and 7-6). A concern with the use of diphtheria toxin based immunotoxins is the prior immunization that patients have had against DT as part of their routine immunizations. Hence, many patients could have pre-formed antibodies to the toxin, which could conceivably blunt its effect. In fact, antibodies to DT and the fusion protein are present in approximately 30% of patients prior to treatment and in 60% of patients after one or more courses of therapy. Nevertheless, the development of anti-DT antibodies in this trial did not impair efficacy or safety of the fusion protein. Seventy patients have been treated thus far on a variety of different dosage schedules, ranging from bolus injection to six-hour infusion, and 47 patients are evaluable for toxicity. Three complete responses have been seen, one each in patients with B-NHL, CTCL, and HD, and seven partial responses have been achieved. Response duration has ranged from 1 to 12+ months.

Solid Tumors ■

Clinical studies with ricin and Pseudomonas exotoxin based immunotoxins have been undertaken in a spectrum of solid tumors including melanoma, breast cancer, and colon cancer (Table 7-7). A particular difficulty inherent in the therapy of solid tumors is the low accessibility of bulk tumor masses to the immunotoxin. Furthermore, while patients with CLL and NHL may be immunosuppressed secondary to their disease, patients with solid tumors may not be intrinsically immunosuppressed and may be more apt to develop HAMA and human anti-toxin antibodies.

Spitler and associates conducted Phase I and II trials using an antimelanoma antibody-ricin A chain immunotoxin (XOMAZYME-MEL). Twenty-two patients were treated on the Phase I trial (Table 7-7).[81] Toxicity included hypoalbuminemia (in 20 patients), weight gain and edema (6 patients), low voltage on EKG (16 patients), nausea, malaise, and fever (Tables 7-5 and 7-6). One patient with pulmonary metastases had a complete response of prolonged duration. Four patients had mixed responses, with a 50% or greater reduction in the area of one or more metastatic lesions. HAMA and HARA formation occurred in 95% of the patients and precluded successful retreatment in the majority of cases. Detailed pharmacologic data are unavailable, but tissue samples of metastatic lesions were obtained from five patients within 24 hours of therapy, and immunoperoxidase staining indicated the presence of ricin A chain and murine immunoglobulin. In a follow-up Phase II trial of 43 patients, 3 partial responses and 10 less sustained responses suggested biological activity of the immunotoxin.[82] A subsequent Phase II trial administered the immunotoxin in conjunction with cyclophosphamide in an attempt to blunt development of an immune response (Table 7-7).[83] Twenty patients with metastatic melanoma were entered on the Phase II trial, and 11 had received prior therapy. Toxicity was notable for nausea and vomiting, fevers, hypoalbuminemia, weight gain, peripheral edema, myalgias, and fatigue (Tables 7-5 and 7-6). One patient developed seizures, neutropenia, and anemia. Because this patient had received prior chemotherapy, the hematological toxicity may have been attributable to cyclophosphamide rather than the immunotoxin. Four patients demonstrated partial responses, and in one case the response continued for over two to three months following therapy. Unfortunately, HAMA and HARA continued to be formed at high rates and cyclophosphamide failed to suppress the immune response. Although cyclophosphamide has low response rates in melanoma, interpretation of response rates is confounded by its concomitant administration.

A Phase I study of a ricin A chain immunotoxin

Table 7–7
Immunotoxins: Clinical Trials in Solid Tumors

Immunotoxin	Disease	Phase	# Pts	Schedule	MTD	HAMA	HARA
Xomazyme-Mel-RTA	MELANOMA	I	22	BOLUS	4000 ug/kg	19/20	19/20
Xomayzme-Mel-RTA	MELANOMA	II	43	BOLUS	2000 ug/kg	N/A	N/A
XMME-001-RTA with Cyclophosphamide	MELANOMA	II	20	BOLUS	400 ug/kg 1000 mg/m2	13/13	13/13
791T/36 = RTA	COLON CA	I	17	BOLUS	1000 ug/kg	16/17	15/17
OVB3-PE	OVARIAN CA	I	23	I.P.	10–15 ug/kg	12/12	12/12 (Anti-PE)
260F9-rRTA	BREAST CA	I	4	BOLUS	300 ug/kg	4/4	3/4
260F9-rRTA	BREAST CA	I	5	C.I.	800 ug/kg	3/5	4/5
Anti-CD5-RTA	GVHD	I/II	34	BOLUS	2800 ug/kg	6/23	6/23

N/A = Not Available

C.I. = Continuous Infusion

I.P. = Intraperitoneal

MTD = Maximum Tolerated Dose

Anti-PE = Anti-Pseudomonas Exotoxin

HAMA/HARA = # of positive patients / total # of patients

was conducted in patients with metastatic colorectal carcinoma (Table 7-7).[55] The monoclonal antibody 791T/36, which recognizes an antigen on the surface of colon carcinoma cells, was conjugated to ricin A chain (XMMCO-791). Seventeen patients were treated with escalating doses of the immunotoxin. Sixteen patients had liver metastases and ten had pulmonary metastases. Pharmacologic analysis indicated that blood levels were obtained for up to 24 hours after a one-hour intravenous infusion.[82] Toxicity included fever, decreases in serum albumin, and flu-like symptoms (Tables 7-5 and 7-6). Reversible proteinuria and mental status changes including fatigue, slurred speech, irritability, and expressive aphasia were unique features of this immunotoxin. Two patients had a reduction in hepatic metastases, three patients had a reduction in supraclavicular metastases, and one patient had a decrease in pulmonary metastases. Sixteen of the patients developed IgM and IgG antibodies against both ricin A chain and the conjugated monoclonal antibody.

An immunotoxin used in breast cancer patients has been associated with more dramatic toxicity. A murine monoclonal antibody, 260F9, directed against an antigen expressed on approximately 50% of breast cancer cells, was conjugated with recombinant ricin A chain. The immunotoxin was administered to patients with metastatic breast cancer by both bolus injection and continuous infusion (Table 7-7).[56,84] Four patients received the bolus injection and developed weight gain, edema, hypoalbuminemia and dyspnea (Tables 7-5 and

7-6). This toxicity occurred even at doses of immunotoxin that were too low to yield detectable binding to the target antigen, and may have been mediated through binding to Fc receptors of monocytes. Peak serum concentrations ranged between 200 and 850 ng/ml, levels which would be cytotoxic *in vitro*. One patient had a clinical response with resolution of a pulmonary nodule. The trial was discontinued early because of neurological toxicity that was observed in the continuous infusion trial. Five patients with refractory breast cancer received the immunotoxin by continuous infusion. Steady-state concentrations of immunotoxin were achieved at 24 hours and were maintained for up to six days. As in other immunotoxin trials, the toxicity included fevers, weight gain, edema, arthralgias, and nausea. Severe neurological toxicity occurred in three patients, including plexopathies which began on the side of previous chest wall irradiation. Subsequently, patients developed sensorimotor neuropathies of the other three extremities. The neuropathies worsened over the following two to three months, to such an extent that the patients were incapable of caring for themselves. During the following six months, the patients recovered their motor function, but had persistent paresthesias. A nerve biopsy in one patient at the time of maximal symptoms revealed axonal loss and segmental demyelination consistent with toxic injury to the Schwann cells. Moreover, the 260F9 Mab was found to intensely stain the nerve sheath by immunoperoxidase staining, suggesting that the

260F9 epitope is present on Schwann cells or myelin. Thus, the major toxicity of this immunotoxin was likely secondary to nonspecific binding of this antibody.

A concern in the immunotoxin therapy of solid tumors is whether the immunotoxin can penetrate the tumor bed and achieve therapeutic blood levels at the site of the malignant cells. One method of directing delivery of the immunotoxin is to administer it directly into a sequestered site. An immunoconjugate between OVB3, a murine monoclonal antibody that reacts with human ovarian cancers, and pseudomonas exotoxin was administered intraperitoneally to 23 patients with refractory ovarian cancer (Table 7-7—LH Pai and DJ Fitzgerald, written communication, 1991). Therapeutic immunotoxin levels were transiently achieved in the peritoneal fluid even at the lowest administered dose of immunotoxin. At higher doses of the immunotoxin, therapeutic serum levels were also detected. As with other immunotoxins, the side-effects included transient elevations of liver enzymes and fever (Tables 7-5 and 7-6). The majority of patients developed abdominal pain, some severe enough to require parenteral narcotics. The dose limiting toxicity was neurological, with two patients developing encephalopathy characterized by confusion, apraxia, and dysarthria several hours after a second dose of 10 ug/kg. Both patients recovered after several months. However, a third patient suffered fatal neurotoxicity after receiving three doses of OVB3-PE at 5 ug/kg. This patient developed a severe encephalopathy with disorientation, myoclonus, dysarthria, seizures, and ultimately coma. On follow-up analysis, OVB3 was determined to be weakly reactive with cells in the molecular layer of the cerebellum. No objective tumor responses were seen.

Immunotoxins may also be used *in vivo* for the therapy of GVHD. The advantage of therapy directed at circulating cells is their ready accessibility to the immunotoxin. An initial report of the efficacy of an anti-CD5 ricin A chain immunotoxin in steroid resistant acute GVHD was followed by a Phase I/II trial in 34 patients with Grade II through IV GVHD who had failed prior steroid therapy (Table 7-7).[85,86] All patients had persistent acute GVHD despite at least five days of steroid therapy. The majority of patients had both visceral and skin involvement. Twenty-five patients received at least 7 of the planned 14 immunotoxin doses and were evaluable for efficacy at day 28. Pharmacokinetic studies revealed that therapeutic blood levels could be achieved with a serum half-life in the range of 1.5 to 3.9 hours. Toxicity included weight gain, hypoalbuminemia, fatigue, fevers, hematuria, and tremors. In 26 patients with evaluable skin disease, 42% demonstrated resolution and 31% were improved. Similarly, 27% of 22 patients with GI involvement showed complete resolution, and 3 of 18 patients with assessable liver involvement demonstrated resolution. In 6 of 7 patients who had flow cytometric analysis of peripheral blood lymphocytes, a reduction in mononuclear cells staining with anti-CD5 and anti-CD3 antibodies was documented beginning within 24 hours of the initiation of therapy. The use of an anti-CD3 antigen, a second T-cell antigen, to track the disappearance of these cells suggested that this phenomenon was not due simply to antigenic modulation.

Where Have We Been? ■

Although anecdotal reports of immunotoxin therapy occurred prior to 1985, this therapeutic modality has been tested in clinical trials only during the past five years. To date, nearly 300 patients worldwide have received immunotoxin therapy. Considering the spectrum of toxins and ligands evaluated thus far, it remains impossible to determine the clinical impact of this therapeutic modality.

However, several conclusions can be drawn. First, immunotoxins have been administered in Phase I/II trials both as bolus injections and as continuous infusions for up to 14 days with tolerable, reversible toxicities occurring in the overwhelming majority of patients. Second, the toxicity profile of systemic symptoms (fever, myalgias, and fatigue) and organ-specific toxicities (hepatic and endothelial damage) significantly differs from the profile observed with conventional chemotherapeutic agents. Indeed, the side effects witnessed with immunotoxin administration are more reminiscent of those observed with cytokine therapy (interleukin-2, tumor necrosis factor, and interferon). Third, clinical responses, albeit transient, have been documented in patients who have either failed standard and salvage chemotherapy regimens or who have no standard therapy available to them. Finally, production of human antibodies directed against the binding ligands and the toxin moieties have confounded the ability to deliver repeated courses of immunotoxin therapy.

It is difficult to determine from many of the reported trials whether serum immunotoxin levels were achieved which were comparable to those reported to the efficacious *in vitro*. Serum half-lives of small ligands such as the Fab and Fv immunoglobulin fragments or growth factors are shorter than those achieved with larger molecules, such as the intact immunoglobulin molecule. Whether these potential differences in clearance will prove clinically important remains unknown. Even more instrumental is the question of whether these small immunotoxins will be better able to reach malignant cells in tumor masses. While this question awaits a definitive answer, preliminary evidence indicates that at least some immunotoxins can penetrate tumor masses. Further work must address the issues of immunotoxin delivery to the targeted cell *in vivo*.

Nevertheless, an analysis of the completed immunotoxin trials permits some conclusions to be drawn. Overall, a remarkably uniform spectrum of toxicities has been seen in patients who have received therapeutic doses of immunotoxins. Tables 7-5 and 7-6 summarize the frequencies with which systemic and organ-specific toxicities were observed in the various trials. These frequencies of occurrence do not reflect the severities of the respective toxicities. As in most Phase I trials, patients treated with these immunotoxins frequently had had extensive prior therapy. Regardless, few severe side effects and only occasional deaths were attributable to the therapy. Fevers, fatigue, nausea, and myalgias were all common side-effects and occurred with a greater frequency than is seen with the infusion of unconjugated monoclonal antibodies. In the majority of trials, hypoalbuminemia was observed, and the presence of capillary leak syndrome was a frequent correlate. The hypoalbuminemia is likely to be secondary to a capillary leak syndrome which has been manifest as weight gain, peripheral edema, and occasional pleural and pericardial effusions at the highest tolerated doses of immunotoxins. Despite the transaminase elevations that have been reported in several trials, it is unlikely that the albumin decreases are secondary to impaired hepatic synthesis in the absence of elevated prothrombin times and partial thromboplastin times that would also be anticipated with impaired synthetic capacity of the liver. Since capillary leak syndrome occurs with so many immunotoxins, it is unlikely to be mediated by nonspecific binding of the antibody to endothelium. Rather, it may be due to direct endothelial damage attributable to the immunotoxin toxic moiety.

The severe neurotoxicity witnessed in two of the trials attests to the potency of these agents *in vivo*, and emphasizes the importance of careful screening of the chosen antibody or ligand to minimize binding to nontargeted tissues. Despite similar nonspecific antibody binding that could be seen when unconjugated monoclonal antibodies were used therapeutically, the reliance of that therapy on weakly cytotoxic endogenous mechanisms may have prevented similar clinical manifestations from becoming evident.

Although immunotoxins are a directed form of cancer therapy, targeted specifically to malignant cells, they are not without systemic effects that can rival those of standard chemotherapeutic agents. There is no convincing evidence that the majority of these nonspecific side-effects are mediated through specific antibody binding. Conceivably, the immunotoxin binds to monocytes through Fc receptors, as has been demonstrated by Weiner and colleagues, and mediates the release of cytokines that can produce the capillary leak syndrome.[84] Nevertheless, immunotoxins containing only the Fab fragments also lead to capillary leak syndromes, suggesting that another mechanism must contribute.

In light of the aforementioned toxicities, it is essential to question whether they represent dose-limiting toxicities that would satisfy the conventional criteria for achievement of a maximum tolerated dose. Although hepatic transaminase elevations of 10 to 20 times normal have been observed in some studies, these abnormalities return to normal within 7–14 days. While late complications of this toxicity could conceivably occur, they are not evident as yet. Similarly, capillary leak syndromes could be potentially hazardous, but the magnitude of capillary leak syndromes reported thus far has proved tolerable to many patients. Therefore, one must question whether many investigators have truly pushed these agents to the maximal tolerated dose. Whether it is necessary to move to higher doses of immunotoxins to observe clinically significant responses in the majority of patients will be determined by on-going Phase II studies.

The responses reported in these preliminary trials have consisted of occasional complete responses and more frequent partial responses. Some of the trials have reported partial responses in patients based on a decrease in the overall tumor volume rather than a 50% decrease in tumor at all sites and may prove to be lesser responses upon traditional restaging. Some complete responses have been fleeting and have not lasted for the four weeks that are required by standard criteria to qualify for a complete response. This issue of staging and definition of response in patients receiving immunotoxin therapy must be resolved in a manner that permits the observed biological activity of these agents to be accurately documented. Furthermore, the majority of patients entered on these trials have been patients with diseases that typically exhibit low response rates to chemotherapy or have been refractory to prior chemotherapeutic regimens. For example, the three complete responses observed with Anti-B4-bR all occurred in patients who relapsed after autologous BMT. The fact that many patients treated with immunotoxins have shown some tumor regression in association with therapy thus strongly suggests the biological activity of these agents. The majority of patients treated have also had prior end-organ toxicity from exposure to chemotherapeutic agents, which could make them more susceptible to the toxicity of immunotoxins.

The rate of HAMA and antitoxin antibody formation, especially in patients with solid tumors, is discouraging. HAMA and antitoxin antibodies are even seen in 25–50% of patients with CLL and NHL who are inherently immunosuppressed by their disease. The use of cyclophosphamide failed to blunt the development of an immune response. The high frequency with which antibody formation has occurred in a group of patients whom we have treated within six months of bone marrow transplantation suggests that the concomitant administration of powerful immunosuppressives like cyclosporine A may need to be tested in an attempt to lessen the immune response.

Where Are We Going? ■

Considering the youth of this field, the initial laboratory and clinical successes merit enthusiasm. Immunotoxins have induced responses in a subset of patients with hematologic malignancies and solid tumors that were resistant to intensive salvage therapy. In fact, the number of partial and complete clinical responses in these "end stage" patients is remarkable. However, the initial high expectations regarding the efficacy of immunotoxin therapy have certainly not yet been realized. Although numerous studies have documented the capacity of immunotoxins to kill 5–6 logs of malignant cells *in vitro,* such dramatic responses have

been rare *in vivo.* If these agents could be delivered effectively to tumor cells in sufficient concentration, then it is possible that many more clinically important and durable responses might be attained. Therefore, an effort to improve immunotoxin therapy is certainly indicated.

We must first achieve the goal of efficient delivery of the immunotoxin to the tumor cell. Accessibility of the immunotoxin to the tumor remains a problem, especially in the case of solid tumors or bulky lymphomatous masses. This has been less of an obstacle for leukemias where the circulating malignant cells are accessible to the immunotoxin. However, the accessibility of circulating cells permits rapid binding of the immunotoxin, preventing both therapeutic blood levels from being achieved and sufficient immunotoxin from being delivered to the bone marrow.

One approach to improving tumor accessibility would be to use these agents in patients who have minimal residual disease following treatment with either standard chemotherapy regimens or after BMT. At present, we are treating patients with B-cell non-Hodgkin's lymphomas with Anti-B4-bR beginning 60 to 100 days after autologous BMT in an effort to treat disease prior to the time it is clinically detectable. When patients who have had a prior relapse of B-cell NHL undergo autologous BMT, the anticipated two-year disease-free survival is approximately 40%.[87] Thus, although all of our transplanted patients are without measurable disease immediately after autologous BMT, 60% of patients will ultimately relapse and must harbor occult disease. The malignant cells remaining in patients after high-dose chemotherapy regimens may reside in sites that are accessible to immunotoxins.

A second approach to increase tumor accessibility would be to administer the immunotoxin concomitantly with other agents that might enhance the expression of the targeted cell surface molecule. For example, the concomitant administration of cytokines, such as γ-interferon, may lead to enhanced expression of the target antigen. Alternatively, agents that might improve vascular permeability may facilitate immunotoxin delivery to the tumor cell.

Once the toxin has accessibility to the malignant cell, the pharmacologic schedule employed to deliver the immunotoxin can be critical in maintaining adequate therapeutic blood levels. *In vitro* studies have shown that prolonged contact between the immunotoxin and the targeted cell can allow for enhanced cytotoxicity through improved internalization of the toxin. Thus, daily bolus injections of the immunotoxin may prove to be less efficacious than extended infusions in which therapeutic blood levels can be maintained for prolonged intervals of time. Moreover, by maximizing the dose of immunotoxin delivered over the first several weeks of therapy, the total dose delivered before HAMA develops potentially may be increased.

Considerable effort must still be directed at ameliorating the nonspecific toxicity of a toxin. By using modified toxins, such as deglycosylated ricin A chain, hepatic uptake of the toxin could be decreased. Since such features of the nonspecific toxicity as fever or capillary leak syndrome may be mediated by cytokine release, either inhibiting the release of those cytokines or blocking their effects may limit the occurrence of systemic side-effects.

The issue of resistance to the cytotoxic effects of immunotoxins is a crucial question that must be addressed. As has been the case with standard chemotherapeutic agents, cell lines have been identified that are resistant to the effects of the protein toxins.[88] Numerous potential mechanisms may account for this resistance, including impaired translocation of the toxin into the target cell, enhanced cleavage of the linker between ligand and toxin in the circulation, or impaired action of the toxin on the ribosome. If one or more of these mechanisms are demonstrated, then attempts to overcome these pathways of resistance must be investigated. Since evidence from clinical studies to date might argue that resistance arises spontaneously, immunotoxins might prove even more efficacious if used earlier in a patient's therapy, prior to the induction of resistance.

Unfortunately, HAMA or antitoxin antibodies develops in over half of the patients treated with immunotoxins. Although it was initially felt that patients with leukemias and lymphomas were inherently immunosuppressed and therefore were unlikely to form HAMA and antitoxin antibodies, our experience with Anti-B4-bR in patients who were immunosuppressed not only from their disease but also from recent bone marrow transplantation suggests otherwise. Moreover, when using conjugates with DT, patients may have prior immunity to diphtheria toxin secondary to immunization. Thus, immunotoxins may need to be administered in conjunction with immunosuppressive agents such as cyclophosphamide or cyclosporine in an effort to curtail the formation of HAMA and antitoxin antibodies. Alternatively, further efforts need to be directed toward the development of chimeric antibodies, humanized antibodies, or Fab fragments as toxin carriers. Vitetta's encouraging experience with reduced HAMA formation in patients receiving a Fab-based immunotoxin, suggests that the potential immunogenicity of the ligand portion of the immunotoxin can be reduced.

To date, preliminary studies with immunotoxins have just begun to explore the potential efficacy of this form of therapy. The cytotoxic activity of these agents has been repeatedly confirmed *in vitro*. The next decade should mark an era of continued advances in this field and will likely see the addition of immunotoxins to the anticancer therapeutic armamentarium.

Acknowledgments. This work is sponsored by National Institutes of Health grant CA-34183. We appreciate the assistance of Walter Blattler of ImmunoGen, Inc. and Jean Nichols of Seragen, Inc. who have kindly provided us with unpublished preclinical and clinical data. Ellen Vitetta of the University of Texas Southwestern Medical Center and David FitzGerald of the National Cancer Institute have graciously provided us with several submitted manuscripts to update the published information already available.

References ■

1. Kohler G, Milstein C. Continuous cultures of fused cells secreting antibody of pre-defined specificity. Nature 1975;256:495.
2. Nadler LM, Stashenko P, Hardy R, et al. Serotherapy of a patient with a monoclonal antibody directed against a human lymphoma-associated antigen. Cancer Res 1980;40:3147.
3. Houghton A, Scheinberg D. Monoclonal antibodies in the treatment of hematopoietic malignancies. S Hematology 1988;25:23.
4. Meeker T, Lowder J, Cleary ML, et al. Emergence of idiotype variants during treatment of B cell lymphomas with anti-idiotype antibodies. N Engl J Med 1985;312:1658.
5. Brown SL, Miller RA, Horning SJ, et al. Treatment of B-cell lymphomas with anti-idiotype antibodies alone and in combination with alpha interferon. Blood 1989;73:651.
6. Ball ED, Bernier GM, Cornwell III GG, McIntyre OR, O'Donnell JF, Fanger MW. Monoclonal antibodies to myeloid differentiation antigen: *In vivo* studies of three patients with acute myelogenous leukemia. Blood 1983;62:1203.
7. Scheinberg DA, Lovett D, Divgi CR, et al. A phase I trial of monoclonal antibody M195 in acute myelogenous leukemia: Specific bone marrow targeting and internalization of radionuclide. J Clin Oncol 1991;9:478.

8. Ritz J, Pesando JM, Sallan SE, et al. Serotherapy of acute lymphoblastic leukemia with monoclonal antibody. Blood 1981;58:141.

9. Dyer MJS, Hale G, Hayhoe FGJ, Waldman H. Effects of CAMPATH-1 antibodies *in vivo* in patients with lymphoid malignancies: Influence of antibody isotype. Blood 1989;73:1431.

10. Dillman RO, Shawler DL, Dillman JB, Royston I. Therapy of chronic lymphocytic leukemia and cutaneous T-cell lymphoma with T-101 monoclonal antibody. J Clin Oncol 1984;2:881.

11. Foon KA, Schroff RW, Bunn PA, et al. Effects of monoclonal antibody therapy in patients with chronic lymphocytic leukemia. Blood 1984;64:1085.

12. Meeker TC, Lowder J, Maloney DG, et al. A clinical trial of anti-idiotype therapy for B-cell malignancy. Blood 1985;65:1349.

13. Hale G, Dyer MJ, Clark MR, et al. Remission induction in non-Hodgkin lymphoma with reshaped human monoclonal antibody CAMPATH-1H. Lancet 1988;2:1394.

14. Scheinberg DA, Straus DJ, Yeh SD, et al. A Phase I toxicity, pharmacology, and dosimetry trial of monoclonal antibody OKB7 in patients with non-Hodgkin's lymphoma: Effects of tumor burden and antigen expression. J Clin Oncol 1990;8:792.

15. Miller R, Oseroff AR, Stratte PT, Levy R. Monoclonal antibody therapeutic trials in seven patients with T-cell lymphoma. Blood 1983;62:988.

16. Waldman TA, Goldman CK, Bongiovanni KF, et al. Therapy of patients with human T-cell lymphotrophic virus I-induced adult T-cell leukemia with anti-Tac, a monoclonal antibody to the receptor for interleukin-2. Blood 1988;72:1805.

17. Sears HF, Herlyn D, Steplewski Z, Koprowski H. Phase II clinical trial of a murine monoclonal antibody cytotoxic for gastrointestinal adenocarcinoma. Cancer Res 1985;45:5910.

18. Steis RG, Carrasquillo JA, McCabe R, et al. Toxicity, immunogenicity, and tumor radioimmunodetecting ability of two human monoclonal antibodies in patients with metastatic colorectal carcinoma. J Clin Oncol 1990; 8:476.

19. Goodman GE, Hellstrom I, Brodzinsky L, et al. Phase I trial of murine monoclonal antibody L6 in breast, colon, ovarian, and lung cancer. J Clin Oncol 1990;8:1083.

20. Elias DJ, Hirschowitz L, Kline LE, et al. Phase I clinical comparative study of monoclonal antibody KS1/4 and KS1/4-methotrexate immunoconjugate in patients with non-small cell lung carcinoma. Cancer Res 1990;50:4154.

21. LoBuglio AF, Saleh MN, Lee J, et al. Phase I trial of multiple large doses of murine monoclonal antibody CO17-1A. I. Clinical aspects. J Natl Cancer Inst 1988;80:932.

22. Divgi CR, Welt S, Kris M, et al. Phase I and imaging trial of indium 111-labeled anti-epidermal growth factor receptor monoclonal antibody 225 in patients with squamous cell lung carcinoma. J Natl Cancer Inst 1991;83:97.

23. Goodman GE, Beaumier P, Hellström I, Fernyhough B, Hellström KE. Pilot trial of murine monoclonal antibodies in patients with advanced melanoma. J Clin Oncol 1985;3:493.

24. Cheung NV, Lazarus H, Miraldi FD, et al. Ganglioside G_{D2} specific monoclonal antibody 3F8: A phase I study in patients with neuroblastoma and malignant melanoma. J Clin Oncol 1987;5:1430.

25. Vadhan-Raj S, Coron-Cardo C, Carswell E, et al. Phase I trial of a mouse monoclonal antibody against G_{D3} ganglioside in patients with melanoma: Induction of inflammatory responses at tumor sites. J Clin Oncol 1988; 6:1636.

26. Dillman RO. Monoclonal antibodies for treating cancer. Ann Int Med 1989;111:592.

27. Dillman RO, Shawler DL, Sobol RE, et al. Murine monoclonal antibody therapy in two patients with chronic lymphocytic leukemia. Blood 1982;59:1036.

28. Hertler AA, Frankel AE. Immunotoxins: a clinical review of their use in the treatment of malignancies. J Clin Oncol 1989;7:1932.

29. Pastan I, Willingham MC, FitzGerald DJ. Immunotoxins. Cell 1986;47:641.

30. FitzGerald D, Pastan I. Targeted toxin therapy for the treatment of cancer. J Natl Cancer Inst 1989;81:1455.

31. Marsh JW, Srinivasachar K, Neville DJ. Antibody-toxin conjugation. Cancer Treat Res 1988;37:213.

32. Wawrzynczak EJ, Thorpe PE. Effect of chemical linkage upon the stability and cytotoxic activity of A chain immunotoxins. Cancer Treat Res 1988;37:239.

33. Vitetta ES, Fulton RJ, May RD, Till M, Uhr JW. Redesigning nature's poisons to create antitumor reagents. Science 1987;238:1098.

34. Preijers FW, Tax WJ, De WT, et al. Relationship between internalization and cytotoxicity of recin A-chain immunotoxins. Br J Haematol 1988;70:289.

35. Glennie MJ, Brennand DM, Bryden F, et al. Bispecific F(ab' gamma)$_2$ antibody for the delivery of saporin in the treatment of lymphoma. J Immunol 1988;141:3662.

36. Derocq JM, Casellas P, Laurent G, Ravel S, Vidal H, Jansen F. Comparison of the cytotoxic potency of T101 Fab, F(ab')$_2$ and whole IgG immunotoxins. J Immunol 1988;141:2837.

37. Kreitman RJ, Chaudhary VK, Waldmann T, Willingham MC, FitzGerald DJ, Pastan I. The recombinant immunotoxin anti-Tac(Fv)-Pseudomonas exotoxin 40 is cytotoxic toward peripheral blood malignant cells from patients with adult T-cell leukemia. Proc Natl Acad Sci USA 1990;87:8291.

38. LoBuglio AF, Wheeler R, Leavitt RD, et al. Pharmacokinetics and immune response to chimeric mouse/human monoclonal antibody (CH17-1A) in man. Proc ASCO 1988;7:111.

39. Hamblin TJ, Cattan AR, Glennie MJ, et al. Initial experience in treating human lymphoma with a chimeric univalent derivative of monoclonal anti-idiotype antibody. Blood 1987;69:790.

40. Siegall CB, FitzGerald DJ, Pastan I. Selective killing of tumor cells using EGF or TGF alpha-Pseudomonas exotoxin chimeric molecules. Sem in Cancer Biol 1990; 1:345.

41. Loberboum-Galski H, FitzGerald DJ, Chaudhary V, Adhya S, Pastan I. Cytotoxic activity of an interleukin-2 Pseudomonas exotoxin chimeric protein produced in *E. coli*. Proc Natl Acad Sci USA 1988;85:1922.

42. Williams DP, Parker P, Bacha P, et al. Diphtheria toxin receptor binding domain substitution with interleukin-2: genetic construction and properties of a diphtheria toxin-related interleukin-2 fusion protein. Protein Engineering 1987;1:493.

43. FitzGerald DJ, Willingham MC, Cardarelli CO, et al. A monoclonal antibody-Pseudomonas toxin conjugate that specifically kills multidrug-resistant cells. Proc Natl Acad Sci USA 1987;84:4288.

44. Lambert JM, Blattler WA, McIntyre GD, Goldmacher

VS, Scott CJ. Immunotoxins containing single-chain ribosome-inactivating proteins. Cancer Treat Res 1988; 37:175.

45. Goldmacher VS, Tinnel NL, Nelson BC. Evidence that pinocytosis in lymphoid cells has a low capacity. J Cell Biol 1986;102:1312.

46. Endo Y, Mitsui K, Motizuki M, Tsurugi K. The mechanism of action of ricin and related toxic lectins on eukaryotic ribosomes. J Biol Chem 1987;262:5908.

47. Olsnes S, Sandvig K. How protein toxins enter and kill cells. Cancer Treat Res 1988;37:39.

48. Youle RJ, Neville Jr DM. Kinetics of protein synthesis inactivation by ricin-anti Thy 1.1 monoclonal antibody hybrids. J Biol Chem 1982;257:1598.

49. Collier RJ. Effect of diphtheria toxin on protein synthesis: Inactivation of one of the transfer factors. J Mol Biol 1967;25:83.

50. Hwang J, Fitzgerald DJ, Adhya S, Pastan I. Functional domains of Pseudomonas exotoxin identified by deletion analysis of the gene expressed in *E. coli*. Cell 1987; 48:129.

51. Calafat J, Molthoff C, Janssen H, Hilkens J. Endocytosis and intracellular routing of an antibody-ricin A chain conjugate. Cancer Res 1988;48:3822.

52. Mecada E, Uchida T, Okada Y. Methylamine stimulates the action of ricin toxin, but inhibits that of diphtheria toxin. J Biol Chem 1981;256:1225.

53. Blewitt MG, Chung LA, London E. Effect of *p*H on the conformation of diphtheria toxin and its implication for membrane penetration. Biochemistry 1984;24:5458.

54. Lambert JM, Blattler WA. Purification and biochemical characterization of immunotoxins. Cancer Treat Res 1988;37:323.

55. Byers VS, Rodvien R, Grant K, et al. Phase I study of monoclonal antibody-ricin A chain immunotoxin XomaZyme-791 in patients with metastatic colon cancer. Cancer Res 1989;49:6153.

56. Gould BJ, Borowitz MJ, Groves ES, et al. Phase I study of an anti-breast cancer immunotoxin by continuous infusion: report of a targeted toxic effect not predicted by animal studies. J Natl Cancer Inst 1989;81:775.

57. Johnson VG, Wilson D, Greenfield L, Youle RJ. The role of the diphtheria toxin receptor in cytosol translocation. J Biol Chem 1988;263:1295.

58. FitzGerald DJ. Construction of immunotoxins using Pseudomonas exotoxin A. Methods Enzymol 1987; 151:139.

59. Kondo T, FitzGerald D, Chaudhary VK, Adhya S, Pastan I. Activity of immunotoxins constructed with modified Pseudomonas exotoxin A lacking the cell recognition domain. J Biol Chem 1988;263:9470.

60. Batra JK, FitzGerald D, Gately M, Chaudhary VK, Pastan I. Anti-Tac(Fv)-PE40: A single chain antibody Pseudomonas fusion protein directed at interleukin-2 receptor bearing cells. J Biol Chem 1990;265:151–198.

61. Hertler AA, Schlossman DM, Borowitz MJ, Blythman HE, Casellas P, Frankel AE. An anti-CD5 immunotoxin for chronic lymphocytic leukemia: enhancement of cytotoxicity with human serum albumin-monensin. Int J Cancer 1989;43:215.

62. Chaudhary VK, FitzGerald DJP, Adhya S, Pastan I. Activity of a recombinant fusion protein between transforming growth factor alpha and Pseudomonas exotoxin. Proc Natl Acad Sci USA 1987;84:4438.

63. Williams DP, Snider CE, Strom TB, Murphy JR. Structure/function analysis of interleukin-2-toxin (DAB486-

IL-2). Fragment B sequences required for the delivery of fragment A to the cytosol of target cells. J Biol Chem 1990;265:118–185.

64. Ball ED, Mills LE, Cornwell GC, et al. Autologous bone marrow transplantation for acute myeloid leukemia using monoclonal antibody-purged bone marrow. Blood 1990;75:1199.

65. Herve P, Cahn JY, Flesch M, et al. Successful graft-versus-host disease prevention without graft failure in 32 HLA-identical allogeneic bone marrow transplantations with marrow depleted T cells by monoclonal antibodies and complement. Blood 1987;69:388.

66. Nadler LM, Takvorian T, Botnick L, et al. Anti-B1 monoclonal antibody and complement treatment in autologous bone-marrow transplantation for relapsed B-cell non-Hodgkin's lymphoma. Lancet 1984;2:427.

67. Preijers FW, De WT, Wessels JM, et al. Autologous transplantation of bone marrow purged *in vitro* with anti-CD7-(WT1-) ricin A immunotoxin in T-cell lymphoblastic leukemia and lymphoma. Blood 1989;74:1152.

68. Preijers FW, De WT, Wessels JM, Meyerink JP, Haanen C, Capel PJ. Cytotoxic potential of anti-CD7 immunotoxin (WT1-ricin A) to purge *ex vivo* malignant T cells in bone marrow. Br J Haematol 1989;71:195.

69. Uckun FM, Gajl PK, Meyers DE, et al. Marrow purging in autologous bone marrow transplantation for T-lineage acute lymphoblastic leukemia: efficacy of *ex vivo* treatment with immunotoxins and 4-hydroperoxycyclophosphamide against fresh leukemic marrow progenitor cells. Blood 1987;69:361.

70. Uckun FM, Kersey JH, Vallera DA, et al. Autologous bone marrow transplantation in high-risk remission T-lineage acute lymphoblastic leukemia using immunotoxins plus 4-hydroperoxycyclophosphamide for marrow purging. Blood 1990;76:1723.

71. Laurent G, Maraninchi D, Gluckman E, et al. Donor bone marrow treatment with T101 Fab fragment-ricin A-chain immunotoxin prevents graft-versus-host disease. Bone Marrow Transplant 1989;4:367.

72. Martin PJ, Hansen JA, Torok SB, et al. Effects of treating marrow with a CD3-specific immunotoxin for prevention of acute graft-versus-host disease [published erratum appears in Bone Marrow Transplant 1989;4:215]. Bone Marrow Transplant 1988;3:437.

73. Filipovich AH, Vallera DA, Youle RJ, et al. Graft-versus-host disease prevention in allogeneic bone marrow transplantation from histocompatible siblings. A pilot study using immunotoxins for T cell depletion of donor bone marrow. Transplantation 1987;44:62.

74. Fulton RJ, Uhr JW, Vitetta ES. *In vivo* therapy of the BCL1 tumor: effect of immunotoxin valency and deglycosylation of the ricin A chain. Cancer Res 1988; 48:2626.

75. Thorpe PE, Wallace PM, Knowles PP, et al. Improved antitumor effects of immunotoxins prepared with deglycosylated ricin A-chain and hindered disulfide linkages. Cancer Res 1988;48:6396.

76. Blakey DC, Watson GJ, Knowles PP, Thorpe PE. Effect of chemical deglycosylation of ricin A chain on the *in vivo* fate and cytotoxic activity of an immunotoxin composed of ricin A chain and anti-Thy 1.1 antibody. Cancer Res 1987;47:947.

77. Blakey DC, Thorpe PE. Effect of chemical deglycosylation on the *in vivo* fate of ricin A-chain. Cancer Drug Deliv 1986;3:189.

78. Shen GL, Li JL, Ghetie MA, et al. The evaluation of four

anti-CD22 antibodies as ricin A chain-containing immunotoxins. Int J Cancer 1988;42:792.

79. Laurent G, Frankel AE, Hertler AA, Schlossman DM,
Casellas P, Jansen FK. Treatment of leukemia patients
with T101 ricin A chain immunotoxins. Cancer Treat Res
1988;37:483.

80. Murphy JR. Diphtheria-related peptide hormone gene
fusions: a molecular genetic approach to chimeric toxin
development. Cancer Treat Res 1988;37:123.

81. Spitler LE, del Rio M, Khentigan A, et al. Therapy of
patients with malignant melanoma using a monoclonal
antimelanoma antibody-ricin A chain immunotoxin.
Cancer Res 1987;47:1717.

82. Spitler LE. Clinical studies: Solid tumors. Cancer Treat
Res 1988;37:493.

83. Oratz R, Speyer JL, Wernz JC, et al. Antimelanoma
monoclonal antibody-ricin A chain immunoconjugate
(XMMME-001-RTA) plus cyclophosphamide in the
treatment of metastatic malignant melanoma: Results of
a phase II trial. J Bio Resp Mod 1990;9:345.

84. Weiner LM, O'Dwyer J, Kitson J, et al. Phase I evaluation of an anti-breast carcinoma monoclonal antibody
260F9-recombinant ricin A chain immunoconjugate.
Cancer Res 1989;49:4062.

85. Kernan NA, Byers V, Scannon PJ, et al. Treatment of
steroid-resistant acute graft-vs-host disease by *in vivo*
administration of an anti-T-cell ricin A chain immunotoxin. JAMA 1988;259:3154.

86. Byers VS, Henslee PJ, Kernan NA, et al. Use of an anti-
pan T-lymphocyte ricin A chain immunotoxin in steroid-
resistant acute graft-versus-host disease. Blood 1990;
75:1426.

87. Freedman AS, Takvorian T, Anderson KC, et al. Autologous bone marrow transplantation in B-cell non-Hodgkin's lymphoma: Very low treatment-related mortality in
100 patients in sensitive relapse. J Clin Oncol 1990;8:784.

88. Goldmacher VS, Anderson J, Schulz ML, Blattler WA,
Lambert JM. Somatic cell mutants resistant to ricin,
diphtheria toxin, and to immunotoxins. J Biol Chem
1987;262:3205.

George D. Webster
Joseph M. Khoury

Continent Urinary Diversion

8

In recent years there has been a surge of enthusiasm in continent urinary diversions. Historically, the impetus to restore lower urinary tract continuity using various bowel segments began in Europe. Couvelaire, in 1951, was the first to use ileum to reconstruct and replace the bladder following cystectomy.[1] Likewise Camey, in 1958, introduced the ureteroileourethrostomy and for the last 30 years has attempted to perfect the pitfalls of urinary reconstruction in his operation.[2] Any operation designed to redirect the urine after cystectomy should be both clinically acceptable to the surgeon and socially and psychologically acceptable to the patient. It must be oncologically appropriate and consider patient survival, anticipated cancer morbidity, possible mechanisms of tumor spread in the pelvis, and the risks to the patient from procedures that often require revision operations. Likewise, patient motivation and aptitude, physical and neurologic disability, and social factors influence the selection of urinary diversion.

The ideal urinary diversion should mimic bladder function as closely as possible. It should achieve a low pressure capacious reservoir to collect and store urine, achieve continence and allow expulsion of urine under voluntary control, protect the upper tracts from obstruction or reflux, and avoid significant shifts of water and electrolytes that may cause metabolic disturbances. By common usage, the term *diversion* applies primarily to the redirection of urine away from the bladder to a skin stoma, but we shall elaborate its use to embrace also those procedures in which the bladder is totally replaced but the urine is still drained through the urethra.

Bricker in the late 1940s was interested in ureteral management following pelvic evisceration for colonic, gynecologic, and urologic malignancies.[3] He initially used ileum and cecum as a continent urinary reservoir, however, continence could not be achieved despite several maneuvers such as imbrication of the external oblique fascia around the pouch stoma, and use of a fascial sling. In 1951, Bricker described the use of an appliance–dependent urinary ileostomy which introduced a new area of acceptability of radical pelvic surgery.

Unfortunately, long-term results, particularly in patients with long life expectancies, were not as favorable as initially anticipated, and this in turn, stimulated the current popularity of continent urinary diversion operations. Nonetheless, the Bricker procedure is still the most widely used form of urinary diversion after cystectomy and remains the standard to which all other diverting

137

procedures must be compared, particularly as continent diversions have had insufficient time to show the development of long-term complications or drawbacks. A number of surgeons, however, are reluctant to perform these operations because they are reportedly associated with a high reoperation rate. A retrospective review of 1,200 standard diversions and 900 continent diversions show the same reoperation rate. Olsson in 1990 prospectively reviewed 22 continent and 51 standard diversions and found no significant difference in reoperation rate as well.[4]

Continent diversions can improve the quality of life after cystectomy, facilitate psychological adjustment, and ease concerns over body image, a factor that might otherwise delay patients in dealing with malignancy. Patient awareness of a continent alternative has spread by word of mouth, by the media, through ostomy associations, and through the requirement that all surgical alternatives be discussed with the patients. This has prompted the urologist to view the development of continent diversion more seriously. Emotional factors aside, social and economic considerations present a need for continent diversions, particularly in some Third World countries where the social taboos of a wet stoma and the cost of ostomy appliances preclude the use of an ileal conduit in most circumstances. The increasing patient desire for a continent diversion is in some respects unfortunate, for it is certainly true that these operations are vastly more complex than the ileal conduit and certainly should not be in the surgical repertoire of the occasional user.

Variables of Continent Urinary Diversion ■

The alternatives to an appliance-dependent urostomy include urinary diversion using the anal sphincter, total bladder replacement, and continent abdominal wall stomas. The ideal continent urinary diversion should attempt to resemble the lower urinary tract in both function and structure. These goals of diversion can be achieved if strict attention is given to the proper selection of bowel and the manner in which it is remodeled, astute management of the ureters, and the type of continence mechanism chosen. The propulsion of intestinal contents in small and large intestine is by peristalsis and mass contraction, respectively, the main stimulus for the activity being distention. Isolated intestinal segments respond to distention with urine in the same fashion, and unacceptably high pressure waves may be generated.[5–8] There is controversy as to which bowel segments provide optimal results. Right colon, ileum and colon, and ileum have been employed and are associated with varying degrees of success. Clinical and experimental data suggest that independent of the intestinal segment chosen, detubularized bowel is preferred to prevent the onset of high pressure phasic contractions that can result in reflux and incontinence. We have shown the advantage of detubularization of both ileal and right colon segments, the incidence and amplitude of contractions being decreased and appearing at higher bladder capacities in the detubularized forms.[5] A detubularized and remodeled capacious ileal segment is the most docile system that can be constructed; however, a relatively docile right colon or ileocolic segment can be fashioned using similar remodeling maneuvers.

The factors determining ureteral management are dependent on whether reflux or obstruction is initially present. Ureteral size, length, and peristalsis also need to be considered as well as the bowel segment selected. Of the many types of ureteral reimplantation techniques, four basic nonrefluxing ureteroenteric anastomoses are commonly used. Tunneled reimplantation into large bowel (Goodwin/Leadbetter)[9,10] or small bowel (LeDuc-Camey),[11] split cuff nipple reimplants,[12] and intussuscepted bowel interpositions[13] appear to prevent reflux and avoid obstruction in approximately 90% of cases. The surgeon should be familiar with all of these techniques since status of the upper tracts will determine the type of reimplantation employed.

An ideal stomal continence mechanism remains to be found. However, in recent times, new modifications based on principles of physics and surgery have been incorporated into stomal reconstruction, causing few long-term complications. Commonly favored continence mechanisms include the ileal intussusception,[14] plication of the ileocecal valve,[15] and the hydraulic ileovalve described by Benchekroun.[16] The continence mechanism in the orthotopic bladder is determined by preservation of the distal sphincter mechanism following cystoprostatectomy. This assumes that the urethral remnant is adequate in length and free of tumor.

Patient Selection and Counseling ■

Preoperative selection criteria for the candidate undergoing a continent urinary diversion is no different from that any other supravesical diversion. A reasonable life expectancy should be anticipated as well as the manual dexterity to perform self-intermittent catheterization. Since many demands are placed on the candidate and the family, compliance and willingness to work with the reconstruction team and enterostomal therapist are crucial to obtain satisfactory postoperative results. Surgical criteria include access to the abdominal cavity, absence of bowel pathology, and the availability of sufficient large and small bowel to create the appropriate urinary reservoir and nipple valves. Radiation therapy is a relative contraindication; however, bowel that has been minimally radiated could pose potential problems as it may compromise the viscoelastic property of the bowel wall, taking longer for the pouch to reach its optimal capacity.[17]

Although obesity is not a contraindication to a continent-cutaneous stoma, it does add considerably to catheterization difficulties if the efferent continent mechanism is not brought through the abdominal wall in the shortest and most direct route, and secured with care to the rectus fascia and skin.

A considerable number of patients may decline a continent diversion in lieu of a simple urinary ileostomy based on an honest reporting to them of the duration of surgery and the hospitalization and the incidence of early and late complications. This dropout rate is certainly better than later dealing with the unhappy, poorly informed patient who has encountered unexpected problems. Boyd and associates[18] addressed the quality of life issues in patients with a wet versus a dry stoma. They compared 100 adults with ileal conduits and 100 adults that had undergone a Kock pouch continent cutaneous diversion. The Kock pouch patients were further stratified into those having a primary diversion or a conversion from a previous ileal conduit. Surprisingly, all groups adapted well to their respective types of diversion, and no significant social or physical restrictions were noted. Patients with a noncontinent form of urinary diversion, however, had negative impact as reflected in self-image, decrease in sexual desire, and all forms of physical contact. The most satisfied group were those that had a wet urostomy and were converted to a continent cutaneous Kock pouch.

Preoperative radiographic studies should include excretory urography and bowel contrast studies in those patients in whom bowel pathology is suspected or in whom prior intestinal surgery may influence one's choice of which bowel segment to use. The patient should be prepared for surgery by both mechanical and antibiotic bowel prep. Dehydration should be avoided by starting intravenous fluids the day before surgery. Those with poor nutrition may require a period of preoperative hyperalimentation. Clear fluids taken in only by mouth are commenced two days prior to surgery and GoLytely, a polyethyline glycol electrolyte gastrointestinal tract lavage solution, is administered the day before surgery. Following transit through the intestinal tract, rectal efflux is generally clear at the termination of this preparation.

Classification of Continent Urinary Diversions ■

There are basically three types of continent urinary diversions, and each is classified based on the location of the continence mechanism. Current clinically acceptable methods are those procedures involving the anal sphincter, bladder replacement *in situ* utilizing the native urethra, and—for those patients in whom this is inappropriate—the use of a continent abdominal wall stoma. A number of techniques have now been reported, each with its proponents and opponents, and it is certainly true to say that at present no one procedure is best.

Continent Diversion with the Anal Sphincter ■

Ureterosigmoidostomy ■

Ureterosigmoidostomy is a classic example of this group of procedures; it was first reported in 1851 when it was performed in a child with ectopia vesicae (exstrophy).[19] In 1911, Coffey introduced the concept of a tunneled ureteral reimplantation into large bowel; however, this did not include a mucosa to mucosa anastomosis nor did it prevent reflux.[20] Subsequently, in the 1950s, Leadbetter[9] and then Goodwin[10] described ureterocolonic anastomoses that were nonrefluxing and involved mucosa to mucosa anastomosis, vastly improving the results. Unfortunately, only about one-third of all patients undergoing ureterosigmoidostomy avoided all major problems, and the incidence of late complications was a direct function of time. Seemingly, the final death knell for ureterosigmoidostomy was the growing evidence of an increased rate of bowel adenocarcinomas at the anastomotic site, with 5% of those with ureterosigmoidostomies likely to develop tumors over a mean of 25 years.[21] This incidence was believed to be due to urinary nitrate products converted by fecal bacteria to active carcinogenic nitrosamines, which act preferentially on intestinal cells. This risk was indeed unfortunate, for the procedure found a particular role in children or young adults with benign disease who otherwise had a long life expectancy. Recognizing the attractions of this internal diversion, however, others have tried to reduce the risk of tumor formation by extracting one of the ingredients from the tumor-forming equation.[22]

Ileocecal Ureterosigmoidostomy ■

Ureteroileocecosigmoidostomy is an attempt to avoid a coloureteral anastomosis and to provide an antireflux ileocecal valve to protect the ureteroileal anastomosis from contact with feces.[22] Thus far no tumors have been reported using this technique, but follow-up has a short history.

Augmented and Valved Rectum ■

Kock has devised a novel surgical procedure in which the rectum is augmented by anastomosing an ileal patch to the anterior rectal wall (Fig. 8-1).[23] In addition, reflux of rectal contents in the colon into the upper urinary tract is prevented by creating a nipple valve formed from intussuscepted sigmoid. The ureters are implanted within the intussuscepted segment. Stool is temporarily diverted using a transverse colostomy, then closed two months later after healing has occurred. Alternatively, in the case of larger aperistaltic ureters that would not fit into a sigmoid intussusception, the sigmoid is left intact after placement of an ileal patch onto the rectum, and the ureters are implanted onto the afferent limb of an intussuscepted

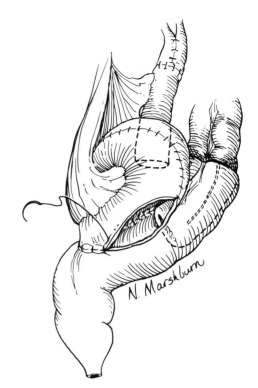

FIG. 8–1 The valved augmented rectum.

ileal nipple, which is anastomosed into the rectum directly. Kock reports a mean rectal reservoir capacity to approximately 800 ml with low pressures, daytime continence, and no nighttime enuresis, with emptying 0–2 times per night.[23]

Ghoneim has performed this operation on 51 patients, and has achieved similar success; however, he emphasizes the importance of longitudinal review to assess the long-term effect on renal function, and whether the incidence of tumor development at the anastomotic site will differ from the standard ureterosigmoidostomy procedure.[70]

Continent Abdominal Stoma ■

The first report of a urinary diversion to a continent abdominal stoma was by Gilchrist and Merrick[24] in 1950, which developed from an anecdotal report of a cecal pouch reservoir with the appendix as a conduit performed in South America in the 1940s. Between 1949 and 1963, they performed 40 ileocecal-ascending colon segment urinary diversions, with a 15% mortality and a 94%

reported continence rate. Other surgeons, however, were unable to reproduce their results, as the efferent unmodified ileocecal valve could not predictably produce continence in the majority of patients. A resurgence of interest followed the successful development of the Kock continent ileostomy for patients undergoing proctocolectomy for ulcerative colitis.[25] The original procedure had no special valvular mechanism and continence depended on low pressure within the pouch and the constricting action of the rectus muscles around the ileum. Continence was unpredictable, so the concept of a nipple valve was introduced, based on a surgical technique originally described by Watsudji in 1899 in the formation of gastrostomies.[26]

The Kock Pouch ■

The idea of an ileal pouch with a continent nipple as inspired by Kock was first applied to the urinary tract by Leisinger in 1976.[27] His successful clinical experience was followed by reports by Madegan,[28] Kock and associates,[14] Ashken,[29] Gerber,[30] and more recently in a large series by Skinner and associates.[31,32] Initially the procedure was beset by a high incidence of problems, mostly related to the efferent nipple, which had a propensity to evaginate, with resultant incontinence, or to become difficult to catheterize. In 1982, Kock described an improved technique for its construction, advocating that the 5 cm long ileal intussusception be secured by 3 rows of intestinal staples.[14] Further stability was added by the use of a fascial or Marlex mesh collar around the base of the ileum where it exited from the intussusception. The collar fixed the pouch and intussusception securely to the anterior abdominal wall fascia, and, in addition to stabilizing the nipple, improved the ability to catheterize the pouch by reducing redundancy between the abdominal wall and the intussusception. Because the mesentery contained within the intussusception was predisposed to evagination, Gerber suggested defatting the mesentery of the intussuscepted portion of the ileum.[30] Skinner and associates[31,32] elaborated on this further by stripping 7–8 cm of mesentery off the ileum at the site of intussusception so as to totally exclude it, a procedure based on the description by Hendren[33] to retain intussusceptions of the ileocecal valve in undiversions. Improved nipple valve stability is ensured by attaching the nipple

to the side wall of the reservoir by one row of staples so that a continuously increasing centripetal force works against the natural extrusion force, which would occur were the attachments not present. Kock has shown that staples become imbedded in the muscular layer of the nipple, completely covered by a regenerating mucosa. Unfortunately, this procedure still provided the nidus for stone formation, a common complication early in the development of this procedure. Skinner recommended the use of modified cartridges wherein the last six staples are removed from the proximal margin of the cartridge.[32]

Bacterial colonization of the urine is common in all catheterizable urinary reservoirs, but pyelonephritis is generally rare, providing an adequate antireflux mechanism is created. Similarly, absorption through the reservoir is not usually a long-term problem, perhaps because the ileal mucosa adapts over time by reduction in villous height, culminating in a nearly flat mucosa with decreased absorptive surface area; only those with impaired renal function are likely to develop hyperchloremic metabolic acidosis.

The Kock pouch procedure continues to be modified, and the technique described here demonstrates the current state of the art. It requires meticulous attention to detail, particularly with respect to the formation of the nipple valves on which the entire success of continence, catheterizability, and prevention of reflux relies. Because of the high learning curve necessitated by this procedure, it is not recommended for the occasional surgeon. Despite suggestions that its performance requires only 1–2 more hours of operating time from the standard ileal conduit, many surgeons find it to be an arduous operation and prefer a two-team approach when it is performed in conjunction with radical cystoprostatectomy.

Since 1983 we have enthusiastically used the Kock pouch technique as a continent cutaneous diversion, orthotopic bladder replacement, and tool for urinary undiversion. Because it is a versatile operation that serves a number of purposes, we have attempted to perfect the procedure. The surgical technique provides for a docile, capacious reservoir which, the majority of the time, will extend into the pelvis or to the abdominal wall. In addition, the antirefluxing nipple is reliable and can protect the upper tracts from further renal impairment. Finally, in our hands, the continence mechanism is dependable and catheterization performed without difficulty.

Technical aspects of the Kock pouch are only

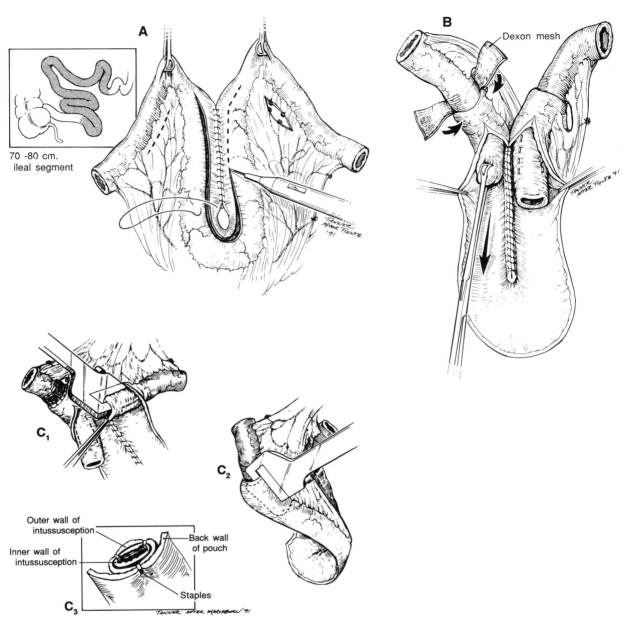

FIG. 8–2 The Kock pouch. **A.** 70–80 cm of ileum are isolated approximately 25 cm proximal to the ileocecal valve. Afferent and efferent limbs are 17 cm long and the pouch is created from two 22-cm segments. The 7–8 cm of mesentery are stripped off of the afferent and efferent limbs and a second opening (window of Deaver) is made a few centimeters away to allow passage of a Marlex strip. **B.** Afferent and efferent continent nipple valves are created. A strip of Dexon mesh is secured around the base of the intussusception, which serves as a collar to fix the limbs to the pouch. **C.** The inner wall of the intussusception is secured with two rows of modified staples at the 10 and 2 o'clock positions using the TA-55 stapler. The back wall of the pouch is secured to the nipple using two rows of unmodified staples (no staples removed from the cartridge) at the 6 o'clock position. **D.** The ureters are anastomosed to the afferent limb using a mucosa-to-mucosa anastomosis, and the pouch closed. **E.** The efferent limb is brought through the abdominal wall and fixed to the rectus fascia using the Dexon collar. A Marlex strip is brought through the window of Deaver supporting the mesentery, thereby avoiding parastomal herniation and providing a direct, straight path for intermittent catheterization.

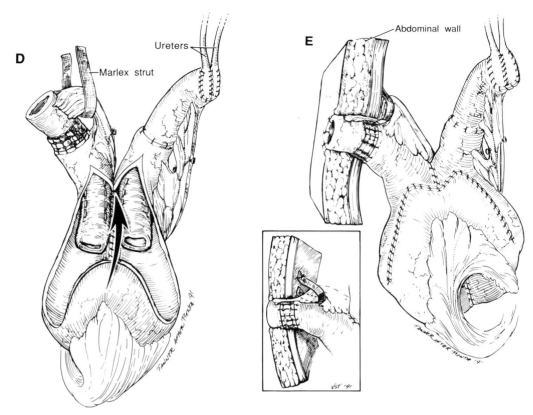

FIG. 8-2   (Continued)

briefly described, as details with current modifications are presented elsewhere.[32] A 70–80 cm length of ileum is isolated, and a 44-cm length at the midportion of the segment is opened along its antimesenteric border and ultimately remodeled to form the reservoir (Fig. 8-2). The antireflux and continence nipples are fashioned by intussusception of the afferent and efferent tubular segments of ileum. A 5–6 cm length nipple is intussuscepted after 8 cm of mesenteric stripping. The nipple is secured by three rows of staples, two through the nipple alone and a third row securing the nipple to the reservoir wall. A collar of Dexon mesh encircles the ileum as it enters the intussusception and is sutured so as to further promote nipple stability and pouch fixation to the abdominal wall. The ureters are stented across the afferent nipple, and the pouch is drained for three weeks by a large-bore catheter through the continent nipple. The pouch is then activated by removal of stents and cathe-

ters after an excretory urogram and a Kock-o-gram confirm no obstruction or extravasation.

Early complications include those of anastomotic urine leakage from the reservoir or uretero-ileal anastomoses, but these are minimized by careful stenting and drainage. Early nipple complications include necrosis or splitting along a staple line, generally ascribed to poor vascular supply and tearing, and manifesting later as reflux or leakage. Leakage can also be due to a short or hypermobile valve, from valve prolapse or valve fistula, which may form at the pin site on the staple line. Difficulty with catheterization can be caused by peristomal hernias or redundancy of the portion of ileum between the abdominal wall and the pouch itself. Late complications include pyelonephritis (1–2%), ureteroileal obstruction (3%), and late ureteral reflux (3%).

Despite the surgical difficulties and the incidence of postoperative problems, most surgeons performing the procedure are enthusiastic, and most patients, even those who have needed one or two revisions, would not trade for an appliance-based urostomy. Skinner reviewed his results in 1988, in 531 patients with Kock pouches, 378 of which were performed in conjunction with radical cystectomy.[32] Perioperative mortality was 1.9%, and operative complications were 16%, although they were higher before technical expertise was acquired. Of 489 patients with Kock pouches and cutaneous stomas, 87 (18%) had urine leakage for any reason. Patient acceptance of the procedure was high, with a 1.5% incidence of conversion to an ileal conduit.[31]

The Kock pouch continues to undergo modifications to improve its reliability and to simplify the surgical technique. One of these modifications includes elimination of the afferent nipple by implantation of the ureters into the afferent limb by either a Camey or split cuff nipple technique, a procedure that is both reliable and considerably short in operative time.[34]

Continent Ileocecal Reservoirs ■

The major criticism of the Kock pouch is that it is a complex, time-consuming operation; however, all recognize its advantages as a capacious low-pressure reservoir with superior bowel dynamics and few or absent phasic contractions. Based on the original work by Gilchrist[24] and because of the simplicity of construction of a right colon reservoir, others continue to improve this procedure either by modifying the ileocecal intussusception to enhance its continence or by colon detubularization or patching with adjacent small bowel to improve reservoir pressure characteristics.

The Gilchrist Ileocecal Reservoir ■

In 1950, Gilchrist described dog investigations and the human trial of an unmodified ileocecal reservoir using slightly over half of the proximal right colon, tunneled reimplants of the ureters into cecum, and a catheterizable ileocutaneous stoma.[24] He later described 40 patients, reporting a 94% complete continence rate with catheterization every 4–6 hours and nightly catheterization, 7% ureteral reflux, 6% reservoir calculi formation, and 4% pyelonephritis.[35] As stated earlier, other surgeons could not reproduce his excellent continence rate.

The Ashken Reservoir ■

The ileocecal valve problem was extensively modified by Ashken in an attempt to improve continence reliability.[36] He initially used an isolated ileocecal segment with the ureters anastomosed to the terminal ileum, protected from reflux by the unmodified ileocecal valve. A separate 5 cm length of ileum was sutured into the open end of the cecum to act as a continence mechanism. However, this method failed, with prolapse of the ileocecal spout valve occurring in three out of seven patients. A modification in which the ileal spout valve was brought through the true ileocecal sphincter similarly failed, as did an ileal spout system fashioned as a flutter valve sewn into the open end of the cecum.[37]

Intussusception of the Ileocecal Valve into Cecum ■

In 1977, a continent cecal reservoir using sutured intussusception of 12 cm of terminal ileum to the ileocecal valve to form a nipple into isolated cecum was described by Zingg and Tscholl.[38] Two of three patients were continent, although devagination of the intussusception at the mesenteric border, similar to that which occurred in the earlier experience of Kock and associates, was reported to be a recurrent problem.

Mansson studied a variety of methods to stabilize the intussuscepted ileocecal valve.[39–41] His final modification uses a 5 cm intussusception of the ileocecal valve with mesenteric exclusion to debulk the intussusception, intestinal staples to secure the nipple valve, and a circumferential rectus fascial strip at the nipple base to stabilize the efferent limb to the skin for catheterization.

This procedure is similar to that described by Webster using the complete right colon and split cuff nipple reimplantation into cecum to prevent reflux.[42] Intussuscepted ileocecal nipple stability was produced by mesenteric exclusion, deep seromuscular coagulation of the intussuscepted serosa to promote fibrosis, three rows of intestinal staples, and a Marlex mesh collar of the efferent limb. Using this technique, the hyperactivity within the nondetubularized right colon segment led to incontinence in three of seven cases, and was controlled using anticholinergic medication.

With further experience the original technique has been modified so that the ileocecal intussusception is performed in an identical fashion with the ileocecal intussusception in a Kock pouch, as reported by Skinner. The entire length of the right colon segment is detubularized and folded on itself to create a pouch, significantly modifying the hyperactivity normally seen in the nondetubularized segments and resolving the problem of spurting incontinence.[42,43] King and associates, attempting to avoid the use of staples, stabilized the intussusception by suturing the intussuscepted nipple to the reservoir wall, using muscle to muscle bonds.[44]

Benchekroun Reservoir ■

Benchekroun has devised a continent urinary reservoir fashioned from 15 cm of nondetubularized right colon with its attached terminal ileum.[16] The ureters were implanted into the terminal ileum with the unmodified ileocecal valve to prevent reflux, and a separate 14 cm segment of ileum on a separate vascular pedicle was isolated and intussuscepted upon itself so that the mucosal surfaces were opposed and the serosal surfaces formed luminal and external surfaces.[16,45] Its construction allows free urine from the pouch to enter between the epithelialized leaves of the intussusception to provide compression along the whole length of the continence mechanism. However, evagination has occurred in 18 of 62 cases, but after revision 58 of 62 patients are continent. High cecal reservoir pressure in the nondetubularized segment was a problem that improved three months postoperatively and was perceived only at filling above 500 ml.

Mainz Pouch ■

Thüroff reported construction of an ileocecal pouch from an open segment of right colon, cecum, and adjacent ileum for continent diversion.[46,47] The pouch so created can be brought to the abdominal wall as a catheterizable stoma relying on an ileoileal intussusception, or to the native urethra, with a prosthetic sphincter for continence. The object of detubularization and patching of the right colon with small intestine was to ablate colonic hyperactivity, and they were moderately successful. Urodynamic evaluation two months postoperatively revealed a mean phasic contractile activity pressure of 63 cm of water, with a mean basal reservoir pressure of 39 cm of water at maximum capacity. An antireflux ureterocolonic an-

astomosis was employed. Six of 12 patients with ileoileal intussusception valve stoma were completely continent, as were an additional three or four patients with a stomal artificial sphincter.

The Mitrofanoff Principle ■

Use of the appendix or an available isolated segment of ureter between the cecal urinary reservoir and the skin was described by Mitrofanoff[48] and further reported by Duckett in the pediatric literature.[49] The catheterizable conduit is narrow and implanted as a submucosal, tunneled nonrefluxing reimplant into the cecal reservoir, as are the afferent ureters. Though a 3–4 cm tunnel was used to prevent reflux, this mechanism failed in 3 of 24 patients. Nonetheless, this procedure is a versatile and seemingly simple one to be considered in the reconstructive armamentarium.

The Indiana Pouch ■

Rowland similarly uses a partially detubularized right colon segment patched with a detubularized section of ileum but relies for continence on a novel technique achieved by plicating the terminal 10 cm of ileum just proximal to the ileocecal valve (Fig. 8-3).[15] Once the pouch has been created and ureters reimplanted by an antireflux method, a 12 French rubber catheter is passed through the terminal portion of the ileum into the pouch to act as a stent over which the plication is performed in two layers, the first layer of interrupted 3–0 silk Lembert sutures placed 8–10 mm apart and the second a running 3–0 silk placed over the first suture line to help reinforce it. At the end of plication the 14 Fr. catheter is held snugly within the sphincter-like reduced lumen of the ileum; however, the segment still can be catheterized with an 18 or 20 Fr. catheter. The stoma is usually brought out through the rectus muscle, and a flushed stoma is created on the abdominal wall. The flexibility of this procedure is that the plicated ileal segment can be adapted for intermittent orthotopic catheterization. The initial volume of the Indiana pouch (500 ml) is greater than the Kock pouch if 25–30 cm of right colon is used, but, despite detubularization, intraluminal reservoir pressures are greater as well. In Rowland's series, no attempt was made to disrupt the tubular configuration of the cecum in the first ten patients undergoing this procedure. Half of the patients ex-

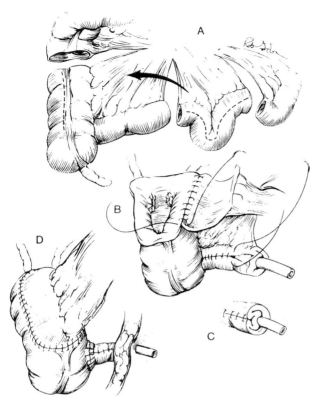

FIG. 8–3 The Indiana Pouch. A low pressure colonic reservoir is created by detubularization and patching with an open ileal segment. The continence mechanism is created by plication of the ileocecal valve and approximately 10 cm of adjacent distal ileum around a 10 Fr. catheter.

perienced incontinence secondary to bolus contractions documented by urodynamic evaluation. These five patients underwent a secondary procedure to prevent these unit contractions and are continent. Rowland's overall daytime continence rate is 93% with 50% of patients dry with once-nightly catheterization, 22% of patients are dry at night without catheterization, and 22% refuse awakening for catheterization and are incontinent at night.

The Florida Pouch ■

Lockhart reports on 170 patients who have underwent a continent urinary diversion using an extended, detubularized right colonic segment as the urinary reservoir, and a plicated distal ileum and

ileocecal valve as a continent catheterizable efferent mechanism. The average reservoir capacity was 747 cc at an average reservoir pressure of 35 cm H_2O. In this series the continence rate, based on a 4–6 hour catheterization program, was 97% with a 1.5% reoperation rate for incontinence. The overall late complication rate was 10% with only 5% necessitating a reoperation for an untoward event.[50]

Orthotopic Bladder Replacement ■

Orthotopic bladder replacement finds its main role in male patients undergoing radical cystoprostatectomy for invasive bladder carcinoma. It is inappropriate management for women with this disease, for an adequate operation in women requires cystourethrectomy. A prerequisite is that a careful dissection and transection of the urethra to be accomplished at the prostatomembranous junction in order to preserve the sphincter mechanism. Obviously any oncologic factors that would dictate a need for urethrectomy contraindicate this approach; such factors appear to exist in approximately 7–10% of patients with bladder cancer undergoing cystoprostatectomy.[51] These patients include those with diffuse carcinoma *in situ,* patients with multifocal bladder tumors, patients with tumors in close proximity to the bladder neck, those with prostatic urethral tumor, and those with advanced disease in whom local pelvic recurrence may be anticipated. However, these actual indications are changing. Levinson and colleagues,[52] after reviewing the records of 200 men who underwent radical cystectomy, noted that significant urethral recurrence (17%) was noted in patients with transitional cell carcinoma involving the prostatic urethra, ducts, or stroma. Patients with solitary tumors, tumors encroaching on the bladder neck, or with carcinoma *in situ,* or multifocal disease not involving the prostate had a low incidence of urethral recurrence (0–4.5%), and were considered appropriate candidates for orthotopic bladder replacement.[52]

In addition to these oncologic factors other features that may mitigate against orthotopic bladder replacement include questionable function of the distal sphincter mechanism either due to preexisting problems or surgical trauma at the time of cystoprostatectomy, female patients, and occasionally anatomic factors. Anatomy is less of a problem now that the range of procedures available has expanded; however, it is notable that a short small bowel mesentery precluded the performance of a Camey operation in approximately 15% of cases. It is probably inadvisable in the aged, infirm individual or the patient unprepared to accept the possibility of continence problems, enuresis, and voiding dysfunction that may require self-catheterization. It is also true to say that these procedures require more refined surgical techniques than the standard cystoprostatectomy and cutaneous urostomy, and should not be performed by the occasional uro-oncologic surgeon.

Currently no consensus exists regarding an optimal orthotopic procedure, and the procedures continue to evolve. Recent developments, including an appreciation of the importance of bowel detubularization and remodeling, and the use of an artificial urinary sphincter, offer further alternatives, even in those patients with sphincter dysfunction.[6] Patients are free of the expense and care of appliance-dependent urostomies and often of catheters as well. Following surgery, patients should understand that gaining control of the new bladder requires some perseverance and fortitude, and sometimes reoperation. Nocturnal enuresis can occur due to an overactive cystoplasty or lack of recruitment of the distal sphincter mechanism. This is best managed by the patient rising to void at least every three hours each night; however, in the event that it persists and the patient is reluctant to rely on a condom catheter, then implantation of an artificial urinary sphincter placed around the bulbous urethra, activated only at night, has proved successful. In the event that incontinence is total, as a result of sphincteric incompetence, an artificial sphincter is the treatment of choice.

The Camey Procedure ■

There is no doubt that Camey has been one of the pioneers in orthotopic diversion, and over 30 years have elapsed since its first performance.[53,54] Currently a 40 cm segment of ileum is selected for mobility to allow the midpoint to be anastomosed to the membranous urethra without tension, and to ensure that the segment is long enough to anastomose to the ureters above the iliac vessels. Camey notes that inability to achieve a tension-free ileourethral anastomosis causes the procedure to be abandoned for an alternative in about 15% of cases.

The ileourethral anastomosis is performed to a 1 cm hiatus on the antimesenteric border of the midpoint of the ileal segment, taking care to avoid injury to the musculature of the membranous urethra by sutures. The ureters are implanted into their respective ileal ends by a LeDuc-Camey 3 cm deepithelialized furrow.[11] All anastomoses are stented for 14 to 16 days; periodic irrigation prevents mucous plugging, and contrast radiograms exclude anatomic leakage before catheter removal.

Camey emphasizes careful dissection of the prostatic apex to preserve the distal sphincter mechanism and preservation of the cavernous nerve to avoid erectile dysfunction. Continence and efficient voiding are the main aims of this procedure. Daytime continence was achieved in 95% of cases performed in the past ten years, though only about 50% of patients have nighttime continence. Sagalowsky reported 80% daytime continence with 100% enuresis.[55] Others have reported even higher daytime incontinence, largely due to the high-pressure contractions in the tubular ileal reservoir. Camey notes peristaltic pressure waves range from 75 to 100 cm of water, but the baseline pressure or compliance of the system is good at its functional capacity. Daytime continence is likely to be partly volitional rather than passive, as a drop of urine forced into the sensitive membranous urethra by the peristaltic waves warns the patient of imminent leakage and induces a strong voluntary temporary external sphincter contraction until the pressure wave passes. Enuresis is probably from a failure of this warning as well as overdistention, and pharmacological ablation has been unsuccessful. Voiding occurs by volitional relaxation of the distal sphincter mechanism and valsalva evacuation. Between 36% and 70% of patients may have sterile urine without prophylaxis. Though ureteral reflux has been seen in about 20% of cases, no stenosis or upper tract deterioration has occurred. In his series the five-year reported survival rate is satisfactory at 56%, with no urethral tumor recurrence in the past 78 cases.

Camey's postoperative complications have declined to 31% over the years, and only one death has been reported since 1970, perhaps due to advances in intensive care, parenteral nutrition, and antibiotics.

The significant possibility of nocturnal enuresis has led by Camey and others to create capacious, low-pressure, docile reservoirs, relying on bowel detubularization and remodeling techniques, often by patching together adjacent open bowel loops.[15,56,57] These procedures can be modified by tapering the bowel segment from the reservoir to the urethra or by prosthetic sphincter to overcome an inefficient distal sphincter mechanism.[15,58]

Ileal Neobladders ■

Melchoir[59] and Hautmann[60] described orthotopic bladder replacement using modified ileal segments in 1988. In the former case, a 40 cm ileal segment is opened on its antimesenteric border, except for its 8 cm proximal segment, which is intussuscepted to create an antirefluxing afferent nipple into which both ureters can be reimplanted. The open ileal segment is then situated in a U shape, anastomosed to the urethral remnant, and closed as a cylindrical detubularized reservoir. Reservoir capacity averaged only 300 ml, requiring voiding originally every two hours, and later every three hours; by six months 95% of the patients had daytime continence, though only 40% had nighttime continence. Morbidity and mortality was similar to the ileal conduit.[59] Hautmann describes a larger ileal reservoir using a 70 cm ileal segment that is completely detubularized. A spherical pouch is fashioned in a W or M shape, anastomosed to the urethra, and the ureters are sewn into the reservoir as tunneled implants. To reduce organized pouch contractions, the bowel is remodeled and closed as a sphere rather than as a cylinder. Initial results are encouraging; reservoir capacity averages 387 ml, with 8 of 11 patients being completely dry day and night, half with nocturia. Three of 11 patients have stress incontinence symptoms during the day.[60]

The Orthotopic Kock ■

Kock modified his pouch so that it could be used as an orthotopic reservoir (Fig. 8-4).[61] It is constructed in the usual fashion using 60 cm of ileum, 44 cm for the reservoir, and 16 cm for the afferent nipple. The reservoir is closed towards the most dependent portion near the urethra. No efferent nipple is constructed; rather, the dependent Kock opening is anastomosed directly to the urethra with approximately six absorbable sutures. The urethral catheter is removed in three weeks if a cystogram and excretory urogram reveal no extravasation. Skinner's results with an orthotopic

Kock pouch parallel those of Melchior, with no daytime incontinence and 50% nighttime incontinence.

Detubularized and remodeled ileal orthotopic reservoirs have the lowest contraction pressures and the highest compliance of all current types of bowel reservoirs; they therefore may be physiologically superior to reservoirs using colon or ileocecal segments. Intrareservoir contraction pressures are generally less than 30 cm of water, usually low enough to avoid forcing urine through a urethral sphincter mechanism with 25–40 cm of water resistance. Colon conduits average 30–40 cm of water contraction pressure and theoretically risk greater incontinence. Any detubularized bowel reservoir may still have contraction sufficient for leakage through a weak native urethral sphincter, in which case an artificial urinary sphincter can be employed.

Orthotopic Ileocecal Segments ■

Ileocecal segments have been used for orthotopic bladder replacement with very good results. Hradec[62] compared various unmodified bowel segments for bladder substitution in 114 patients, and, using urodynamics, felt that ileocecal or sigmoid colon segments had greater capacity, more complete evacuation, and greater flow rates than ileal bladders. Although intrareservoir pressures are higher in colonic or ileocecal reservoirs than ileal reservoirs, even with Heineke-Mikulicz remodeling, the relative simplicity of construction has led to several varieties of reservoirs that differ in technique of remodeling, ureteral implantation, and antireflux mechanism. Each has its own advantages and disadvantages, and patient selection and surgeon preference largely dictate choice.

Unmodified Ileocecal Segments ■

Gil-Vernet,[63] Khafagy[64] and Alcini[65] reported their results with unremodeled ileocecal segments. In each case ureters were implanted directly into the terminal ileum of the segment, and the unmodified ileocecal valve acted as the antireflux mechanism. The urethra was anastomosed directly to the cecum, with continence achieved by an intact external sphincter mechanism. Gil-Vernet reported excellent results in 26 patients with good capacity,

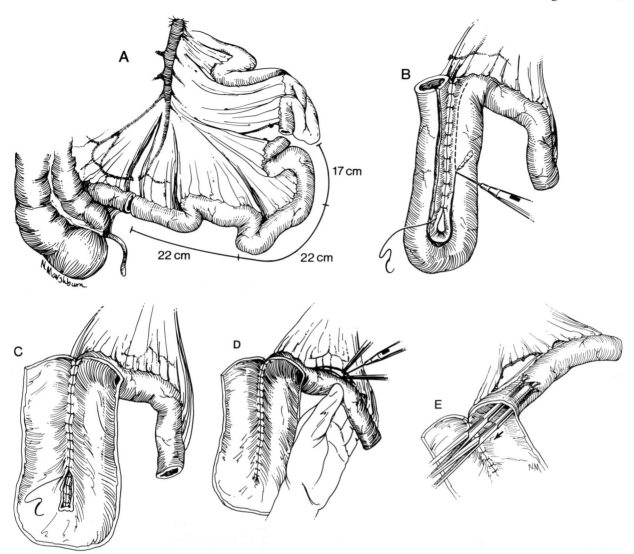

FIG. 8–4   A. Approximately 60 cm of ileum are isolated on its mesentery. **B.** The distal 44 cm of bowel is folded into a U configuration. A side-to-side serosal anastomosis is completed using a continuous suture. The U is then opened using electrocautery. **C.** A full-thickness running suture line reinforces the serosal layer to form the ileal plate. **D.** Two mesenteric windows are created in the still intact 17 cm bowel segment. The 8 cm window should be located just proximal to the ileal plate. One vascular arcade proximal to it, a second window 1 cm wide is formed. **E.** Two small Babcock clamps are passed halfway up the stripped ileum. The ileal wall is grasped from within and intussuscepted to form a nipple approximately 5 cm in length.

(Figure 8–4 con't on following pages)

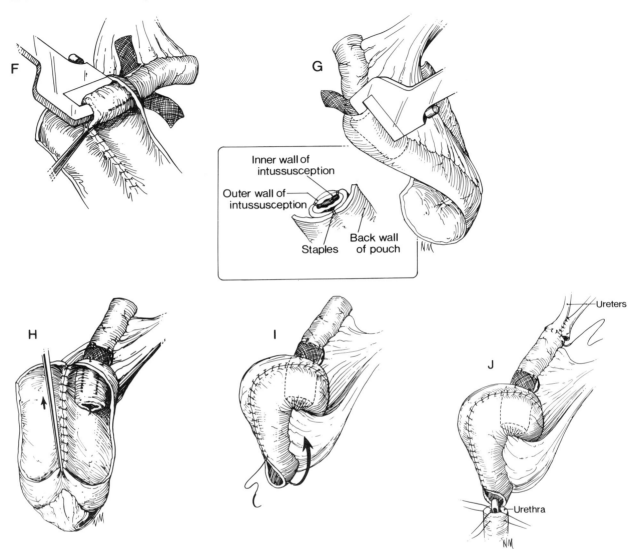

FIG. 8–4 (*Continued*) **F.** Three rows of staples are used to fix the nipple in place. Two rows are placed from "inside the pouch" and fixed the nipple to itself. The fourth row fixes the nipple to the back wall of the pouch (see Fig. G). A 1 cm strip of Dexon mesh is then passed through the previously created mesenteric window and sutured in place. **G.** The third back row of staples fixes the nipple to the back wall of the pouch. **H and I.** Once the Dexon collar is sutured in place, the pouch is folded on itself and closed in two continuous layers. **J.** The open lower end of the pouch is approximated to the pelvic floor so that the length of the afferent ileal limb necessary for ureteroileal anastomosis without tension can be ascertained and any redundant ileal limb excised. A Wallace-type spatulated stented end-to-end ureteroileal anastomosis is performed. The urethral anastomosis is now performed between the membranous urethra and the residual opening at the inferior aspect of the pouch using interrupted sutures. A 20–24 Fr. Foley catheter inserted per urethra across the anastomosis completes pouch construction.

volitional voiding every 4–5 hours, satisfactorily emptying, and a forceful stream.[63] He emphasized that the ileum between the cecum and ureters should be under no tension so as to preserve the antireflux geometry of Bauhin's valve and that cecostomy or appendicostomy should be used for defunctionalization during the healing phases.

Khafagy[64] studied 130 of his patients with carcinoma of the bilharzial bladder. He reported a 15% mortality, mostly due to sepsis, and five patients with fistulae. Most patients had extreme urinary frequency during the early postoperative period. After 12 months 74% of patients voided every two hours or longer. Eighty-two percent of patients reported daytime continence, though 76% of patients had nocturnal enuresis. Bladder capacity exceeded 350 ml and urodynamics demonstrated no vesicoureteral reflux in ten of ten patients studied, and all voided by abdominal straining.

Alcini[65] reported technical aspects similar to those of other investigators in his 26 cases and further noted that his complications of pelvic abscesses and urinary fistulae might be due to preoperative radiation therapy, which has since been discontinued. He reported that all his patients were continent by day, and all patients had nocturnal enuresis to varying degrees for two years postoperatively, which gradually diminished.

Remodeled Ileocolonic Pouch Bladder Replacement Procedures ■

The recently reported Mainz pouch,[46,47] LeBag,[56] and the Indiana pouch[15] typify these procedures. In each, the bowel segment is remodeled by detubularization and adjacent open large and small intestinal plates are combined to form the pouch. This technique is performed in a further effort to inhibit troublesome mass contractions in the distended bowel segment that we have previously noted may lead to incontinence or reflux. In each of these procedures, the exiting bowel segment may be either anastomosed to the residual urethra or brought to the skin surface of the abdominal wall as a continent cutaneous stoma. Suffice it to say here that these remodeling techniques are reported to have achieved their goal, that is, to modify the pressure characteristics within the reservoir. Fluoroscopic evaluation has shown that spontaneous contractions of the large bowel portion are dampened or cancelled by the small bowel

segment of the reservoir; however, it is important to know that these contractions are not in fact lost. In the Mainz pouch series, urodynamics four to eight weeks after surgery revealed that maximum reservoir pressures of 45–90 cm of water (mean, 63 cm of water) were still attained. Basal reservoir pressure between these phasic peristaltic contractions is, however, generally low, and those high-pressure contractions usually only occur at maximum fill, so if a capacious reservoir is constructed, pressures remain relatively low in the functional range of the pouch. Urodynamics in "LeBag" showed the capacity to range from 400–700 ml with the full resting pressure being 20–45 cm of water and low amplitude contractions at capacity remaining below 45 cm of water.

Orthotopic Colonic Reservoirs ■

Right Colocystoplasty Bladder Replacement ■

Camey,[53] Deleveliotis,[66] Hradac,[62] Reddy,[69] and other groups have reported that unmodified colon segments anastomosed to the urethra exhibit very high pressure contractions, which are propagated by the tubular shaped bowel, and lead to incontinence. Zinman and Libertino[67] have recently reported on techniques for right colocystoplasty bladder replacement. This procedure utilizes a nondetubularized right colon segment anastomosed to the membranous urethra or residual apical prostatic capsule. The ureters are anastomosed to the ileal tail, relying on the reinforced ileocecal valve for reflux prevention. Zinman comments on the preservation of the apical prostatic capsule or cuff as aiding in the anastomosis, facilitating potency, and sparing and improving the effectiveness of the continence mechanism. In commenting on this procedure criticisms may be leveled at those very features that actually render this a simple procedure—the inefficient antireflux prevention of the ileocecal valve, the possible "cancer sparing" preservation of the apical prostatic cuff, and the lack of detubularization of the segment—which many would say are responsible for the high incidence of enuresis that occurred in Zinman's series. Alternatively, Goldwasser[57] modified the above technique in seven patients by employing the entire right colon, including the proximal transverse colon as far as the middle colic vessels, to provide a capacious storage reservoir.

The entire segment, except for the most dependent 8 cm of cecum is detubularized and remodeled. The ureters are implanted into the reservoir itself, and the dependent cecum is anastomosed to the membranous urethra. Of seven patients, one was totally incontinent, presumably due to distal sphincter damage, but the other six voided every three to six hours during the day and night and experienced no incontinence. Reservoir capacity varied from 400 to 900 ml, with 20–35 ml residual urine, and voiding occurred by relaxation of the pelvic floor with abdominal valsalva.

Bladder Replacement Together with Artificial Urinary Sphincter Implantation ■

After a decade of improvements and prosthetic design and surgical implantation techniques, the artificial urinary sphincter has achieved an established role in the management of intractable urinary incontinence, and it was natural for this role to be expanded to include patients undergoing total lower urinary tract reconstruction in which the device is implanted around an intestinal neourethra.[58,68] Although certainly less desirable than use of the native urethra and sphincter mechanisms, this alternative does considerably expand the scope for bladder replacement. Exquisite care is necessary to avoid complications such as erosion and infection of the device, and the incidence of revision surgery is high.

Conclusions ■

Contemporary reconstructive urology will see more demands placed on it by patients as quality of life factors such as body image, self-esteem, and sexuality take on a more important role in urologic-oncology. Patients now know that the urostomy bag is not the only alternative to urinary diversion, and will seek more cosmetically appealing options. The field of continent urinary diversion has certainly not matured to the point where any one of these procedures or options can be considered best. Success relies on careful patient selection with particular regard to capabilities, expectations, and prognosis. All of these continent urinary diversions require a strong commitment by a motivated patient to comply with appropriate postoperative instruction and timely review as dictated. Proper patient selection therefore is the key to success and minimal complications. Meticulous surgical technique is needed to achieve the goals of a low-pressure, docile, and capacious reservoir, a stable, functional continence mechanism, and reflux prevention. Most of the aforementioned procedures can attain these goals, and often procedure selection depends on the individual surgeon's philosophy and past experiences, successes, and failures. Eventually, a preferred technique may develop, but in the meantime, it is highly desirable that the operating surgeon be acquainted with features of each of these procedures in order to be versatile when intraoperative circumstances dictate a change. The ultimate role of each of these techniques will be dependent on the results of long-term follow-up in large series with good scientific reporting. Nonetheless, continent diversion procedures have widespread application in improving the quality of life in patients undergoing cystectomy.

References ■

1. Couvelaire PR. Le reservoir ileal de substitution apres la cystectomie totale chez l'homme. J d'Urologie Med Chur 1951;2:408–417.
2. Lilien OM, Camey M. 25 year experience with replacement of the human bladder (Camey Procedure). J Urol 1984;132:886.
3. Bricker EM. Bladder substitution after pelvic evisceration. Surg Clin North Am 1950;30:1511–1521.
4. Slowin KM, Benson MC, Wechsler MH, and Olsson CA. Accepted AUA abstract #844. J Urol (suppl) 1990;143(4):339A.
5. Goldwasser B, Barrett DM, Webster GD, et al: Cystometric properties of ileum and right colon in patients following bladder augmentation, substitution and replacement. J Urol 1987;138:1007–1010.
6. Light JK, Engelman UH: Reconstruction of the lower urinary tract: observations on bowel dynamics and the artificial urinary sphincter. J Urol 1985;133:594–597.
7. Sidi AA, Reinber Y, Gonzales R. Influence of intestinal segment and configuration on outcome of augmentation enterocystoplasty. J Urol 1986;136:1201.
8. Hedlund H, Lindstrom K, Mansson W. Dynamics of a continent cecal reservoir for urinary diversion. Br J Urol 1984;56:366.
9. Leadbetter WF. Consideration of problems incident to performance of ureteroenterostomy: Report of a technique. J Urol 1951;65:818.
10. Goodwin WE, Harris AP, Kaufman JJ, et al: Open, transcolonic ureterointestinal anastomosis: A new approach. Surg Gynecol Obstet 1953;97:295.
11. LeDuc A, Camey M, Teillac P. An original antireflux ureteroileal implantation technique: Long-term follow-up. J Urol 1987;137:1156–1158.

12. Kirby RS, Turner-Warwick R. Substitution Cystoplasty. In: King LR, Stone AR, Webster GD, eds. Bladder reconstruction and continent urinary diversion. Chicago: Yearbook Medical Publishers, 1987:61.

13. King LR. Protection of the Upper Tracts in Undiversion. In: King LR, Stone AR, Webster GD, eds. Bladder reconstruction and continent urinary diversion. Chicago: Yearbook Medical Publishers, 1987:142.

14. Kock NG, Nilson AE, Nillson LO, Nolen LJ, Philipson BM. Urinary diversion via a continent ieal reservoir: Clinical results in 12 patients. J Urol 1982;128:469–475.

15. Rowland RG, Mitchell ME, Bihrle R. The cecoileal continent urinary reservoir. World J Urol 1985;3:185–190.

16. Benchekroun A. Continent cecal bladder. Br J Urol 1982;54:505–506.

17. Ahlering TE, Kanellos A, Boyd SD, Lieskovsky G, Skinner DG, Bernstein L. A comparative study of perioperative complications with Kock pouch urinary diversion in highly irradiated versus nonirradiated patients. J Urol 1988;139:1202–1204.

18. Boyd SD, Feinberg SM, Skinner DG, Lieskovsky G, Baron B, Richardson, J. Quality of life survey of urinary diversion patients: Comparison of ileal conduits vs. continent Kock ileal reservoirs. J Urol 1987;138:1386–1389.

19. Simon J. Ectopia vesicae (absence of the anterior walls of the bladder and pubic abdominal parietes): Operation for diverting the orifices of the ureters into the rectum; temporary success; subsequent death; autopsy. Lancet 1852;2:568.

20. Coffey RC. Physiologic implantation of the severed ureter or combination bile-duct into the intestine. JAMA 1911;56:397–402.

21. Spence HM, Hoffman WW, Fosmine GP. Tumor of the colon as a late complication of ureterosigmoidostomy for exstrophy of the bladder. Br J Urol 1979;51:466.

22. Rink RC, Retik AB. Ureteroileocecosigmoidostomy and Avoidance of Carcinoma of the Colon. In: King LR, Webster GD, Stone AR, eds. Bladder replacement and continent urinary diversion. Chicago: Yearbook Medical Publishers, 1987:252–286.

23. Kock NG, Ghoneim MA, Lycke KG, Mahran MR. Urinary diversion to the augmented and valved rectum: Preliminary results with a novel surgical procedure. J Urol 1988;140:1375–1379.

24. Gilchrist RK, Merrick JW, Hamlin HH, et al. Construction of a substitute bladder and urethra. Surg Gynec Obstet 1950;90:752–760.

25. Kock NG. Intra-abdominal "reservoir" in patients with permanent ileostomy: Preliminary observations on a procedure resulting in fecal "continence" in five ileostomy patients. Archives of Surgery 1969;99:233–235.

26. Watsudji H. Eine Combiniente Anwendung des Hacker- und Fontan'scher Verfahrens bei der Gastrostomie. Mitt'd Med Gesellszh du Tokyo 1899;13:879.

27. Leisenger JH, Sauberli H, Schauwecker H, et al. Continent ileal bladder: First clinical experience. Eur Urol 1976;2:8.

28. Madigan MR. The continent ileostomy and the isolated ileal bladder. Ann R Coll Surg Engl 1976;58:62.

29. Ashken MH. Urinary reservoirs. In: Ashken MH, ed. Urinary diversion. New York: Springer Verlag, 1982:112.

30. Gerber A. The Kock continent ileal reservoir for supravesical urinary diversion: An early experience. Am J Surg 1983;146:15–19.

31. Skinner DG, Lieskovsky GR, Boyd SD. Continuing experience with the continent ileal reservoir (Kock pouch) as an alternative to cutaneous urinary diversion: An update after 250 cases. J Urol 1987;137:1146–1150.

32. Lieskovsky G, Skinner DG, Boyd SD. Complications of the Kock pouch. Urol Clin North Am 1988;15:195.

33. Hendren WH. Reoperative ureteral reimplantation: Management of the difficult case. J Ped Surg 1980;15:770–785.

34. Camey M. Bladder replacement by ileocystoplasty following radical cystectomy. World J Urol 1985;3:161–166.

35. Sullivan H, Gilchrist RK, Merricks JW. Ileocecal substitute bladder: Long-term follow-up. J Urol 1973;109:43–45.

36. Ashken MH. An appliance-free ileocecal urinary diversion: Preliminary communications. Br J Urol 1974;46:631–638.

37. Ashken MH. Urinary Cecal Reservoir. In: King LR, Stone AR, Webster GD, eds. Bladder reconstruction and continent urinary diversion. Chicago: Yearbook Medical Publishers, 1987:238.

38. Zingg E, Tscholl R. Continent cecoileal conduit: Preliminary report. J Urol 1977;118:724–728.

39. Hedlund H, Lindstrom K, Mansson W. Dynamics of a continent cecal reservoir for urinary diversion. Br J Urol 1984;56:366–372.

40. Mansson W, Colleen S, Sundin T. Continent cecal reservoir in urinary diversion. Br J Urol 1984;359:65.

41. Mansson W, Colleen S, Sundin T. The continent cecal reservoir for urinary diversion. World J Urol 1985;3:173–178.

42. Webster GD, Bertram RA. Continent catheterizable urinary diversion using the ileocecal segment with stapled intussusception of the ileocecal valve. J Urol 1986;135:465–469.

43. Norlen L, Trasti H. Functional behavior in a continent ileum for urinary diversion: An experimental and clinical study. Scand J Urol Neph 1978;49:33–35.

44. King LR, Robertson CN, Bertram RA. A new technique for the prevention of reflux in those undergoing bladder substitution or undiversion using bowel segments. World J Urol 1985;3:194–196.

45. Benchekroun A. The ileocecal continent bladder. In: King LR, Webster GD, Stone AR, eds. Bladder reconstruction and continent urinary diversion. Chicago: Yearbook Medical Publishers, 1987:224.

46. Thüroff JW, Alken P, Riedmiller H, Engelmann U, et al. The Mainz pouch (Mixed augmentation ileum and zecum) for bladder augmentation and continent diversion. J Urol 1986;136:17–26.

47. Thüroff JW, Aiken P, Riedmiller H, Engelmann U, et al: The Mainz pouch (mixed augmentation ileum n' Zecum) for bladder augmentation and continent diversion. World J Urol 1986;136:179–184.

48. Mitrofanoff P. Cystostomie continente trans-appendiculaire dans le traitement des vessies neurologiques. Chir Pediatr 1980;21:297–305.

49. Duckett JW, Snyder HM. Use of Mitrofanoff principle in urinary reconstruction. World J Urol 1985;3:191–193.

50. Lockhart JL, Pow-Sang JM, Persky L, Kahn P, Helal M, Sanford E. A continent colonic urinary reservoir: The Florida pouch. J Urol 1990;144:864–876.

51. Schellhammer PF, Whitmore WF. Transitional cell carcinoma of the urethra in men having cystectomy for bladder cancer. J Urol 1976;115:56–59.

52. Levinson AK, Johnson DE, Wishnow KI. Indications for urethrectomy in an era of continent urinary diversion. J Urol 1990;144:73–75.

53. Camey M. Bladder replacement by ileocystoplasty following radical cystectomy. Seminars in Urol 1987;5:8–14.

54. Camey M. Bladder replacement by ileocystoplasty following radical cystectomy. World J Urol 1985;3:161–166.

55. Sagalowsky AI. Experience with the ileal bladder (Camey procedure) and cecoileal reservoirs for continent urinary diversion. Seminars in Urol 1987;5:28–45.

56. Light JK, Engelmann VH. LeBag: Total replacement of the bladder using an ileocolonic pouch. J Urol 1986;136:27–31.

57. Goldwasser B, Barrett DM, Benson AC. Bladder replacement with use of a detubularized right colonic segment: Preliminary report of a new technique. Mayo Clinic Proc 1986;61:615–621.

58. Light JK, Scott FB. Total reconstruction of the lower urinary tract using bowel and the artificial urinary sphincter. J Urol 1984;131:953–956.

59. Melchoir H, Spehr C, Knopf-Wagemann I, et al. The continent ileal bladder for urinary tract reconstruction after cystectomy: A survey of 44 patients. J Urol 1988;139:714–718.

60. Hautmann RE, Egghart G, Frohneberg D, Miller K. The ileal neobladder. J Urol 1988;139:39–42.

61. Kock NG, Ghonheim MA, Lycke KG, Mahran MR. Replacement of the bladder by the urethral Kock pouch: Functional results, urodynamics and radiological features. J Urol 1989;141:1111–1116.

62. Hradec EA. Bladder substitution: Indications and results in 114 operations. J Urol 1965;94:406–417.

63. Gil-Vernet JM. The ileocolic segment in urologic surgery. J Urol 1965;94:418–426.

64. Khafagy MM, el-Kalany M, Ibrahim A, Safa M, et al. Radical cystectomy and ileocecal bladder reconstruction for carcinoma of the bladder. Br J Urol 1987;160:60–63.

65. Alcini E, d'Addessi A, Giustacchini M, et al. Bladder reconstruction after cystectomy: Use of ileocecal segment in 3-loop ileal reservoir. Urol 1988;31:10–13.

66. Deleveliotis A, Macris SG. Replacement of the bladder with an isolated segment of sigmoid: Achievement of physiological urination in patients with carcinoma of the bladder. J Urol 1961;85:564–568.

67. Zinman L, Libertino JA. Right colocystoplasty for bladder replacement. Urol Clin N Am 1986;13:321.

68. Engelmann UH, Light JK, Scott FB. Use of the artificial urinary sphincter with lower urinary tract reconstruction and continent urinary diversion: Clinical and experimental studies. In: King LR, Webster GD, Stone AR eds. Bladder reconstruction and continent urinary diversion. Chicago: Yearbook Medical Publishers, 1987:321–335.

69. Reddy PK, Lange PH, Fraley EE. Bladder replacement after cystoprostatectomy: Efforts to achieve total continence. J Urol 1987;138:495–499.

70. Ghoneim MA. Urinary diversion to the modified rectal bladder (the augmented and valved rectum): An anal sphincter-controlled bladder substitute. In: King LR, Webster GD, Stone AR eds. Bladder reconstruction and continent urinary diversion, 2nd Edition. Chicago: Yearbook Medical Publishers, in press.

Dan L. Longo
Vincent T. DeVita, Jr.

The Use of Combination Chemotherapy in the Treatment of Early Stage Hodgkin's Disease

9

Introduction ■

One principle that emerged from preclinical animal models in anticancer drug development and has been proven time and again in the application of combination chemotherapy programs to patients with cancer is that curability is inversely related to tumor burden.[1] There are a number of clinical situations in which radiation therapy has been used because it was the first available effective therapy. For example, the treatment of early stage (stage I and II) testicular cancer often involved surgical removal of the involved testis followed by radiation therapy delivered to the paraaortic and ipsilateral inguinal nodes in a "hockey stick" field.[2] More recently, however, with the development of combination chemotherapy programs effective in advanced stages of testicular cancer, combination chemotherapy has become the treatment of choice in early stages of testicular cancer, as well.[3,4]

Similarly, radiation therapy has been the treatment of choice for early stages of Hodgkin's disease. The stages that have been considered "early stage," however, have been transformed over the years since the development of effective combination chemotherapy programs. For example, radiation therapy was originally used to treat all patients except those with stage IV disease. Yet it

was apparent that radiation therapy alone was not very effective in patients with stage IIIB disease. Stage IIIB disease therefore became defined as advanced stage disease.

Subsequently, the results of treating patients with stage IIIA disease were felt to be inadequate and anatomic substages of IIIA disease were created to separate patients who responded well to irradiation and those who did not.[5-7] Good prognosis patients had disease limited to the upper abdomen or limited splenic involvement while poor prognosis patients had lower abdominal node involvement or extensive splenic involvement. The addition of combination chemotherapy to radiation therapy appeared to improve the treatment outcome when compared to radiation therapy alone.[8-10] Combined modality therapy, however, is associated with substantially increased toxicity over the use of a single modality. Finally, it was shown that combination chemotherapy alone was superior to radiation therapy[11] and was comparably effective to combined modality therapy[12,13] in patients with stage IIIA disease regardless of the anatomic substage. Therefore, today anatomic substaging of stage III disease is unnecessary and the treatment of choice for all stage III patients, like stage IV patients, is combination chemotherapy.

These developments have left patients with

stage I and II as those considered to have "early stage" disease; such patients are generally treated with total nodal or subtotal nodal irradiation. However, even some subsets of stage II patients are not appropriately treated with radiation therapy alone. For example, patients with massive mediastinal involvement will have a 50–74% relapse rate when treated with radiation therapy alone.[14,15] Furthermore, patients with stage IB and IIB disease who have two of three or all three B symptoms have a worse prognosis than other patients of similar stage treated with radiation therapy alone. Other adverse prognostic factors such as extranodal disease, involvement of three or more nodal groups, elevated erythrocyte sedimentation rate, male sex, advanced age, and mixed cellularity histology have also been reported.[16,17] Thus, some fraction of early stage patients has been separated out, and combined modality therapy has been advocated to optimally control the disease. As experience with the treatment of Hodgkin's disease accumulates, therefore, radiation therapy is the treatment of choice for a smaller and smaller fraction of patients.

Adding chemotherapy to radiation therapy in early stage Hodgkin's disease patients improves disease control; however, overall survival is not significantly higher in patients treated with combined modality therapy.[15,18–21] Usually disease-free survival is about 10%–20% better for patients receiving combined modality therapy, but about 10%–20% of such patients die from secondary acute leukemia related to the use of chemotherapy with radiation therapy together[22,23] or from secondary solid tumors related to the use of radiation therapy.[24] A recent prospective randomized study from Stanford suggests that at least the addition of combination chemotherapy may permit the reduction in radiation fields. Horning and colleagues found that patients receiving involved field radiation therapy plus six cycles of VBM (vinblastine, bleomycin, methotrexate) combination chemotherapy had somewhat better freedom from progression and comparable survival to those treated with total or subtotal nodal radiation fields.[21] Most of the 67 patients in this study had stage IA or IIA disease. It is not yet clear whether VBM—which, to our knowledge, has not been tested in advanced stage disease or in the absence of radiation therapy—would be effective adjuvant therapy in the subgroup of stage IIB patients felt by the Stanford group to require combined modality treatment. The virtue of the VBM regimen is said to be its limited toxicity. It spares fertility and is thought to be less carcinogenic than MOPP. Yet ABVD has

the same virtues[25,26] plus the advantage of having been shown to be as effective as MOPP chemotherapy in advanced stage patients.[27] It is therefore unclear what advantages VBM plus radiation therapy might have over other regimens combined with radiation therapy.

An even more important question relates to whether the results of combined modality therapy are better than would be obtained using chemotherapy alone. Most investigators recognize that one should not use two modalities where one is sufficient.

Combination Chemotherapy vs Combined Modality Therapy in Early Stage Hodgkin's Disease ■

Two prospective randomized studies have examined whether combined modality therapy is superior to combination chemotherapy alone in patients with early stage Hodgkin's disease. Investigators at the University of Maryland Cancer Center randomized 36 patients with stage IB to IIIA disease to receive extended field radiation therapy followed by MOPP combination chemotherapy or to receive MOPP alone.[28] With a median follow-up of over six years, no significant differences occurred between the combined modality group (75% of patients alive and free of disease) and the group treated with MOPP alone (80% of patients alive and free of disease). However, overall toxicity of the two regimens was different. Viral and fungal infections occurred more frequently in the combined modality group. Four of the 17 patients treated with combined modality therapy had toxicities related to the use of radiation therapy: constrictive pericarditis produced limited exercise capacity in two patients, and two patients developed hypothyroidism. There were three second neoplasms: two squamous cell lung cancers (one on each arm of the study) and one acute leukemia in a patient who had received both radiation and chemotherapy. The study is too small to lead to sweeping conclusions; however, there is no evidence that combined modality therapy is more efficacious than combination chemotherapy alone, and it appears to be associated with more late toxicities.

Pavlovsky and his colleagues performed a prospective randomized study in clinical stage I and II patients with Hodgkin's disease, comparing CVPP (cyclophosphamide, vincristine, procarbazine, prednisone) chemotherapy alone to CVPP chemotherapy with involved-field radiation therapy administered between the third and fourth cycles of chemotherapy.[29] Although patients were said to be clinically staged, this examination did not include lymphography in about one-third of the patients. The majority of the patients who did not receive lymphograms were staged by abdominal CT scanning. Patients were not taken to exploratory laparotomy. Thus, it is likely that a considerable fraction of the patients (probably about one-third) had advanced stage disease. Another caveat in interpreting this study is that the cyclophosphamide and vinblastine were given only once per cycle (intravenously on day 1). This is half as frequent as the usual administration of these agents to patients with Hodgkin's disease. Indeed, the median nadir of the white blood cell count with CVPP therapy was 4,100 cells/cu mm. Thus, the chemotherapy was administered in attenuated doses. Both of these features (clinical staging and chemotherapy dose attenuation) would tend to bias the study in favor of the combined modality arm. Nevertheless, in the patients without poor prognostic factors (which in this study included age greater than 46, more than three sites of disease or large mediastinal mass)—which accounted for about 63% of the patients—those randomized to receive CVPP alone had an 88% complete response rate, 77% seven-year disease-free survival, and 92% overall survival at seven years. Patients without poor prognostic factors who received combined modality therapy had a 97% complete response rate, 70% seven-year disease-free survival, and 91% overall survival at seven years. No significant differences existed between dose-attenuated CVPP alone and dose-attenuated CVPP plus involved-field radiation therapy. The treatment outcome in patients with bulky mediastinal disease favored the use of combined modality therapy in this patient subset.

Thus, these studies provide no evidence that combined modality therapy is superior to combination chemotherapy alone in the treatment of early stage Hodgkin's disease.

Lessons from Pediatric Hodgkin's Disease ∎

Pediatric Hodgkin's disease has generally been managed in a distinct fashion from adult Hodgkin's disease for two main reasons: first, children appear to be at a significantly higher risk of developing overwhelming sepsis after splenectomy than adults, and second, radiation therapy to growing bones induces premature fusion of the epiphyseal plates and bone growth retardation. For these reasons, the pediatric oncologists have been pioneers in the use of clinical staging (rather than exploratory laparotomy) and the application of combination chemotherapy to all stages of Hodgkin's disease.

The first reported experience with combination chemotherapy in early stage Hodgkin's disease was from the National Cancer Institute (NCI) project located in Uganda, where there were limited diagnostic and radiotherapy facilities.[30] Forty-eight clinical early stage Ugandan children with Hodgkin's disease were treated with MOPP combination chemotherapy; 42 (88%) achieved a complete response and 75% of the children were alive and free of disease at eight years.

Henry Ekert and his colleagues in Australia and New Zealand have also demonstrated the efficacy of an approach based on the use of combination chemotherapy in clinically staged children.[31] They have treated 38 children with stage I or II Hodgkin's disease with MOPP[32] or ChlVPP[6] (chlorambucil, vinblastine, procarbazine, prednisone). Thirty-seven of these children (97%) obtained a complete response to therapy; one patient relapsed and was induced into a durable second remission by salvage therapy. Two patients tragically died of preventable deaths: fatal graft-vs-host disease after transfusion of nonirradiated blood products. The overall survival was 94% and the disease-free survival was 97%. It is difficult to imagine how combined modality therapy could improve upon these results with optimally delivered combination chemotherapy. Indeed, these results strongly suggest that combination chemotherapy is the treatment of choice for early stages of Hodgkin's disease.

Combination Chemotherapy vs Radiation Therapy in Early Stage Hodgkin's Disease ∎

Two prospective randomized studies compare the efficacy of radiation therapy and combination chemotherapy in early stage Hodgkin's disease. Cimino and colleagues[32] randomized 89 patients with pathological stage IA or IIA disease to receive subtotal nodal radiation therapy or six cycles of MOPP chemotherapy. Complete response was obtained in all patients treated with radiation therapy and in 40 of 44 (91%) patients treated with MOPP. With a median follow-up of five years, the disease-free survival and overall survival of patients treated with radiation therapy was 74% and 94%, respectively. For patients treated with MOPP, disease-free and overall survival were 73% and 87%, respectively. There were no significant differences between the two arms. Relapse on both arms was more common in patients with massive mediastinal disease. The authors raised the concern that patients relapsing from chemotherapy-induced complete remission might be less responsive to salvage therapy since their survival from the time of relapse was 45%, compared to 76% for the group relapsing from radiation therapy. This difference was not statistically significant because of the small numbers of relapsed patients. However, since relapses from radiation therapy tended to occur later than relapses from chemotherapy, the observed differences could be explained entirely by differences in median follow-up of relapsed patients. As would be expected, infertility was a problem for more patients treated with MOPP chemotherapy. All the men were azoospermic and half the women developed amenorrhea after MOPP therapy compared with 0% and 10%, respectively, after irradiation.

At the NCI, we began a prospective randomized trial comparing subtotal nodal radiation to MOPP in early stage Hodgkin's disease in 1978. The study population included 136 patients with stage IA, IB, IIA, IIB, or IIIA$_1$ Hodgkin's disease. Patients were taken to exploratory laparotomy to complete their staging in most cases (92%). Patients with peripheral stage IA disease (usually defined as stage I disease located above the clavicles) were treated with radiation therapy since their survival with this approach is 95% or better in most series. Patients with stage IA (central), IB, IIA, IIB, and IIIA$_1$ were randomized to receive subtotal nodal radiation therapy (mantle and paraaortic fields) or MOPP combination chemotherapy precisely as it was administered to patients with advanced stage disease.

Eighty-one patients were treated with radiation therapy; 30 patients with peripheral stage IA disease and 51 patients randomized to receive radiation therapy. In most studies of the effects of radiation therapy in the treatment of early stage Hodgkin's disease, peripheral IA patients are included. Thus, when we examine the treatment outcome of patients with early stage Hodgkin's disease treated with radiation therapy by Eli Glatstein and his colleagues at the NCI, we see the results depicted in Figure 9-1.[33] The disease-free

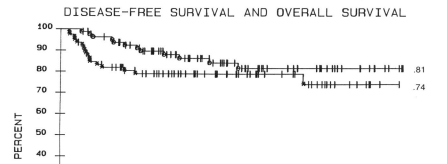

EARLY STAGE HODGKIN'S DISEASE: RADIATION THERAPY
DISEASE-FREE SURVIVAL AND OVERALL SURVIVAL

Legend: * DFS   o SURVIVAL
          17/79 failed   12/81 failed

FIG. 9–1 Kaplan-Meier plot of disease-free (*) and overall survival (o) of all patients who received radiation therapy on the NCI early stage Hodgkin's disease study (30 nonrandomized peripheral IA plus 51 randomized central IA, IB, IIA, IIB, or IIIA$_1$ patients).

survival at ten years is 74% and the overall survival is 81%. These results are completely comparable to the best results in the literature. This point is not a trivial one since not all radiation therapists achieve the same excellent results as those reported from Stanford with radiation therapy alone. Reputable academic treatment centers have reported relapse rates from radiation therapy twice as high as those observed at Stanford. It is an accepted notion that alterations in schedule and reductions in doses during the administration of combination chemotherapy programs compromise efficacy. It has been less commonly acknowledged that there are also important technical factors in the administration of excellent radiation therapy that make an impact on the results. The Patterns of Care study documented that relapse rates for stage IIA Hodgkin's disease varied from 14% to 39% at different institutions and that over one-third of randomly reviewed portal films failed to encompass the known extent of disease.[34,35] When the portal films were adequate, the results were excellent. When disease was left out of the treatment portal, relapse rates were high. Thus, Figure 9-1 confirms that the NCI treatment outcome from radiation therapy alone is as good as could be expected anywhere in the world.

In the randomized portion of the NCI study, pa-tients with stages IA (central), IB, IIA, IIB, and IIIA$_1$ were randomized to receive radiation therapy or chemotherapy. Forty-nine of the 51 patients (96%) who received radiation therapy achieved a complete remission, but 17 (35%) of the complete responders relapsed, 7 within the treatment portals, 5 outside a treatment portal, and 5 both within and outside a treatment portal. Ten (20%) patients randomized to receive radiation therapy have died, 7 with Hodgkin's disease and 3 free of Hodgkin's disease. Fifty-two of the 54 evaluable patients (96%) who were randomized to receive MOPP chemotherapy achieved a complete response. Seven (13%) patients relapsed, all in previously involved sites of disease. Four (7%) patients have died—three with Hodgkin's disease and one free of disease. Figure 9-2 shows the disease-free survival of the complete responders on the randomized portion of the study. The 10-year disease-free survival of MOPP-treated patients is 86%; for radiation therapy-treated patients, the 10-year disease-free survival is 60%. The difference between these curves is statistically significant in favor of MOPP treatment ($P_2 = 0.009$). Figure 9-3 shows the overall survival for all randomized patients. The 10-year overall survival for MOPP-treated patients is 92%; the 10-year overall survival for radiation therapy-treated patients is 76%.

FIG. 9–2 Kaplan-Meier plot of disease-free survival of patients randomized to receive MOPP (*) or radiation therapy (o) who achieved complete response on the NCI early stage Hodgkin's disease study. Disease-free was significantly higher among patients treated with MOPP chemotherapy.

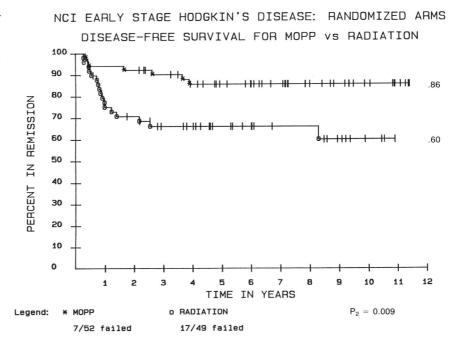

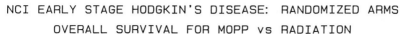

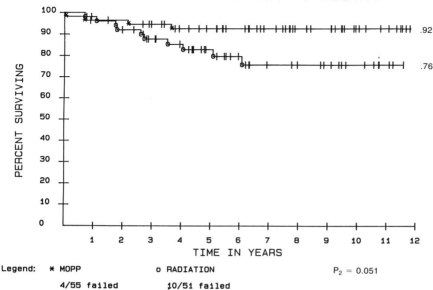

NCI EARLY STAGE HODGKIN'S DISEASE: RANDOMIZED ARMS

OVERALL SURVIVAL FOR MOPP vs RADIATION

Legend: * MOPP   o RADIATION $P_2 = 0.051$

4/55 failed   10/51 failed

FIG. 9–3 Kaplan-Meier plot of overall survival of patients randomized to receive MOPP (*) or radiation therapy (o) on the NCI early stage Hodgkin's disease study. MOPP-treated patients had a survival advantage of borderline statistical significance.

The difference between the curves is on the borderline for statistical significance in favor of MOPP treatment ($P_2 = 0.051$).

The study by Cimino and colleagues[32] raised the concern that patients relapsing from a MOPP-induced complete response might be more refractory to salvage therapy than those relapsing after radiation therapy. In our study, eight of 17 patients (47%) relapsing after radiation therapy are alive and free of disease after salvage therapy. Three of the seven (43%) patients relapsing from a MOPP-induced complete response are alive and free of disease after salvage therapy. Thus, although the number of patients in our study is also small, we do not at this time see evidence that relapsed patients are more refractory to salvage therapy if their primary treatment was combination chemotherapy.

Analysis of prognostic factors demonstrated that the advantage of MOPP over radiation therapy was highly significant in two groups of patients: those with massive mediastinal involvement and those with stage IIIA$_1$ disease. All eleven such patients treated with MOPP are alive and free of disease in their first remission. On the other hand, six of the eight patients with massive mediastinal or stage IIIA$_1$ disease who randomized to receive radiation therapy have relapsed and five have died ($P_2 = 0.0004$ for disease-free survival;

$P_2 = 0.0015$ for overall survival—both in favor of MOPP). When these two subsets of patients are excluded from both arms of the randomized study, the differences between MOPP and radiation in disease-free (Fig. 9-4) and overall survival (Fig. 9-5) are no longer significant. Thus, in the subsets of patients generally treated with radiation therapy today, MOPP combination chemotherapy and radiation therapy are equally effective.

Toxicity Trade-Offs in Making the Treatment Decision ■

In light of two prospective randomized studies suggesting that radiation therapy and combination chemotherapy are comparably effective in patients with stage I and II Hodgkin's disease, it is important to consider the relative risks associated with each treatment approach and weigh these factors in the treatment decision.

Patients for whom radiation therapy is a treatment option must undergo exploratory laparotomy, since there is no enthusiasm for irradiating clinically staged patients. If there were reliable ways of evaluating the spleen and upper abdomen for Hodgkin's disease involvement, this situation

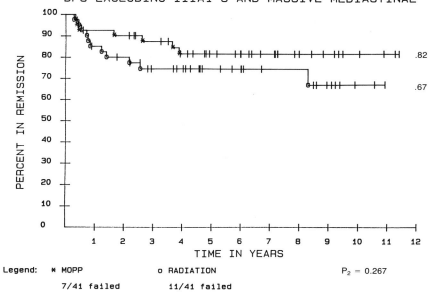

FIG. 9–4 Kaplan-Meier plot of disease-free survival of patients randomized to receive MOPP (*) or radiation therapy (o) who achieved a complete response, omitting those with either massive mediastinal involvement or stage IIIA₁ disease. The difference between MOPP and radiation therapy is no longer statistically significant when these two patient subsets are excluded from the analysis.

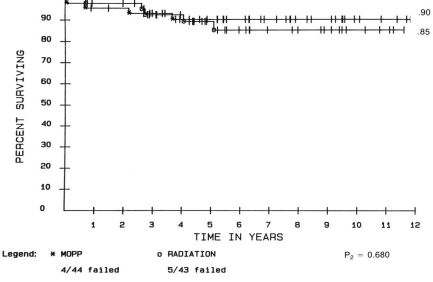

FIG. 9–5 Kaplan-Meier plot of overall survival of patients randomized to receive MOPP (*) or radiation therapy (o), omitting those with either massive mediastinal involvement or stage IIIA₁ disease. The difference between MOPP and radiation therapy is no longer significant when these two patient subsets are excluded from the analysis.

could change. At the moment, however, the use of radiation therapy as the sole treatment modality implies invasive staging. There is a 1–3% mortality rate from the splenectomy procedure and 10–15% of patients have serious perioperative morbidity (infection, bleeding, wound dehiscence). Another small fraction of patients have chronic postoperative problems, some requiring repeat operations (*e.g.*, obstruction from adhesions). The long-term sequelae of splenectomy are mainly related to infection (reviewed by Bookman and Longo[36]). About 28% of splenectomized Hodgkin's disease patients get one or more serious infections within the first six years after the operation, generally in the setting of salvage chemotherapy after radiation relapse.[37] Patients are particularly susceptible to the pneumococcus, and to a lesser extent Staphylococcal species and gram negative organisms. Splenectomized patients cannot respond to polysaccharide vaccines such as pneumovax; thus, patients should receive it before splenectomy or not at all. Recently it has been claimed that patients who undergo splenectomy are at an increased risk of developing secondary acute leukemia.[38,39] If patients who are taken to exploratory laparotomy are more commonly treated with combined modality therapy in these series, the association is spurious. On the other hand, if splenectomy is an independent risk factor for developing secondary acute leukemia, we should stop staging patients with exploratory laparotomy. Unfortunately, none of the papers reporting the association of splenectomy and acute leukemia provide sufficient data to evaluate whether this is a finding we should take seriously. It is important to note that the problems associated with exploratory laparotomy are a consequence of attempting to make the patient a candidate for radiation therapy treatment. On average, about a third of patients taken to laparotomy will have undergone the procedure in vain since disease will be found in the abdomen and those patients will require chemotherapy treatment in spite of the laparotomy.

Radiation therapy is generally less toxic acutely than most combination chemotherapy programs, with the possible exception of ChlVPP. Myelosuppression may occur, but is generally mild. Mucositis and esophagitis may occur in a minority of patients. The most troublesome toxicities associated with the use of radiation therapy are late toxicities. Many patients develop ageusia, and most patients produce considerably less saliva after treatment. This problem can lead to dental caries. An occasional patient has persistent xerostomia. The majority of Hodgkin's disease patients treated with radiation develop thyroid dysfunction. In the NCI randomized study, 47 of the 68 living patients (69%) evaluable for toxicity who were treated with radiation therapy are on synthroid due to thyrotropin elevations or low thyroxine levels. This poses a problem that is not insignificant. Too vigorous thyroid replacement with the maintenance of thyrotropin levels that are too low can result in accelerated bone demineralization and osteoporosis. Too little thyroid replacement can result in hypothyroidism, goiter, and even thyroid neoplasia 20 years or more following treatment. Acute pulmonary problems can occur if a substantial fraction of lung tissue receives the mantle-field dose of radiation therapy. Steroids are probably helpful in acute radiation pneumonitis. It is important to avoid high FIO2 if possible since oxygen can make the radiation pneumonitis considerably worse. Late lung sequelae of radiation injury include fibrosis, scarring, and loss of lung volume. This problem is rare with modern radiation technique. Cardiac problems are also rare with equally weighted anterior and posterior treatment ports; however, if anteriorly weighted ports are used, a significant fraction of patients may develop constrictive pericarditis in the first decade after treatment that may require pericardial stripping to alleviate. Some loss of ventricular function independent of the pericardial disease has also been seen in this setting. Radiation therapy does not lead to infertility unless the gonads receive significant scatter irradiation. Generally, fertility is preserved.

The major reason to fear radiation therapy is the development of second solid tumors. At 15 years after treatment, 13% of patients will have developed a second solid tumor, and it appears that the risk continues to increase with time.[24] Radiated patients appear to be at significantly increased incidence of lung cancer, melanoma, breast cancer, thyroid cancer, sarcomas, and gastric cancer. Although patients treated with radiation therapy alone have a low risk of developing secondary acute leukemia, about one-third of radiation-treated patients will relapse and require combination chemotherapy for optimal disease control. The comparable survival of patients treated with radiation therapy and combination chemotherapy is due at least in part to the fact that a substantial fraction of the patients relapsing after radiation therapy received salvage chemotherapy. Thus, the fraction of patients that received combined modality therapy is at an increased risk of secondary acute leukemia, which may affect up to 10% of patients in the first decade after treatment, but the risk declines after that time.[23] The magnitude of the leukemic risk is considerably smaller than the risk of other second tumors. Appropriate surveillance may detect the second tumors at a more treatable stage. So far, however, there is no evidence that patients treated with combination chemotherapy alone are at an increased risk of second solid tumors, and the risk in radiated patients does not seem to be increased by the use of chemotherapy.

A major drawback to using MOPP combination chemotherapy is that it produces more nausea and vomiting and myelosuppression than radiation therapy acutely. However, there is evidence that ChlVPP combination chemotherapy is equally effective in patients with advanced stage disease and is considerably better tolerated. By inference and according to the experience reported by Ekert in children with clinical early stage disease, ChlVPP should be effective in adults with clinical early stage disease who have an extraordinary fear of nausea and vomiting. The major chronic toxicity of concern with MOPP chemotherapy is infertility, which affects nearly 100% of men and the majority of women over age 26. Interviews with patients who entered the NCI randomized study suggested that this toxicity may affect only a fraction of patients. Among the 21 men evaluated who were treated with MOPP chemotherapy, only four wanted children. Among 30 women treated with MOPP, ten desired to have children and six were successful. Nevertheless, for individual patients in whom fertility status is an overriding concern, ABVD chemotherapy appears considerably less toxic to both the male and female gonads and, by inference, is as effective as MOPP chemotherapy. Thus, primary fertility-sparing chemotherapy is a valid option for this patient subset.

The concern about secondary acute leukemia in patients treated with MOPP is virtually without basis. The major risk of acute leukemia is in patients who are treated with combined modality therapy and those who receive multiple courses of induction therapy or maintenance therapy. The leukemic risk from six cycles of MOPP combination chemotherapy is very low. Pedersen-Bjergaard and colleagues[40] showed that there is a dose threshold for the small leukemic risk associated with chemotherapy alone and that threshold generally begins at about eight cycles of MOPP. In 27 years of using the regimen at the NCI, we have seen only a single case of acute leukemia occurring in a patient who received only six cycles of MOPP chemotherapy. However, if a particular patient's fear of acute leukemia is greater than fear of second solid tumors, one can recommend ABVD chemotherapy, which is considerably less leukemogenic even when combined with radiation therapy. The risk of leukemia from ABVD alone is very near zero and may be as low as the risk of leukemia from radiation therapy alone. The use of ABVD has the virtue of sparing the patient the late risk of secondary solid tumors.

Conclusions and Treatment Recommendations ■

There appears to be consensus that patients with peripheral stage IA Hodgkin's disease should receive radiation therapy, a mini-mantle field for presentations above the diaphragm and an inverted-Y for presentations below the diaphragm. For patients who have massive mediastinal involvement, most investigators would recommend treatment with combined modality therapy, though some have suggested that the results may be as good with primary radiation therapy followed by salvage chemotherapy for the 50–74% of patients who relapse. If one wishes to maximize the chances that the first treatment will cure the patient, primary combined modality therapy is probably the treatment of choice.

For patients with clinical advanced stage disease with or without B symptoms, primary combination chemotherapy is the treatment of choice. A minority of patients (~15%) with slowly responding nodal disease might benefit from involved field radiation therapy after a clinical complete response has been achieved with combination chemotherapy. However, routine use of radiation therapy in patients with advanced stage disease has been shown to be ineffective at lowering relapse rates in prospective randomized trials.[13,41]

For patients with clinical early stage disease and B symptoms, the choice would seem to be straightforward—primary combination chemotherapy. If one is considering the use of radiation therapy, the patient would need to undergo the acute and chronic morbidity of exploratory laparotomy, and the probability that such a patient actually has advanced stage disease is about 50%. Even in the event that the exploratory laparotomy confirms the absence of advanced stage disease, many radiation therapy groups recommend that patients with stage IIB disease receive combined modality therapy. It makes no sense to subject such patients to the risks and toxicities of laparotomy and the toxicities associated with radiation therapy, combination chemotherapy, and combined modality therapy. The strategy that minimizes the risk of toxicity and maximizes the chances for cure is primary combination chemotherapy without taking the patient to laparotomy. If fertility is a major consideration, ABVD chemotherapy would seem the best choice.

For patients with clinical early stage disease without B symptoms, there are more choices of management approaches. Combination chemotherapy with MOPP, MVPP, ChlVPP, ABVD, MOPP/ABVD, or MOPP/ABV hybrid programs would be highly likely to cure the patient. Indeed, it cannot be said that any other approach is more likely to result in cure. On the other hand, if the fear of chemotherapy side-effects is overwhelming, such patients can undergo staging laparotomy and splenectomy risks and have about a 75% chance of being found to have pathological stage IA or IIA disease. Stage IA or IIA disease can be managed with radiation therapy alone. This patient has avoided chemotherapy risks and accepted laparotomy and radiotherapy risks. On the other hand, the patient has a 25% chance of being found to require combination chemotherapy for treatment of advanced stage disease after laparotomy. In such a circumstance, undergoing laparotomy has added its risk to the toxicities of chemotherapy. Furthermore, for the one-third of irradiated patients who relapse, chemotherapy will be required to control the disease. Thus, another 25% of the patients who undergo laparotomy will require chemotherapy. So about half the people who are taken to laparotomy will need chemotherapy anyway (25% with advanced disease at laparotomy and 25% treated with radiation therapy who relapse). Again it would appear that primary chemotherapy after clinical staging would be a reasonable strategy to maximize the chances for long-term disease control and minimize toxicities. ABVD would be the best choice if the problem of infertility was of paramount importance.

References ■

1. DeVita VT Jr. The relationship between tumor mass and resistance to chemotherapy: implications for surgical adjuvant treatment of cancer. Cancer 1983;1209:51.
2. Hussey DH, Luk KH, Johnson DE. The role of radiation therapy in the treatment of germinal cell tumors of the testis other than pure seminoma. Radiology 1977; 175:123.
3. Einhorn LH. Adjuvant therapy of testis cancer. In: Salmon SE, ed. Adjuvant therapy of cancer VI. Philadelphia: WB Saunders, 1990:471–474.
4. Horwich A, Dearnaley DP, Nicholls J, Jay G, Mason M, Harland S, Peckham MJ, et al. Effectiveness of carboplatin, etoposide, and bleomycin combination chemotherapy in good-prognosis metastatic testicular nonseminomatous germ cell tumors. J Clin Oncol 1991;9:62–69.
5. Golomb HM, Sweet DL, Ultmann JE, Miller JB, Kinzie JJ, Gordon LI. Importance of substaging of stage III Hodgkin's disease. Sem Oncol 1980;7:136–143.
6. Stein RS, Golomb HM, Mauch P, Hellman S, Wiernik PH, Ultmann JE, Rosenthal DS. Anatomic substages of stage IIIA Hodgkin's disease: a collaborative study. Ann Intern Med 1980;92:159–165.
7. Hoppe RT, Cox RS, Rosenberg SA, et al. Prognostic factors in pathologic stage III Hodgkin's disease. Cancer Treat Rep 1982;66:743–749.
8. Mauch P, Goffman T, Rosenthal DS, Canellos GP, Come SE, Hellman S. Stage III Hodgkin's disease: improved survival with combined modality therapy as compared with radiation alone. J Clin Oncol 1985;3:1166–1173.
9. Prosnitz LR, Cooper D, Cox EB, et al. Treatment selection for stage IIIA Hodgkin's disease patients. Int J Radiat Oncol Biol Phys 1985;11:1431–1436.
10. Willett CD, Linggood RM, Meyer J, et al. Results of treatment of stage IIIA Hodgkin's disease. Cancer 1987;59:27–35.
11. Lister JA, Dorreen MS, Faux M, Jones AE, Wrigley PFM. The treatment of stage IIIA Hodgkin's disease. J Clin Oncol 1983;1:745–749.
12. Crowther D, Wagstaff J, Deakin D, et al. A randomized study comparing chemotherapy alone with chemotherapy followed by radiotherapy in patients with pathologically staged IIIA Hodgkin's disease. J Clin Oncol 1984;2:892–897.
13. Grozea PN, DePersio EJ, Coltman CA Jr, et al. A Southwest Oncology Group study: chemotherapy versus chemotherapy plus radiotherapy in stage III Hodgkin's disease. Rec Results Cancer Res 1982;80:83–91.
14. Lee CK, Bloomfield CD, Goldman AI, Levitt SH. Prognostic significance of mediastinal involvement in Hodgkin's disease treated with curative radiotherapy. Cancer 1980;46:2403–2409.
15. Hoppe RT, Coleman CN, Cox RS, Rosenberg SA, Kaplan HS. The management of stage I-II Hodgkin's disease with irradiation alone or combined modality therapy: the Stanford experience. Blood 1982;59:455–465.
16. Crnkovich MH, Leopold K, Hoppe RT, Mauch PM. Stage I to IIB Hodgkin's disease: the combined experience at Stanford University and the Joint Center for Radiation Therapy. J Clin Oncol 1987;5:1041–1049.
17. Crnkovich MJ, Hoppe RT, Rosenberg SA. Stage IIB Hodgkin's disease: the Stanford experience. J Clin Oncol 1986;4:472–479.
18. Hagemeister FB, Fuller LM, Velasquez WS, et al. Stage I and II Hodgkin's disease: involved-field radiotherapy versus extended-field radiotherapy versus involved-field radiotherapy followed by six cycles of MOPP. Cancer Treat Rep 1982;66:789–798.
19. Nissen NI, Nordentoft AM. Radiotherapy versus combined modality treatment of stage I and II Hodgkin's disease. Cancer Treat Rep 1982;66:799–803.
20. Anderson H, Deakin DP, Wagstaff J, et al. A randomized

study of adjuvant chemotherapy after mantle radiotherapy in supradiaphragmatic Hodgkin's disease PS IIA-IIB: a report from the Manchester Lymphoma Group. Br J Cancer 1984;49:695–702.

21. Horning SJ, Hoppe RT, Hancock SL, Rosenberg SA. Vinblastine, bleomycin, and methotrexate: an effective adjuvant in favorable Hodgkin's disease. J Clin Oncol 1988;6:1822–1831.

22. Coleman CN, Williams CJ, Flint A, et al. Hematologic neoplasia in patients treated for Hodgkin's disease. N Engl J Med 1977;297:1249–1252.

23. Blayney DW, Longo DL, Young RC, et al. Decreasing risk of leukemia with prolonged follow-up after chemotherapy and radiotherapy for Hodgkin's disease. N Engl J Med 1987;316:710–714.

24. Tucker MA, Coleman CN, Cox RS, et al. Risk of second cancers after treatment for Hodgkin's disease. N Engl J Med 1988;318:76–81.

25. Viviani S, Santoro A, Ragni G, et al. Gonadal toxicity after combination chemotherapy for Hodgkin's disease. Comparative results of MOPP versus ABVD. Eur J Cancer Clin Oncol 1985;21:601–605.

26. Valagussa P, Santoro A, Fossati-Bellani F, et al. Second acute leukemia and other malignancies following treatment for Hodgkin's disease. J Clin Oncol 1986;4:830–837.

27. Bonadonna G, Zucali R, Monfardini S, et al. Combination chemotherapy of Hodgkin's disease with adriamycin, bleomycin, vinblastine, and imidazole carboximide versus MOPP. Cancer 1975;36:252–259.

28. O'Dwyer PJ, Wiernik PH, Stewart MB, Slawson RG. Treatment of early stage Hodgkin's disease: a randomized trial of radiotherapy plus chemotherapy versus chemotherapy alone. In: Cavalli F, Bonadonna G, Rozencweig M, eds. Malignant Lymphomas and Hodgkin's Disease: Experimental and Therapeutic Advances. Boston, Martinus Nijhoff, 1985:329–336.

29. Pavlovsky S, Maschio M, Santarelli MT, et al. Randomized trial of chemotherapy versus chemotherapy plus radiotherapy for stage I-II Hodgkin's disease. J Natl Cancer Inst 1988;80:1466–1473.

30. Olweny CLM, Katongole-Mbidde E, Kiive C, et al. Childhood Hodgkin's disease in Uganda: A 10-year experience. Cancer 1978;42:787–792.

31. Ekert H, Waters KD, Smith PJ, Toogood I, Mauger D. Treatment with MOPP of ChlVPP chemotherapy only for all stages of childhood Hodgkin's disease. J Clin Oncol 1988;6:1845–1850.

32. Cimino G, Biti GP, Anselmo AP, et al. MOPP chemotherapy versus extended-field radiotherapy in the management of pathological stages I-IIA Hodgkin's disease. J Clin Oncol 1989;7:732–737.

33. Longo DL, Glatstein E, Duffey PL, et al. Radiation therapy versus combination chemotherapy in the treatment of early stage Hodgkin's disease: seven-year results of a prospective randomized trial. J Clin Oncol 1991;9.

34. Hanks GE, Kinzie JJ, White RL, et al. Patterns of Care outcome studies: results of the national practice in Hodgkin's disease. Cancer 1983;51:569–573.

35. Kinzie JJ, Hanks GE, Maclean CJ, Kramer S. Patterns of Care study: Hodgkin's disease relapse rates and adequacy of portals. Cancer 1983;52:2223–2226.

36. Bookman MA, Longo DL. Concomitant medical illness in patients treated for Hodgkin's disease. Cancer Treat Rev 1986;13:77–111.

37. Coker DD, Morris DM, Coleman JJ, et al. Infection among 210 patients with surgically staged Hodgkin's disease. Am J Med 1983;75:97–109.

38. Van der Velden JW, Van Putten WL, Guinee VF, et al. Subsequent development of acute nonlymphocytic leukemia in patients treated for Hodgkin's disease. Int J Cancer 1988;42:252–255.

39. Kaldor JM, Day NE, Clarke EA, et al. Leukemia following Hodgkin's disease. N Engl J Med 1990;322:7–13.

40. Pedersen-Bjergaard J, Specht L, Larsen SO, et al. Risk of therapy-related leukaemia and preleukaemia after Hodgkin's disease. Relation to age, cumulative dose of alkylating agents, and time from chemotherapy. Lancet 1987;ii:83–88.

41. Glick J, Tsiatis A, Chen M, et al. Improved survival with MOPP-ABVD compared to BCVPP ± radiotherapy for advanced Hodgkin's disease: 6-year ECOG results (abstract 1392). Blood 1990;76:350a.

Thomas H. Shawker
Jeffrey A. Norton
Edward H. Oldfield

The Use of Intraoperative Ultrasound During Cancer Surgery

10

Intraoperative ultrasound imaging is one of the newest and most promising applications of ultrasound technology.[1,2] In skilled hands, it can shorten and simplify surgery and increase the chances of a favorable surgical outcome for the cancer patient. Using its broadest definition, intraoperative ultrasound is any use of ultrasound technology in the operating room. It could therefore be said to encompass techniques and equipment ranging from nonimaging continuous-wave Doppler probes and ultrasonic cauteries to the new ultrasound endoscopy and angiographic units. For the purposes of this chapter, however, a more narrow and more commonly accepted definition will be used—intraoperative ultrasound is the employment of an ultrasound transducer directly on or near a surgically exposed organ to obtain a real-time ultrasound image.

Ultrasound images are produced from transducers consisting of one or more piezoelectric crystals that both generate an ultrasound beam and receive an echo back. Ultrasound sound waves, at a frequency of 2–10 MHz, are focused as a beam and sent into the body as a pulse. This high frequency ultrasound beam is propagated through the body as a pressure wave. During its passage, the beam interacts with organs and tissues in the body. Where it encounters a tissue interface, that is, a region where two adjacent tis-

sues differ in their density or elasticity, part of the beam is reflected back to the transducer. The returning reflection or echo strikes the transducer crystal and by piezoelectric effect generates a small electrical pulse. This pulse, along with others reflected from different structures the beam encounters in its trip through the body, is displayed on a television monitor in shades of gray corresponding to the magnitude of the returning echo. The gray scale assignment is dependent on the degree of tissue interface mismatch. For instance, the boundary between two adjacent organs would generate a stronger mismatch and therefore a higher intensity reflection (whiter on the image) than the structures comprising the parenchyma of a large organ such as the liver. By measuring the time elapsed from the generation of the beam to the time of the returning echo, the ultrasound scanner displays the returning echo at the correct tissue depth on the television monitor.

Ultrasound images display only soft tissues; at ultrasound frequencies beam transmission is stopped completely by air and bone. The more inhomogeneous the tissue the greater the echo-producing characteristics. Structures such as fluid-filled cysts that have few or no internal interfaces are displayed on the video monitor as echo free (hypoechoic) or black with no white echoes. Some very homogeneous solid tumors, such as lymphomas, will also have few areas of acoustic mismatch, and the interior of the tumor will either be echo-free or have relatively few internal echoes. By contrast, other tumors, such as a sarcoma with areas of necrosis, generate areas of high acoustic mismatch that produce ultrasound images that have many internal echoes of varying amplitude (hyperechoic or echogenic).

The equipment used in intraoperative ultrasound is generally the same as that used in non-intraoperative studies. These units or "scanners" have gray-scale displays and use real-time sector or real-time linear transducers. "Real-time" transducers generate a "real-time" image on the video monitor. By continually sweeping the beam back and forth, either mechanically or electronically, these transducers generate a continuous or "fluoroscopic" image of the soft tissues on the television monitor. A wide range of transducer formats, designs, and frequencies is available.

When considering the selection of ultrasound equipment for intraoperative use, the first and major consideration is the type of transducer needed.[3] If the transducer cannot be placed in the exposed surgical area or if it does not give adequate resolution at the required depth, then the intraoperative ultrasound study will fail. Transducers are chosen based on the depth of penetration required and on the physical shape and size of the transducer that can be used in the exposed surgical field. For most intraoperative applications, transducers with a frequency range of from 5 to 10 MHz are used. The higher the frequency, the better the resolution but the poorer the penetration into tissue. For most intraoperative applications, the depth of penetration needed is relatively short, generally less than 4 cm, so high-frequency transducers can be employed. For instance, to examine a relatively thin organ like the pancreas, one might choose a 7 or 10 MHz transducer. In other organs, lower frequency transducers, such as 5 MHz, are required in order to achieve more depth of penetration. This is true, for example, in intraoperative scanning of the liver where penetration to the center of the organ is essential to find a deep, centrally located primary or metastatic lesion.

Sterilization is either by gas sterilizing the transducer itself or by enclosing the transducer in a sterile transparent plastic wrap.[4] Sterile warm saline is then used in the operating field to ensure good acoustic coupling of the transducer with the exposed tissue. The transducer can be applied directly on the surface of the exposed organ or the operating field can be flooded with saline and the transducer immersed in the saline and held several centimeters away from the organ.

The equipment needed for intraoperative ultrasound is identical to the equipment used in radiology departments for clinical scanning. All these units are portable and can be brought to the operating room. Intraoperative ultrasound functions best when it is performed as a joint effort between a surgeon, an ultrasound technologist, and an ultrasonographer, generally a radiologist with a special interest and expertise in ultrasound imaging. A surgeon who wishes to use intraoperative ultrasound must become comfortable with the images, must recognize the normal anatomy as seen with ultrasound, and must learn to distinguish neoplasms from the surrounding tissue. A degree of hand-eye coordination also must be acquired so that the ultrasound transducer can be skillfully applied to an exposed organ while observing the video monitor. Equipment maintenance and upgrading, record keeping, film archiving, and an advanced knowledge of ultrasound instrumentation, physics, and image interpretation are some of the skills that an ultrasound technologist and ultrasonographer bring to the operating room to ensure a successful study.

Although it is difficult to generalize about the value of intraoperative ultrasound because of its broad scope and many uses, several comments on its benefits can be made. In general, intraoperative ultrasound can detect lesions unsuspected on preoperative imaging or by surgical inspection. More often, intraoperative ultrasound is used to locate precisely a lesion that is not palpable or visible but that is known to be present from preoperative imaging. It helps to characterize a focal abnormality by displaying it as cystic or solid, necrotic or hemorrhagic, and shows areas of calcification. Once a focal lesion is visualized, its size, extent, and relationship to the normal surrounding anatomy is demonstrated. Intraoperative ultrasound can direct the surgeon to the lesion, showing the best surgical approach, or when necessary, it can guide a biopsy needle, shunt, or drain to the appropriate area.[5] At times, intraoperative ultrasound is also useful at the conclusion of surgery to confirm that the operative procedure achieved its objectives. Machi and Sigel,[6] reviewing their experience using intraoperative ultrasound during 2299 operations from 1979 to 1988, found that they could summarize intraoperative ultrasound benefits into four categories—(1) for the acquisition of new information not otherwise available; (2) as a complement to, or replacement for, operative radiography; (3) for guiding surgical manipulation; and (4) for confirming the completion and success of the operation. Based on the occurrences of one or more of these benefits, Machi and Sigel judged operative ultrasonography to be useful in 2103 of their 2299 operations (91.5%) by reducing surgical tissue dissection, reducing operating time, decreasing the need for operative radiography, and enabling surgeons to devise new surgical procedures.

Intraoperative ultrasound has been applied to virtually every soft tissue area of the body. Some applications, such as in neurosurgery or in liver surgery, are now becoming well-established operating room procedures. Others, such as scanning the kidneys or major blood vessels, are less often employed but are potentially equally useful. Although intraoperative ultrasound has been used in many different types of surgery and for many different causes, there are four organs in which this technique is having a major influence on the conduct of cancer surgery. These organs are the brain, spinal cord, liver, and pancreas.

Brain ■

Most intraoperative ultrasound examinations of the brain are performed using 3 to 7.5 MHz transducers. The higher frequencies are used for more superficial masses, the lower frequencies for deeper lesions. Because of the rounded contour of the brain and because of the limited cranial windows often used in modern neurosurgery, sector scanners, with their smaller contact surface, are preferable to larger linear array transducers in most situations. For lesions that are located superficially and that are too large to be included in the narrow angle of a sector transducer, a high frequency linear array transducer with its larger area of surface contact may be preferable. If only a sector transducer is available, a water bag can be interposed between the transducer and the brain surface, moving the transducer away from the brain so that a superficial lesion will be projected in a larger portion of the image sector.[7] Intraoperative ultrasound can be performed either with the transducer placed directly on the dura or with the transducer gently placed on the exposed brain after opening the dura. The quality of the image is comparable with either technique. It is often advantageous to scan before opening the dura to de-termine if the size and the location of the craniotomy is adequate to gain access to an underlying tumor. A needle, guided by ultrasound, can also be used to drain and decompress fluid collections before duratomy to prevent transcranial herniation of the brain under pressure.[8] Saline irrigation on the dura or the exposed brain must be used to ensure good transducer to soft tissue contact. It is possible also to scan through a burr hole, but this requires an in-line scanhead ("end-firing transducer") to fit in the limited opening of the burr-hole. Generally, burr-hole scanning is less satisfactory than scanning through a craniotomy because of the limited scanning area for the transducer.[9]

Using gray-scale intraoperative ultrasound, the normal brain is relatively hypoechoic. Sulci, ventricular walls, bone, and the choroid plexus appear hyperechoic or echogenic. White matter cannot be differentiated from gray matter. Fluid-filled areas, such as the ventricles, arachnoidal cysts, or cystic cavities in tumors, such as low-grade gliomas, are shown as hypoechoic regions, more echo-free than the brain substance. Intraoperative orientation is accomplished by identification of major landmarks such as the ventricle system and cerebral major fissures. One of the problems encountered in performing examinations through a craniotomy is that the cerebral anatomy as visualized with intraoperative ultrasound may be at a different angle or perspective than the standard views generated by preoperative CT and MR imaging.[10] It can be difficult to define an area of pathology in relationship to the normal anatomy and in relation to the CT and MR images. On the other hand, the instantaneous images seen as the transducer is moved help to compensate for the lack of a standardized presentation of the cerebral anatomy. The transducer should be turned, scanning in at least two planes, to identify all structures. Echodense normal brain structures, such as a distorted sulcus, can be confused with a tumor if seen from only one view.[11] Scanning at right angles to the original image plane generally will show the difference between a spherical tumor and the linear echo of a sulcus.

The primary oncological application of intraoperative ultrasound in the brain is to find and precisely localize subcortical tumors. It does this extremely well. In a recent study of 52 intracerebral masses, which included 23 primary and 10 metastatic brain tumors, ultrasound visualization was accomplished in all cases with no false positive or no false negative studies.[12] In another study of 45 lesions, including 16 metastatic and 29 primary brain tumors, in no instance did intraoperative ultrasound fail to depict a lesion previously identified by CT.[13] Real-time ultrasound in the neurosurgical operating room, therefore, ensures that the surgeon will find almost all tumors. As a corollary, if a craniotomy has been correctly centered over the tumor, the tumor should be visible on intraoperative ultrasound. Failure to visualize a tumor on initial scanning suggests that the craniotomy may need to be extended to expose the tumor properly for excision.

It now appears that all intracranial tumors are of increased echo density (echogenic) compared with the adjacent normal brain (Figs. 10-1 and 10-2). Areas of calcifications within the tumor are seen as even more echogenic focal areas with posterior shadowing; fluid spaces in the tumor are hypoechoic, or free of internal echoes (Fig. 10-2). The appearance on ultrasound of the many different types of brain tumors is similar. Therefore the images are nonspecific and cannot reliably indicate a histological diagnosis. Generally, low-grade astrocytomas appear relatively homogeneous on intraoperative ultrasound, while anaplastic astro-cytomas are more inhomogeneous.[14] Certain low-grade primary brain malignancies and metastases appear sharply demarcated from the normal brain, while high-grade primary brain tumors often have less-defined margins.[8] In low-grade gliomas, areas of increased echogenicity without shadowing correspond to areas of pathologic enhancement on contrast CT. In high-grade (malignant) gliomas most echogenic areas without shadowing correspond to areas of necrosis.[15] Intraoperative ultrasound cannot differentiate between types of primary tumor or reliably distinguish a primary from a metastatic tumor.

While the sonographic appearance of brain tumors is nonspecific for tumor type, intraoperative ultrasound can add information on tumor characterization in addition to that provided by CT. It is generally agreed that the results of treatment of primary and metastatic brain tumor are better when there has been complete tumor resection with the least disturbance to normal tissue before the administration of radiation or chemotherapy. If intraoperative ultrasound is to be helpful in monitoring the completeness of tumor removal, it is important that it accurately depict the full extent of a tumor. Generally the size of a lesion as seen with intraoperative ultrasound closely correlates with the size of the lesion as seen on preoperative CT. In a recent study of 22 patients in which the volume of tumor measured on preoperative CT was compared to the volume measured at intraoperative ultrasound, LeRoux and colleagues found a close correlation between the size of the tumor depicted on intraoperative ultrasound and the size calculated from the CT study.[16] In some patients in this series, intraoperative ultrasound demonstrated the tumor margin more clearly and with greater correspondence to the operative findings than was seen on the preoperative CT, thus maximizing the extent of resection. Visualization of tumor margins on intraoperative ultrasound is independent of enhancement of tumor following contrast injection on the preoperative CT.[13,14] In those instances where there is contrast enhancement on CT, the size of the tumor on intraoperative ultrasound correlates closely with the contrast-enhancing areas.[16] In those tumors that do not enhance following contrast injection or that are poorly seen on CT, intraoperative ultrasound can still precisely delineate the tumor. In one study of 45 lesions, including 16 metastatic and 29 primary brain tumors, there were 12 instances where intraoperative ultrasound was felt to yield more information than the preoperative CT.[13] In

FIG. 10–1 Intraoperative ultrasound of the brain showing an echogenic 1.5 cm diameter intracerebral melanoma metastasis (white arrowheads), lying 1 centimeter deep to the cortical surface. All brain tumors, both primary and secondary, appear echogenic (white) compared with the adjacent normal brain. This lesion also has a slightly lucent center (hypoechoic) possibly because of early central necrosis. (All ultrasound images are still-frame prints obtained from video tapes of the intraoperative ultrasound examinations.)

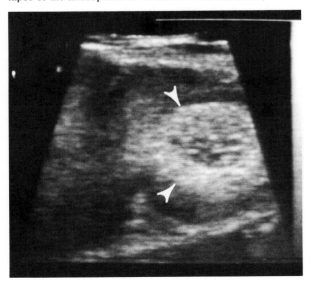

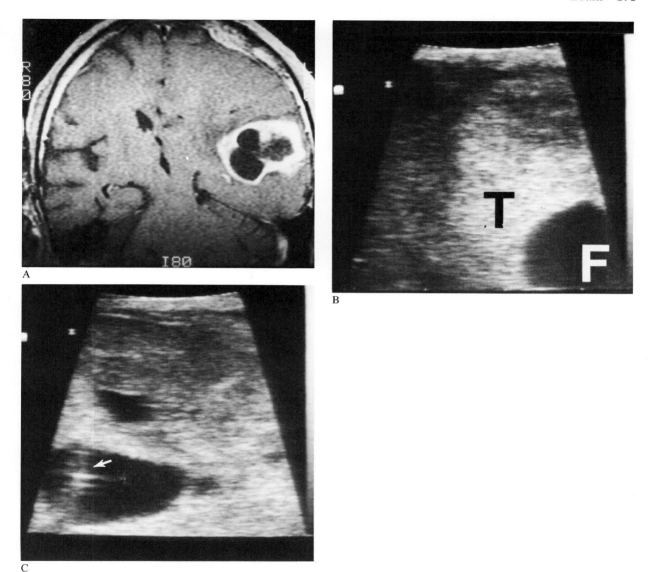

FIG. 10–2   A. Preoperative Gd-DTPA-enhanced T1-weighted MR (600/20) shows a lobular, heterogeneously enhancing mass in the left temporal lobe with central areas of low signal intensity consisting of fluid. The low signal area in the brain surrounding the tumor is peritumoral edema. **B.** Intraoperative ultrasound shows part of the tumor (T) as a well-demarcated echogenic mass against a background of low-level echoes that presumably represent peritumoral edema. The echo-free region, (F), represents one of the central fluid regions in this glioma. **C.** A drainage needle has been inserted into one of the fluid areas under ultrasound guidance and is visible within the fluid (arrow).

these instances, intraoperative ultrasound clearly showed lesions that had appeared on CT as either poorly marginated areas of low attenuation or as a "mass effect" with poor definition of tumor margins and with little or no contrast enhancement. In each of these 12 patients, intraoperative ultrasound revealed abnormal hyperechoic areas which represented solid tumors that were clearly distinguishable from the surrounding brain.

Because virtually any change in brain tissue is displayed as an echogenic area on ultrasound, non-neoplastic alteration in neural tissue adjacent to a brain neoplasm theoretically should make its borders more difficult to see. Many brain tumors are accompanied by edema of the surrounding brain. Peritumoral cerebral edema caused by an intracranial tumor may be visible as an area of slightly increased echogenicity during intraoperative ultrasound imaging. Smith and colleagues[17] found that in each of ten patients, the white matter adjacent to a tumor had a diffusely echogenic appearance that they attributed to edema. The echogenic tumor, however, was always visible within the area of edema, and in only a few patients did the surrounding echogenic brain edema make it slightly more difficult to map the precise extent of a moderately echogenic tumor. Almost all individuals using intraoperative ultrasound have commented that either the peritumoral edema is not visible or, if visible, it is less echogenic than tumor and therefore does not interfere with tumor visualization.[8,12,13,16,18] On the other hand, non-edematous changes in the brain surrounding a tumor cause some difficulty in distinguishing tumor margins. In 9 of 22 patients in whom tumor volumes from preoperative CT were compared to volumes determined by intraoperative ultrasound, intraoperative ultrasound overestimated the tumor size.[16] All nine patients had received previous surgery and radiation. LeRoux and associates postulated that peritumor echogenic gliosis contiguous with the echogenic tumor made the tumor appear larger by ultrasound. Echogenic hemorrhage next to a tumor also could be confused with tumor. Generally, therefore, intraoperative ultrasound depicts the size and margins of most tumors accurately. In rare instances when there is surrounding edema or hemorrhage, and in previously treated lesions with peritumoral gliosis, intraoperative ultrasound may overestimate lesion size. Intraoperative ultrasound rarely, if ever, underestimates brain tumor volume.

As almost all solid tumors have appeared echogenic compared to the brain, intraoperative ultrasound is of only limited use in differential diagnosis; its primary use is in tumor localization and intraoperative guidance. When the tumor is visualized, the surgeon, by scanning from different areas on the brain surface, can find the shortest and safest route through the brain to the tumor. Critical areas of the brain can thus be avoided. Localization with ultrasound reduces operating time and diminishes the risk of damage to normal brain tissue. Accurate identification of cysts within the tumor permits decompression under ultrasound guidance by needle drainage before resection (Fig. 10-2).[19] Furthermore, the removal of deep tumors can be monitored as resection proceeds. Rescanning at intervals and the use of cottonoid markers to chart the progress and accuracy of the incision can guide the surgeon directly, and accurately, to a deep tumor.[20] By scanning after tumor resection, intraoperative ultrasound can establish whether the tumor has been completely removed by showing absence of residual tumor.[21] If resection is not feasible, ultrasound can be used to guide a biopsy needle into the lesion to obtain diagnostic tissue, facilitating an accurate biopsy by showing the best area for sampling. It also can facilitate accurate placement of ventricular and cyst catheters for shunting or for drug administration. When doing a needle biopsy or placement of a catheter under ultrasound guidance, the area is continuously scanned as the needle is advanced. By properly angling the transducer towards the needle, it is possible to follow the needle or to see the needle tract entering the target area. For low-grade gliomas and metastases, the most accurate biopsies are obtained by directing the needle to areas of increased echogenicity that correspond to tumor areas of contrast enhancement on CT.[15] In contrast, with higher grade gliomas, echogenic areas in the center of the tumor may correspond to areas of tumor necrosis and be unrewarding sites for biopsy. The most consistent results with these tumors are obtained by directing the biopsy needle to the inner portion of the echogenic tumor margin.[22] After the biopsy, the area should be rescanned before closing. Visualization of an echogenic focus that develops a few minutes after biopsy indicates a biopsy-induced hemorrhage.[23] The extent and significance of hemorrhage also can be determined by using intraoperative ultrasound.

Intraoperative ultrasonography has a unique and important role in the operative treatment of patients with cerebral neoplasms. The technique is reliable and rapid and has nearly eliminated unguided brain exploration searching for subcortical lesions. While the efficacy of ancillary techniques is always difficult to measure, in one large study in which intraoperative ultrasound was used to facilitate resection of 136 brain tumors, intraoperative ultrasound was found of value in 66 (49%) of cases[24] by significantly expediting or aiding the surgical procedure. In other words, the procedure would have been more difficult to perform without sonography, or intraoperative ultrasound demonstrated that the goals of the procedure had not been achieved and allowed the surgeon to take alternative action. As examples of the latter circumstance, intraoperative ultrasound detected residual tumor after complete resection had been attempted or detected hematomas that developed after tumor resection or biopsy.

Not only is intraoperative ultrasound useful, it is also safe. In one series of 91 patients in whom intraoperative ultrasound was used, no intraoperative complications and no postoperative infections were attributed to the use of intraoperative ultrasound.[12] Intraoperative ultrasound permits faster, safer, and more accurate surgical treatment of cerebral neoplasms. It is already considered to be an essential technique in the modern neurosurgical operating room.

Spinal Cord ■

Intraoperative ultrasound of the spinal canal, introduced approximately a decade ago,[25,26] has had no less an impact on operative neurosurgery than intraoperative ultrasound scanning of the brain. Like cranial ultrasound, spinal intraoperative ultrasound is used to detect and locate spinal masses before opening the dura, to determine tumor size and position in relation to the spinal cord, dura, and nerve roots, and to identify cysts or fluid compartments (Fig. 10-3). Unlike its use with the brain, intraoperative ultrasound of the spinal canal and spinal cord is always conducted at a shallow depth. Higher frequency transducers, generally ranging from 7.5 to 10 MHz, which offer higher resolution are used.[27]

Usually ultrasound is performed from the posterior approach with the patient prone following a laminectomy, but it also can be done from an anterior approach to the spine after removal of part or all of one or more vertebral bodies. In the prone patient, following removal of one or more laminae,

and before opening the dura, the surgical cavity is filled with warm saline and the transducer is introduced in the saline pool and held 1–3 cm from the posterior dural surface. The extent of extramedullary or intramedullary masses and their relationship to the spinal cord and dura is determined with ultrasound imaging before disturbing the delicate contents of the spinal canal. By imaging the lesion, it is possible to obtain information that can be used to select the site of the dural opening. Once the dura is opened, the procedure is repeated, again filling the surgical field with warm saline and immersing the tip of the transducer, holding it 1–3 cm from the spinal cord. By using this saline bath technique, the transducer never needs to touch the dura or the spinal cord and therefore the possibility of mechanical distortion and damage to the cord or dura is avoided. Because all transducers give their best resolution in their focal zone, generally a few centimeters from the transducer, the saline pool technique also helps to position the spinal cord into the area of maximal resolution of the transducer, avoiding the lower resolution and artifacts that would be produced if the transducer were directly applied to the dural surface or the spinal cord. The saline pool technique requires the prone position for cervical laminectomy; it is impossible to adequately image the spinal cord with the patient in a sitting or lateral position in which the technique of pooling the saline is not possible.[28]

Using ultrasound, it is possible to identify the dorsal and ventral dural surfaces, the dorsal and ventral subarachnoid spaces, the spinal cord, and the central canal. The cervical and thoracic segments of the spinal cord are similar in appearance, although the thoracic cord has a slightly rounder shape.[29] The dorsal and ventral surfaces of the spinal cord are seen as highly reflective structures against the background of cerebrospinal fluid that surrounds them, or with the dura opened, against the saline pool. The spinal cord produces uniform, low-level echoes. A reflective structure often is seen in the mid to ventral part of the spinal cord, the "central echo complex," which represents either the central canal or the base of the anterior median fissure.[30,31] The dorsal arachnoid septations and the denticulate ligaments also are seen commonly within the subarachnoid space. The spinal cord tapers at the conus medullaris. Iatrogenically introduced materials, such as Gelfoam, pantopaque, and cottonoid pledgets, are clearly visible in the subarachnoid space as echogenic foci (Fig. 10-4).[29]

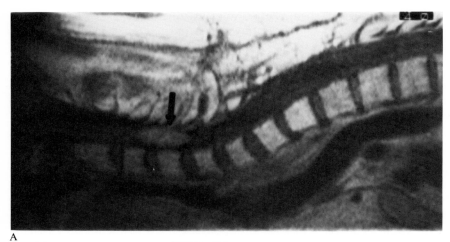

A

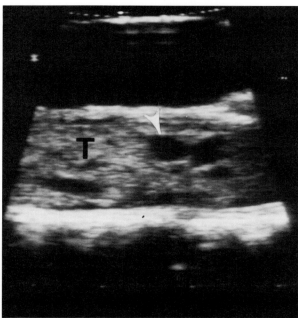

B

FIG. 10–3 A. A preoperative Gd-DTPA-enhanced T1-weighted MR (400/20) shows an oval-shaped density in the center of the cord (arrow). **B.** Intraoperative ultrasound demonstrates an echogenic intramedullary tumor (T), subsequently found to be an ependymoma. Immediately adjacent to the tumor are two echo-free intramedullary cystic spaces (arrowhead).

Except for cystic areas, intramedullary spinal cord tumors tend to be hyperechoic, like those in the brain, although occasionally they may be isoechoic to the adjacent cord. For instance, gliomas may be echogenic or isoechoic to the cord; ependymomas are almost always hyperechoic (Fig. 10-3). When hyperechoic tumor is encountered a sharp margin shows at the interface between the tumor and the adjacent cord. The cranial and caudal extent of intramedullary hyperechoic or echogenic tumor can be confidently determined and located for resection or biopsy. For those intramedullary tumors that are isoechoic, or that have an echo texture so similar to that of the adjacent normal cord that they are hard to see, other signs, such as focal expansion of the spinal cord with associated narrowing of the adjacent subarachnoid space and absence of the normally visible central echo complex, can help to localize the lesion. In a study of 21 patients with intradural spinal lesions,[30] the central echo complex was disrupted or disappeared in all 5 with intramedullary

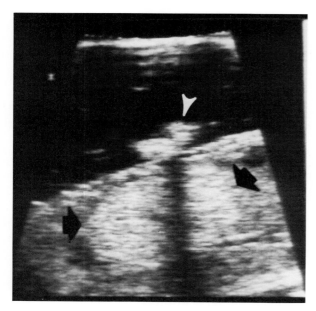

FIG. 10–4 Intraoperative ultrasound image of the spinal cord shows a well-defined hyperechoic intramedullary hemangioblastoma (arrows). A cottonoid pledget (arrowhead) has been placed on the posterior surface of the cord to indicate the center of the tumor.

lesions, but was present in the remaining 16 patients with extramedullary lesions. By scanning directly over the intact dura or the spinal cord, the surgeon is assured that he or she is directly at the site of the lesion seen on preoperative imaging studies. In a recent study of 14 patients with intramedullary spinal cord neoplasms,[32] intraoperative spinal sonography accurately localized all tumors, often revealing the need for rostral or caudal extension of the initial laminectomy.

Many intramedullary tumors—astrocytomas, ependymomas, and hemangioblastomas—have adjacent or intratumoral intramedullary fluid collections or cysts (Fig. 10-3).[32] These "cysts" may be multiple and show fine septations. Intraoperative ultrasound can help to distinguish between communicating syringomyelia and a syrinx associated with an adjacent echogenic tumor[33] and can help to clarify the etiology of an indeterminate appearance on preoperative MR imaging. For instance, in one patient in whom a primary low-grade astrocytoma was reported on preoperative MR imaging as showing a cystic space with a solid nodule, intraoperative ultrasound demonstrated an almost entirely solid mass with a localized intramedullary cyst that corresponded to the area of presumed solid tumor.[34] In 14 intramedullary spinal cord tumors, intraoperative ultrasound was found to be as accurate as preoperative imaging in the evaluation of solid neoplasms, and was superior to computed tomography and magnetic resonance imaging for delineating cystic components of neoplasms.[32]

Intramedullary lesions can be precisely located for biopsy. For those masses that are hard to distinguish from the adjacent spinal cord, a biopsy site is chosen at the site of maximal cord enlargement. When the intramedullary tumor is echogenic compared with the adjacent cord, the biopsy is obtained directly from the tumor visualized by ultrasound, avoiding any adjacent or intratumoral cystic spaces. Intraoperative ultrasound, therefore, improves the chances of obtaining a diagnostic biopsy of intramedullary lesions.

There are also advantages in visualizing extramedullary masses. Intradural extramedullary masses—meningiomas, neurinomas, ependymomas, and metastases—lying adjacent to the cord are usually easily visible as round to oval homogeneous echogenic masses outlined against the sharp margin of the spinal cord and surrounding CSF.[35] They tend to be more echogenic than the spinal cord and can therefore be easily distinguished from it.[36] Cord displacement or compression also can be visualized. Ultrasound is especially useful for extramedullary masses that are anterior to the spinal cord and that are not visible by direct inspection. In this circumstance, intraoperative ultrasound can show the exact location and size of the mass and eliminate the need to retract the cord or the thecal sac.[37] Periodic motion of the spinal cord due to transmitted pulsations from the anterior spinal artery may be seen with ultrasound when the artery is compressed between a ventral extramedullary mass and the spinal cord.[38] Extradural masses appear as homogeneous echogenic masses that displace the dura and the spinal cord. On occasion, ultrasound reveals that a mass that was thought to be exclusively extradural has some degree of intradural extension.[35] With extradural masses and intradural extramedullary masses, intraoperative ultrasound can help one to judge the extent of bone removal necessary for adequate exposure to accomplish total tumor removal before opening the dura, assess the degree of spinal cord compression, and monitor the adequacy of decompression after removal of the tumor.[37]

Liver ■

Computerized tomography, preoperative ultrasound, magnetic resonance imaging and the widespread use of tumor markers have markedly increased the ability to detect early hepatic primary and metastatic neoplasms. Small hepatomas and patients with several liver metastases are more and more frequently being referred for surgical management. For a successful enucleation or resection of primary or metastatic hepatic cancers, the surgeon must be able to locate the lesion precisely, determine if resection is feasible, and, if it is, determine the magnitude of the resection required.

Intraoperative ultrasound can accurately localize intrahepatic neoplasms for resection or biopsy; assess the possible involvement of hepatic or portal veins by tumor; characterize unsuspected liver lesions found at surgery; establish the relationship between a tumor and the intrahepatic vascular structures; and generally facilitate the surgical resection of a mass by defining the exact site and boundaries of the lesion in relation to the intrahepatic vessels and ducts (Fig. 10-5).[39,40–42] Intraoperative ultrasound can detect primary or secondary liver tumors that were unsuspected on preoperative imaging and are not palpable or visible at the time of surgery (Table 10-1).[43,44] For instance, Clarke and associates[45] recently compared the accuracy of preoperative computed tomography and preoperative and intraoperative ultrasound in a prospective study of 54 patients undergoing resection of hepatic neoplasms. The preoperative imaging results were compared to the surgical findings and intraoperative ultrasonography. A total of 167 lesions were seen by intraoperative ultrasound, which found 25% to 35% additional lesions compared with the preoperative ultrasound study and CT. Most importantly, 40% of the lesions demonstrated by intraoperative ultrasound were neither visible nor palpable at surgery. Modern preoperative imaging techniques are remarkably good, but small focal lesions (less than 1 cm in diameter) may not be detected. For example, in one study, intraoperative ultrasound detected 13 of 40 liver neoplasms less than 1 cm in diameter that had not been detected by preoperative imaging and were not palpable at surgery.[46]

With its ability to image the liver directly at surgery, it is not surprising that the information intraoperative ultrasound provides influences the surgical decision.[39] In a recent study to evaluate the influence of intraoperative ultrasound on the surgery of primary and secondary liver tumors, Parker and colleagues[47] found that intraoperative ultrasound affected the operative management in 22 of 45 operative episodes (49%). They concluded that intraoperative ultrasound was superior to both preoperative CT and surgical exploration in assessing both the feasibility and the extent of resection required for primary and secondary hepatic cancers. In their study of 42 patients with liver tumors who underwent 45 exploratory operations, intraoperative ultrasound was the most sensitive indicator of the number of lesions present in the liver. By displaying hepatic venous anatomy and its relationship to a tumor, intraoperative ultrasound helped to determine if resection was feasible and, if so, how best to approach the surgery. In another study involving 77 patients operated on on 79 occasions for hepatocellular carcinoma, it was found that intraoperative ultrasound gave supplemental information in about a third of the time (26 cases).[48] In 21 of these 26 instances, the intended surgical procedure was altered because of information found on intraoperative ultrasound. On 7 occasions, the preoperative imaging had suggested that a surgical resection was possible, but intraoperative ultrasound indicated more extensive and inoperable intrahepatic disease. On 2 occasions, intraoperative ultrasound indicated the need to perform a more extensive resection than had been planned, and in the remaining 12 instances, intraoperative ultrasound localized the lesion sufficiently to permit a lesser resection (8 subsegmentectomies, 4 segmentectomies) than originally considered.[48]

Intraoperative ultrasound of the liver is most often performed with a 5 to 7 MHz linear array transducer, or with a 5 MHz sector transducer when a large view is needed or when there are deep-seated lesions. The transducer is applied directly on any part of the saline-moistened surface of the exposed liver. For most instances, it is generally advisable to use some systematic scanning technique to examine the entire liver rather than scanning only in the area of a suspected tumor. On the gray-scale display, the normal liver appears as a homogeneous low echo-amplitude matrix, punctuated by linear densities with fluid in the center that represent the normal hepatic and portal vein branches. The normal intrahepatic veins should be systematically identified and are generally easily visible as they course toward the inferior vena cava. The portal veins have more echogenic walls than the hepatic veins and can be followed into the liver parenchyma from the hilum. The three hepatic veins identify the four sectors of the liver and

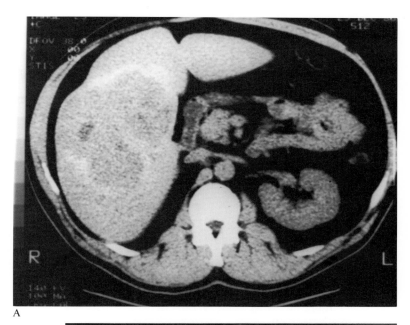

A

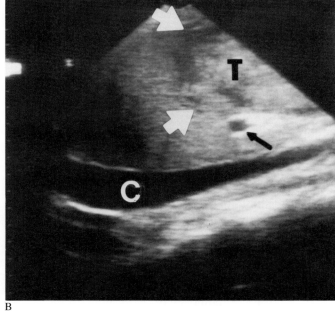

B

FIG. 10–5 **A.** Preoperative post-contrast CT shows a hepatoma within the right lobe of the liver. **B.** Longitudinal intraoperative ultrasound scan shows a large homogeneous tumor (T, white arrows) occupying the right lobe. The portal vein (black arrow) is seen in cross-section immediately adjacent to the tumor. (C, Inferior Vena Cava)

identification of the intrahepatic portal venous system defines the eight liver segments.[46] By identifying the intrahepatic vessels, it is possible to map out a particular segment on the surface of the liver for a subsequent segmentectomy.[46,49]

Tumors, either primary or secondary, will appear as either focal areas of lower echo amplitude or focal areas of higher amplitude against the normal liver background. In a few instances, a tumor will be "isoechoic," that is, its echo pattern will be equal to the surrounding liver. In these instances, the tumor will generally be detectable by a thin hypoechoic rim and by its mass effect on adjacent intrahepatic vascular structures. An ultrasound guided needle biopsy can be performed by visualizing the lesion and directing a needle,

Table 10–1
Sensitivity and Specificity of Preoperative CT and Intraoperative Ultrasound Imaging (IOUS) in the Detection of Primary and Metastatic Liver Tumors

Study	No. of Patients	No. of Tumors	Type of Tumor†	Sensitivity (%)* CT	IOUS	Specificity (%)* CT	IOUS
Igawa, et al[50]	83	83	H	97.6	96.4	NA‡	NA
Castaing, et al[53]	98	126	H 25 M 27	66	78.5	93	100
Machi, et al[64]	84	46	M	47.8	97.8	92.5	94
Makuuchi, et al[52]	152	203	H	89.6	99	NA	NA
Hayashi, et al[56]	45	NA	H	67	94	100	92
Parker, et al[47]	42	89	M 31 N 11	77	98	NA	NA
Russo, et al[65]	70	73	M	42.8	92.8	96.6	96.6
	574						

Note: In all instances, the imaging studies were verified by the findings at surgery.

*Sensitivities and Specificities as reported by authors

†H = Hepatomas, M = Metastatic Tumors. For mixed series, the number of patients affected in the series is given after the tumor type.

‡NA = Not available

under ultrasound guidance, into the lesion (Fig. 10-6). This procedure may be valuable in those instances where there is an atypical appearance to a lesion. For instance, in one series of 37 patients with suspected liver tumors, 3 cases of atypical tumors required an intraoperative ultrasound guided biopsy to establish their benign nature and avoid resection.[42]

Much of the initial work and the continuing interest in using intraoperative ultrasound during the surgery of hepatocellular carcinoma has come from Japan, where hepatomas are a common diagnosis.[40,50,51] Resection of hepatocellular carcinoma is especially difficult when there is concomitant cirrhosis because the tumor may not be palpable within the abnormally hard liver. In cirrhotic patients with underlying marginal liver function, partial hepatic resection rather than extensive lobectomies are often preferred. In this situation, intraoperative ultrasound becomes essential in order to detect the primary tumor and to delineate the surrounding intrahepatic anatomy so that an adequate liver-sparing resection can be performed.

The accuracy of intraoperative ultrasound in

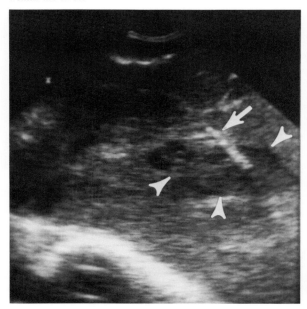

FIG. 10–6 Intraoperative ultrasound of the right lobe of the liver shows a biopsy needle (arrow) that has been inserted under ultrasound guidance into a tumor (arrowheads) deep within the liver.

visualizing hepatocellular carcinoma is very good. In a large series of 152 patients with small tumors (less than 5 cm in diameter), intraoperative ultrasound detected 198 of a total of 203 hepatomas for a sensitivity of 99%.[52] Sixty of these 152 patients had hepatomas smaller than 2 centimeters in diameter, and 65% of the 203 hepatomas were not palpable at surgery. Although intraoperative ultrasound has shown a high sensitivity for detecting liver tumors, no imaging technique is perfect. There may be tumors or tumor involvement of intrahepatic veins that may not be detected with intraoperative ultrasound.[53] To improve sensitivity, recent efforts have been directed toward using contrast agents, injected at the time of surgery, in an attempt to increase lesion visibility.[54] The application of the newer color-flow Doppler units to intraoperative use, with their simultaneous display of intrahepatic vasculature in color and tumors in gray scale, should also yield additional information.[55] At a minimum, color-flow imaging should make identification and evaluation of intrahepatic vessels easier, and possibly improve lesion detectability by showing tumor neovascularity.

Besides detecting the primary hepatoma, intraoperative ultrasound is useful for determining extent, that is, for detecting venous involvement and additional intrahepatic metastases. Hepatomas spread through the portal venous system. As the tumor grows, it enters an adjacent portal vein radicle and can spread to other areas supplied by that portal vein. At each bifurcation, tumor fragments may break off and be carried distally to lodge and grow as daughter nodules. Small intrahepatic metastases (less than 1 cm in diameter) are being detected with increasing frequency with intraoperative ultrasound. Gozzetti and associates[42] found small, 0.8 to 2 cm, intrahepatic metastases in 5 of his 19 patients undergoing surgery for hepatocellular carcinoma. These lesions were not palpable and were located at some distance from the main tumor. In another series of 45 patients, subsequently found to have 18 metastatic nodules, intraoperative ultrasound was found to have a sensitivity of 94% and a specificity of 92% for detecting these lesions.[56] This study also proves that visualization with intraoperative ultrasound is not dependent on tumor vascularity since four of the nodules found with intraoperative ultrasound were avascular or hypovascular hepatocellular carcinomas that both preoperative hepatic angiography and CT had failed to demonstrate.[56]

The intrahepatic veins should be identified and located in relationship to the tumor in order to aid in resection and to examine the vessels themselves for tumor involvement. If segmental surgery is planned, the segment can be delineated further by identifying the hepatic veins that anatomically border the segments. The relationship and distance between a tumor and the intended resection line should be determined to ensure that all of the tumor will be removed. Any abrupt interruption of a vessel or the presence of echogenic tumor thrombi within the vein lumen indicates vascular invasion by the tumor. Using intraoperative ultrasound during surgery for hepatomas, Igawa detected tumor thrombi within the portal vein in 9 of 13 patients (69.2%).[50] When vascular invasion is detected, the surgical approach must be modified accordingly.[42] One case of hepatoma has been reported in which intraoperative ultrasonography revealed a tumor thrombus in the epiploic vein of the adhering omentum.[57]

Intraoperative ultrasound also can be used to detect and inject the portal vein of the tumor-containing liver segment in order to outline that particular liver segment.[58] In those instances when cirrhosis of the liver precludes doing a lobectomy for hepatoma, it may be more desirable to perform a more limited resection such as a segmentectomy or subsegmentectomy.[50] Because there are no good anatomic landmarks for the hepatic sections on the surface of the liver, it may be necessary and helpful to use intraoperative ultrasound guidance to facilitate anatomical identification. One technique has been to outline a segment or subsegment by injecting the supplying portal vein with a stain. Under direct visualization with intraoperative ultrasound, the portal vein branch leading to the involved segment or subsegment is located and a needle is inserted. A dye, such as indigo carmine, is injected. Within minutes, the dye stains the liver parenchyma supplied by that portal branch and an outline of the limits of that segment becomes visible on the liver surface.[50] At that point the segment can be marked on the liver surface with an electrocautery. Another technique is to insert, under ultrasound guidance, a 6-F balloon catheter into a supplying portal vein branch.[59] By inflating the balloon, it is possible to stop the portal venous blood flow to the target segment, diminishing the amount of bleeding encountered during resection as well as the postoperative lymphatic discharge associated with manipulation of the liver hilus.[50]

A growing number of investigators have shown that surgical resection of hepatic colorectal metastases significantly improves long-term survival in selected patients.[60] Intraoperative ultrasound techniques are valuable for accurately monitoring curative resection of large colorectal metastases requiring anatomical procedures such as right hepatic trisegmentectomy, bisegmentectomy, and hepatic lobectomy. Although preoperative imaging of the patients with computed tomography, ultrasound, or magnetic resonance imaging can demonstrate the size and the extent of tumor, these preoperative imaging techniques do not define the tumor in relationship to the normal tissue planes. If a metastasectomy is to be performed, intraoperative ultrasound will show the size of the lesion, its depth from the liver surface, and any intervening or adjacent blood vessels that may need to be avoided or ligated. Ultrasound guided segmentectomies, permitting resection of a wide margin of healthy tissue around a tumor in a controlled anatomical fashion, have also been advocated as a reasonable compromise between major resection and metastasectomy for small tumors.[61] Segmentectomies can be performed by identifying the hepatic and portal veins that outline the segment or by staining the segment with dye injections into the portal vein. In assessing the resectability of colorectal metastases, intraoperative ultrasound criteria include the proximity of the major portal and hepatic venous structures, the exclusion of simultaneous minimal metastatic disease in the remaining parenchyma, and the distinction between marginal resectability and resectability for cure along the proposed parenchymal dissection plane.[62]

In addition to visualizing and aiding the resection of metastases known to be present through preoperative imaging, intraoperative ultrasound can also detect liver metastases unsuspected on any preoperative imaging and not palpable at the time of surgery. Intraoperative ultrasound can detect lesions less than 1 centimeter in diameter and miliary-type neoplastic infiltrate that are difficult to detect on preoperative imaging.[63] It cannot be emphasized enough that, when searching for liver metastases, it is important that intraoperative ultrasound be used systematically to scan the entire liver. Such a study should normally take no more than about 10–15 minutes. In one study where intraoperative ultrasound was used in this fashion during 84 colorectal cancer operations, in 10 cases (11.9%), intraoperative ultrasonography identified 14 previously unrecognized metastatic tumors. All these tumors were less than 2 cm in size and none was palpable. In this study, the sensitivity of intraoperative ultrasound in detecting metastatic liver

lesions (97.8%) was significantly superior to that of preoperative ultrasound (41.3%), computed tomography (47.8%), and surgical exploration (58.7%), while the specificity of each test was comparable (approximately 90%).[64] In another study of 70 patients undergoing surgery for colorectal carcinoma, Russo and colleagues[65] observed that seven of 13 (53.9%) metastatic liver lesions in 10 patients could only be found by using intraoperative ultrasound. None of these lesions diagnosed by intraoperative ultrasound were palpable or visible at the time of surgery, or had been detected on the preoperative workup. All were very small—ranging from 4 to 16 mm in diameter.

Several other applications of intraoperative ultrasound in the liver appear promising. Recently, intraoperative ultrasound has been used to monitor hepatic resections in pediatric patients. In five pediatric patients with primary liver tumors, the information derived from intraoperative ultrasound changed the operative strategy in all, despite extensive preoperative evaluations.[66] Another new technique that uses intraoperative ultrasound imaging is cryosurgery.[67] Cryosurgery has a number of advantages that make it particularly appealing in the treatment of liver cancer; however, a major problem that delayed the clinical application of hepatic cryosurgery was the lack of a precise means of monitoring the freezing process *in situ*. Preliminary work with dog livers had shown that the entire freezing and thawing cycle could be monitored easily using real-time ultrasound.[68] This was substantiated when Ravikumar and associates[69] used cryosurgery with intraoperative ultrasound monitoring in ten patients to treat multiple unresectable hepatic metastases from colorectal carcinoma. Freezing was monitored by ultrasound, which visualized frozen tumor as a hyperechoic rim with posterior acoustic shadowing. Tumor response was documented by pathologic findings, progressive fall of carcinoembryonic antigen levels, and computed tomographic scan evidence of necrosis and shrinkage of tumor.

In one study where intraoperative ultrasound was used for screening of liver metastases, a sensitivity of approximately 98% was achieved for intraoperative ultrasound detection.[64] Obviously, the more extensive the preoperative workup and the more it is performed with high quality "state-of-the-art" diagnostic imaging equipment, the fewer unsuspected lesions will be found by intraoperative ultrasound at surgery. Imaging technology continues to evolve rapidly so it is difficult to assemble data about the sensitivity of any imaging modality before it is out of date. For instance, MR imaging of the liver is still too new to be placed correctly in the perspective of other imaging techniques or to be compared with intraoperative ultrasound; its role is still evolving.[70] Nevertheless, it is fairly certain that intraoperative ultrasound will remain, if not the best, certainly one of the best techniques for imaging intrahepatic neoplasms, especially for small, less than 1 cm, lesions. Intraoperative ultrasound also has one great advantage over all other imaging systems; it locates a tumor at the most important time, when it is immediately under the surgeon's hand, and shows the tumor in direct relationship to the surrounding intrahepatic and surface anatomy of the liver.

Pancreas ■

After transecting the gastrocolic omentum and exposing the pancreas, an intraoperative ultrasound examination of the pancreas can be performed with a high frequency transducer placed either directly on the exposed organ or held a centimeter away within an abdomen cavity filled with warm saline. Using saline and holding the transducer away from the pancreas often gives better images as it puts the organ in the focal zone of the transducer rather than close to the scanning head where reverberation artifacts are common. This positioning also avoids any distortion of the gland and surrounding anatomy that may arise with direct contact. Following an initial saline bath examination, the saline can be removed and the pancreas rescanned with direct contact and palpation to confirm and localize any abnormalities. As with intraoperative scanning of the liver, a systematic approach to scanning should be used. The pancreas should be examined from the head to the tail in both longitudinal and transverse orientation. The pancreatic tail may be difficult to reach, although there are small transducers now available that fit in the operator's hand and can be used to visualize this area if it has not been surgically mobilized.

The normal pancreas appears as a uniform echogenic structure lying in front of the splenic vein. The normal pancreatic duct is seen as a 2–3 mm tubular fluid-filled structure in the center of the pancreas bordered by densities representing the walls of the duct. Fatty infiltration or previous pancreatitis will degrade the uniformity of the parenchyma and the pancreatic texture will appear patchy and inhomogeneous. Focal areas of calcification from pancreatitis will appear as high echo-amplitude focal areas with posterior acoustic shadowing. Generally, focal lesions, pancreatic tumors, and pancreatitis appear as areas of altered echo amplitude and are frequently hypoechoic compared to the pancreas. If a possible lesion is encountered, the transducer should be turned 90° and the lesion scanned in the opposite plane to ensure that it is a true lesion, that is, that it is round in all directions.

In inflammatory disease, intraoperative ultrasound can provide additional and useful information such as the size and appearance of the pancreatic duct, locate and estimate the wall thickness of a pseudocyst, detect nonpalpable intrapancreatic fluid collections and abscesses, and direct any needle aspirations of fluid collections.[71,72] Nonpalpable pseudocysts as small as 2 cm in diameter can be located and intraoperative ultrasound used to guide needle aspiration.[73]

The long-term survival for adenocarcinoma of the pancreas continues to remain dismal because surgery frequently reveals advanced, unresectable tumor. At present, intraoperative ultrasound cannot reliably distinguish between adenocarcinoma of the pancreas and pancreatitis, especially since these two conditions are frequently found together. The role of intraoperative ultrasound in adenocarcinoma of the pancreas is generally to assist in establishing the diagnosis, in selecting the optimal site for biopsy, and in the staging for possible resection by visualizing tumor margins and secondary effects of the tumor. In one review of 22 patients suspected of having cancer of the pancreas, referred to surgery either because of painless jaundice or because of a pancreatic mass seen on preoperative imaging, Plainfosse and colleagues[74] reported that intraoperative ultrasound assisted palpation to find 7 cancers that were not visualized with preoperative imaging. These particular cancers were generally small, less than 15 mm in diameter. In this same series, cancer was excluded in one patient when both palpation and intraoperative ultrasound found no tumor. In 11 patients with tumor, 3 were seen with intraoperative ultrasound to have invasion of the adjacent veins precluding further efforts at resection. In the remaining 8 of 11 patients, intraoperative ultrasound showed no venous involvement and resection was performed. Four patients had their liver metastases confirmed with intraoperative ultrasound and in two instances intraoperative ultrasound identified small liver metastases that had not been suspected preoperatively and were not palpable at surgery.

The common bile duct can usually be seen in the pancreatic head as a fluid-filled tubular structure. It is especially easy to image when dilated. In exploratory surgery for common duct obstruction, ultrasound imaging can exclude small intraductal stones and suggest pancreatitis when the pancreas is hyperechoic and tumor if the mass is hypoechoic, particularly if tumor infiltration of the duct wall is visible.[75] A stone impacted in the distal common bile duct is relatively easy to see, appearing as an echogenic foci with posterior shadowing. If no stone is found, the ultrasound appearance of the distal dilated common bile duct can also be helpful in establishing a diagnosis of carcinoma. Many of the criteria for the appearance of the distal duct described for operative cholangiography can be applied to the appearance of the duct on ultrasound. An abrupt cut-off of the distal common bile duct, for example, is more suspicious for cancer than for pancreatitis. Sigel and associates[76] summarized the ultrasound signs associated with malignant obstruction of the common bile duct as the presence of common bile duct dilation, the absence of stones in the distal duct, and an abrupt or "shelf-like" termination of the duct. Small, nonpalpable cancers in the pancreatic head can be localized, even if not palpable. Rifkin and colleagues[77] reported two cases in which patients presented with painless jaundice but had normal pancreatic heads on preoperative imaging with conventional ultrasound and computed tomography. At surgery no tumor was palpable in either case, but intraoperative ultrasound demonstrated small, 5 mm and 1 cm, tumors.

Focal hypoechoic masses around the distal end of a dilated common bile duct and possible small tumors in the pancreatic head can be biopsied under ultrasound guidance. With direct imaging, it is possible to avoid a dilated common bile duct and to direct a needle directly into a suspicious area. In general, and for the pancreatic head in particular, intraoperative ultrasound has made needle biopsy of the pancreas a safer procedure than it has been in the past.[78] Before intraoperative ultrasound imaging, blind biopsy of the pancreas ran the risk of an inadvertent puncture of an obstructed duct with the risk of leakage and the development of a pancreatic fistula, abscess, or pseudocyst. This problem can be avoided by using intraoperative ultrasound to select a site that is well away from any dilated pancreatic ducts or major blood vessels.[78]

Intraoperative ultrasound also can assist in determining resectability for cancer of the pancreas. In 1980, Lane showed that it was possible to image infiltration of the portal vein by adenocarcinoma, using ultrasound to determine the feasibility of Whipple pancreaticoduodenectomy or the necessity of a palliative bypass procedure. He also found that he could visualize the level of tumor growth in relation to the biliary ducts so that the optimal palliative drainage procedure could be planned.[79] By visualizing the various branches of the portal system, intraoperative ultrasound can eliminate the need for a long and unavailing dissection of the tumor.[80,81] Encasement or invasion of these portal branches is one of the deciding factors determining the feasibility of a pancreaticoduodenectomy or whether the tumor is to be considered nonresectable and only a palliative bypass procedure performed. On intraoperative ultrasound, encasement may be suggested when tumor is seen adjacent to the vein wall, when there is narrowing of the vein at that point, and when there is lack of the normal distention of that vein segment with respiration.[78] At times, actual tumor thrombus can be seen within the vein lumen.[79]

Intraoperative ultrasound therefore is useful in establishing the diagnosis of cancer of the pancreas and helpful in evaluating its spread. Although cancer of the pancreas is typically hypoechoic, it also may be isoechoic or hyperechoic and therefore difficult to distinguish from normal pancreas or from pancreatitis.[75] On the other hand, pancreatic islet cell tumors have been found to be much more distinct on ultrasound imaging, appearing as round, homogeneous, hypoechoic masses within the pancreas (Fig. 10-7). Intraoperative ultrasound is having a major influence on the surgery of islet cell tumors, especially insulinomas, since in many cases it is capable of detecting tumors that have not been localized by preoperative imaging and are not visible or palpable at surgery.[75,82–84]

Insulinomas are diagnosed by finding an inappropriately elevated serum insulin level in the presence of a low blood glucose level. The search for these elusive, generally small, tumors can be frustrating. Preoperative imaging with CT, ultrasound, and MR generally will only visualize large tumors. Small, 1 cm diameter islet cell tumors are often not detected. Selective arteriography, frequently considered the best preoperative imaging technique, may only localize about 50% of pan-

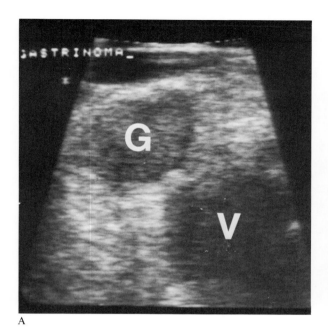
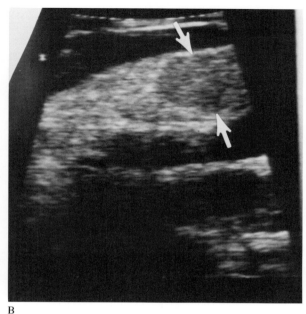

A   B

FIG. 10–7   Islet cell tumors of the pancreas. **A.** Transverse intraoperative ultrasound scan through the pancreatic head shows a 1.1 × 1.4 cm intrapancreatic gastrinoma (G) in close proximity to the superior mesenteric vein (V), seen in cross-section. **B.** Transverse intraoperative ultrasound scan shows a 1 cm diameter insulinoma (arrows) within the body of the pancreas.

creatic insulinomas.[85] Despite various attempts at preoperative localization, insulinomas remain undetected in at least 10–20% of patients.[86] In a review of 36 adult patients who were surgically treated for insulinomas at the Mayo Clinic from 1982 through 1987, the sensitivities of tumor localization using arteriography, computed tomography, and preoperative and intraoperative ultrasonography were 53%, 36%, 59%, and 90%, respectively.[86] In this series, 29 patients underwent intraoperative ultrasonography, and each patient's insulinoma was identified with a combination of ultrasound imaging and intraoperative palpation, with nonpalpable tumors being imaged in four patients. In 18 patients (62%), information obtained from intraoperative ultrasound appeared to influence the surgical management. Based on their data, investigators at the Mayo Clinic no longer recommend performing preoperative angiography, CT, or MR imaging to detect an insulinoma and suggest that preoperative and intraoperative ultrasound alone is sufficient.[87]

In patients with negative preoperative imaging studies, we have found portal venous sampling to be helpful.[85] Detecting an elevated insulin level from one of the pancreatic veins will reveal the ap-

proximate location of the insulinoma within the pancreas. An elevated insulin level in the splenic vein or from branches draining the body and tail of the pancreas indicates a distal lesion. Even if an insulinoma is not palpable, visible, or detectable with intraoperative ultrasound, a positive sampling from this area suggests that the surgeon can perform a distal pancreatectomy with a high probability of success.[88] An elevated insulin level detected from the veins draining the pancreatic head, however, can be a more difficult surgical situation when the insulinoma is not visible. Localization of pancreatic head insulinomas with intraoperative ultrasound is critical because if the lesion is visible, the tumor can be enucleated under ultrasound guidance and a proximal pancreaticoduodenectomy or a total pancreatectomy avoided.[83] In a recent report of 12 consecutive patients with occult insulinomas, that is, with negative preoperative ultrasound, CT, and selective pancreatic angiography, portal venous sampling correctly predicted the location in nine (75%) and that no tumor would be found in one.[88] In this same series, intraoperative ultrasound correctly identified 10 of the 11 insulinomas that were found including 5 tumors in the pancreatic head that were not visible or palpable. Occult tumors in the pancreatic head were enucleated under ultrasound guidance. The size of the lesion, its depth from the pancreatic surface and its relationship to major vessels and ducts were noted with intraoperative ultrasound before enucleation was performed. Intraoperative ultrasound was then used to monitor the progress of the enucleation. Occult tumors in the pancreatic body and tail were also enucleated unless they were in close proximity to the pancreatic duct, in which case a distal pancreatectomy was performed. The combination of intraoperative ultrasound, surgical palpation, and portal venous sampling found insulinomas in 11 of the 12 patients with occult insulinoma that were removed for cure.[88]

About 70% to 80% of gastrinomas, the next most common islet cell tumor after insulinoma, are malignant. Preoperative localization is even more difficult than insulinomas because many are quite small and they may be extrapancreatic in location, occurring frequently in the wall of the duodenum.[85,89] In this location, they may be difficult to separate from bowel on preoperative angiography, CT, or ultrasound. Intraoperative ultrasound can visualize gastrinomas, but generally with less success than insulinomas. In one series of 10 pancreatic insulinomas and 4 gastrinomas, intraoperative ultrasound visualized 9 of 10 insulinomas but only one of the gastrinomas.[90] We detected 23 gastrinomas in 19 patients in our series of 36 consecutive laparotomies for gastrinomas. Intraoperative ultrasound was found to be equal to palpation in its ability to localize gastrinomas. Gastrinomas that were successfully imaged by intraoperative ultrasound were significantly larger than gastrinomas that were not imaged. Twelve extrapancreatic duodenal wall gastrinomas were found in nine patients, and palpation was more sensitive than intraoperative ultrasound at localizing these small tumors. One patient had a pancreatic gastrinoma enucleated that would not have been found without intraoperative ultrasound.[91] Intraoperative ultrasound, therefore, is useful in gastrinomas as it can occasionally detect nonpalpable tumors or distinguish tumor from normal pancreas when there is an area suspicious to palpation. In those instances when gastrinomas are visualized in the pancreas, they appear as focal hypoechoic to isoechoic masses, similar to insulinomas. Intraoperative ultrasound does not appear to be useful for detecting duodenal wall gastrinomas. The combination of a fluid and gas filled lumen and normally inhomogeneous bowel wall limits the ability of intraoperative ultrasound to detect small intramural tumors.

Conclusion ■

In addition to these four organs where intraoperative ultrasound has had a major influence in cancer surgery, intraoperative ultrasound has been found helpful in other areas of the body. For instance, intraoperative ultrasound has been used during urological surgery to locate small nonpalpable renal cell carcinomas[92] and testicular tumors.[93] In 30 cases of early gastric carcinoma, intraoperative ultrasound was found to be more accurate than palpation in detecting intramural spread and lateral extension along the stomach wall.[94] In 60 operations for lung cancer, intraoperative ultrasound was found to be valuable for detecting direct cardiovascular invasion of tumor, lymph node metastasis, and liver metastasis.[95] In this study, the accuracy of operative ultrasound in diagnosing the presence or the extent of cardiovascular invasion by lung cancer was 91.7% (22 of 24 operations), which was significantly higher than preoperative studies (62.5%), including computed tomography and angiography. Operative ultrasound provided the capability of depicting lymph nodes as small as 3 mm. More lymph nodes were detected with operative ultrasound than with computed tomography; however, the sensitivity and specificity of operative ultrasound in determining lymph node metastasis were 82.4% and 67.3%, respectively. The information provided by operative ultrasound regarding cardiovascular invasion and lymph node and liver metastasis was considered helpful in selecting the type of surgical procedure and in avoiding unnecessary tissue dissection. A similar evaluation of the aorta to exclude invasion and the detection of possible abnormal lymph nodes has also been done with intraoperative ultrasound during surgery for esophageal carcinoma.[94]

The primary accomplishment of intraoperative ultrasound is to expedite surgical performance. Increasingly, however, intraoperative ultrasound is changing the outcome of some operations, improving the results over what could be accomplished without ultrasound imaging. For example, finding an additional nonpalpable liver metastasis or identifying a nonpalpable pancreatic islet cell tumor are situations where intraoperative ultrasound clearly alters the ultimate surgical result. More recently, new operative approaches that were not possible without intraoperative ultrasound have been developed, such as using ultrasound to find and inject a feeding portal vein to outline a liver segment. Undoubtedly, as more and more experience is gained with intraoperative ultrasound, many new and exciting applications will be developed in the field of cancer surgery.

References ■

1. Mittelstaedt CA, Staab EV, Drobnes WE, Daniel EB. The intraoperative uses of real-time ultrasound. Radiographics 1984;4:267–282.
2. Vincent LM, Mittelstaedt CA. Intraoperative abdominal ultrasound. In: Sanders RC, Hill M, eds. Ultrasound annual 1984. New York: Raven Press, 1984:95–120.
3. Shawker TH, Bradford M, Norton JA: Intraoperative ultrasound: guidelines for the sonographer. J Diagnostic Med Sonography 1988;4:126–129.
4. Shawker TH, Bradford MH, Norton JA. Equipment considerations for intraoperative ultrasound. J Diag Med Sonography 1988;4:49–54.
5. Machi J, Sigel B, Kurohiji T, Zaren HA, Sariego J. Operative ultrasound guidance for various surgical procedures. Ultrasound Med Biol 1990;16:37–42.
6. Machi J, Sigel B. Overview of benefits of operative ultrasonography during a ten year period. J Ultrasound Med 1989;8:647–652.
7. Boyd MC, Steinbok P, Cooperberg PL. Intraoperative localization of intracranial lesions with real-time ultrasound. Can J Neurol Sci 1985;12:31–34.
8. Rogers JV 3d, Shuman WP, Hirsch JH, Lange SC, Howe JF, Burchiel K. Intraoperative neurosonography: application and technique. AJNR 1984;5:755–760.
9. Gooding GA, Boggan JE, Powers SK, Martin NA, Weinstein PR. Neurosurgical sonography: intraoperative and postoperative imaging of the brain. AJNR 1984;5:521–525.
10. Merritt CR, Coulon R, Connolly E. Intraoperative neurosurgical ultrasound: transdural and transfontanelle applications. Radiology 1983;148:513–517.
11. Pasto ME, Rifkin MD. Intraoperative ultrasound examination of the brain: possible pitfalls in diagnosis and biopsy guidance. J Ultrasound Med 1984;3:245–249.
12. Quencer RM, Montalvo BM. Intraoperative cranial sonography. Neuroradiology 1986;28:528–550.
13. Knake JE, Chandler WF, Gabrielsen TO, Latack JT, Gebarski SS. Intraoperative sonographic delineation of low-grade brain neoplasms defined poorly by computed tomography. Radiology 1984;151:735–739.
14. Enzmann DR, Wheat R, Marshall WH, Bird R, Murphy-Irwin K, Karbon K, Hanbery J, Silverberg GD, Britt RH, Shuer L. Tumors of the central nervous system studied by computed tomography and ultrasound. Radiology 1985;154:393–399.
15. Hatfield MK, Rubin JM, Gebarski SS, Silbergleit R. Intraoperative sonography in low-grade gliomas. J Ultrasound Med 1989;8:131–134.
16. LeRoux PD, Berger MS, Ojemann GA, Wang K, Mack LA. Correlation of intraoperative ultrasound tumor volumes and margins with preoperative computerized tomography scans. An intraoperative method to enhance tumor resection. J Neurosurg 1989;71:691–698.
17. Smith SJ, Vogelzang RL, Marzano MI, Cerullo LJ, Gore RM, Neiman HL. Brain edema: ultrasound examination. Radiology 1985;155:379–382.
18. Enzmann DR, Britt RH, Lyons TL, Carroll B, Wilson DA, Buxton J. High resolution ultrasound evaluation of experimental brain abscess evolution: comparison and computed tomography and neuropathology. Radiology 1982;54:95–102.
19. Rubin JM, Dohrmann GJ. Intraoperative neurosurgical ultrasound in the localization and characterization of intracranial masses. Radiology 1983;148:519–524.
20. Voorhies RM, Bell WO, Patterson RH, Gamache FW Jr. Cottonoid as an acoustical marker for intraoperative ultrasound scanning. J Neurosurg 1984;60:438–439.
21. Shkolnik A, Tomita T, Raimondi AJ, Hahn YS, McLone DG. Work in progress. Intraoperative neurosurgical ultrasound: localization of brain tumors in infants and children. Radiology 1983;148:525–527.
22. McGahan JP, Ellis WG, Budenz RW, Walter JP, Boggan J. Brain gliomas: sonographic characterization. Radiology 1986;159:485–492.
23. Lillehei KO, Chandler WF, Knake JE. Real-time ultrasound characteristics of acute intracerebral hemorrhage as studied in the canine model. Neurosurgery 1984;14:48–51.
24. Rubin JM, Dohrmann GJ. Efficacy of intraoperative ultrasound for evaluating intracranial masses. Radiology 1985;157:509–511.
25. Dohrmann GJ, Rubin JM. Intraoperative ultrasound imaging of the spinal cord: syringomyelia, cysts, and tumors—a preliminary report. Surg Neurol 1982;18:395–399.
26. Rubin JM, Dohrmann GJ. Work in progress: intraoperative ultrasonography of the spine. Radiology 1983;146:173–175.
27. Gooding GA, Berger MS, Linkowski GD, Dillon WP, Weinstein PR, Boggan JE. Transducer frequency considerations in intraoperative US of the spine. Radiology 1986;160:272–273.
28. Chadduck WM, Flanigan S. Intraoperative ultrasound for spinal lesions. Neurosurgery 1985;16:477–483.
29. Quencer RM, Montalvo BM. Normal intraoperative spinal sonography. Am J Roentgenol 1984;143:1301–1305.
30. St. Amour TE, Rubin JM, Dohrmann GJ. The central canal of the spinal cord: ultrasonic identification. Radiology 1984;152:767–769.
31. Montalvo BM, Skaggs PH. The central canal of the spinal cord: ultrasonic identification. Letter to the editor. Radiology 1985;155:535–536.
32. Platt JF, Rubin JM, Chandler WF, Bowerman RA, DiPietro MA. Intraoperative spinal sonography in the evaluation of intramedullary tumors. J Ultrasound Med 1988;7:317–325.
33. Hutchins WW, Vogelzang RL, Neiman HL, Fuld IL, Kowal LE. Differentiation of tumor from syringohydromyelia: intraoperative neurosonography of the spinal cord. Radiology 1984;151:171–174.
34. Rubin JM, Aisen AM, DiPietro MA. Ambiguities in MR imaging of tumoral cysts in the spinal cord. J Comput Assist Tomogr 1986;10:395–398.
35. Montalvo BM, Quencer RM. Intraoperative sonography in spinal surgery: current state of the art. Neuroradiology 1986;28:551–590.
36. Rubin JM, DiPietro MA, Chandler WF, Venes JL. Spinal ultrasonography. Intraoperative and pediatric applications. Radiol Clin North Am 1988;26:1–27.
37. Quencer RM, Montalvo BM, Green BA, Eismont FJ. Intraoperative spinal sonography of soft-tissue masses of the spinal cord and spinal canal. Am J Roentgenol 1984;143:1307–1315.
38. Rubin JM, Dohrmann GJ. The spine and spinal cord dur-

ing neurosurgical operations: real-time ultrasonography. Radiology 1985;155:197–200.

39. Rifkin MD, Rosato FE, Branch HM, Foster J, Yang S, Barbot DJ, Marks GJ. Intraoperative ultrasound of the liver: An important adjunctive tool for decision making in the operating room. Ann Surg 1987;205:466–472.

40. Makuuchi M, Hasegawa H, Yamazaki S. Intraoperative ultrasonic examination for hepatectomy. Jpn J Clin Oncol 1981;11:367–390.

41. Bismuth H, Castaing D. Operative ultrasound of the liver and biliary ducts. New York: Springer-Verlag, 1985.

42. Gozzetti G, Mazziotti A, Bolondi L, Cavallari A, Grigioni W, Casanova P, Bellusci R, Villanacci V, Labo G. Intraoperative ultrasonography in surgery for liver tumors. Surgery 1986;99:523–529.

43. Nagasue N, Kohno H, Chang YC, Galizia G, Hayashi T, Yukaya H, Nakamura T. Intraoperative ultrasonography in resection of small hepatocellular carcinoma associated with cirrhosis. Am J Surg 1989;158:40–42.

44. Roh MS. Hepatic resection for colorectal liver metastases. Hematol Oncol Clin North Am 1989;3:171–181.

45. Clarke MP, Kane RA, Steele G Jr, Hamilton ES, Ravikumar TS, Onik G, Clouse ME. Prospective comparison of preoperative imaging and intraoperative ultrasonography in the detection of liver tumors. Surgery 1989; 106:849–855.

46. Traynor O, Castaing D, Bismuth H. Peroperative ultrasonography in the surgery of hepatic tumours. Br J Surg 1988;75:197–202.

47. Parker GA, Lawrence W Jr, Horsley JS 3d, Neifeld JP, Cook D, Walsh J, Brewer W, Koretz MJ. Intraoperative ultrasound of the liver affects operative decision making. Ann Surg 1989;209:569–577.

48. Bismuth H, Castaing D, Garden OJ. The use of operative ultrasound in surgery of primary liver tumors. World J Surg 1987;11:610–614.

49. Castaing D, Kunstlinger F, Habib N, Bismuth H. Intraoperative ultrasonographic study of the liver. Methods and anatomic results. Am J Surg 1985;149:676–682.

50. Igawa S, Sakai K, Kinoshita H, Hirohashi K. Intraoperative sonography: clinical usefulness in liver surgery. Radiology 1985;156:473–478.

51. Igawa S, Kinoshita H, Sakai K. Clinical significance of intraoperative sonography on hepatectomy in primary carcinoma of the liver. World J Surg 1984;8:772–777.

52. Makuuchi M, Hasegawa H, Yamazaki S, Takayasu K, Moriyama N. The use of operative ultrasound as an aid to liver resection in patients with hepatocellular carcinoma. World J Surg 1987;11:615–621.

53. Castaing D, Emond J, Kunstlinger F, Bismuth H. Utility of operative ultrasound in the surgical management of liver tumors. Ann Surg 1986;204:600–605.

54. Takada T, Yasuda H, Uchiyama K, Hasegawa H, Shikata J. Contrast-enhanced intraoperative ultrasonography of small hepatocellular carcinomas. Surgery 1990; 107:528–532.

55. Sukigara M, Koga K, Komazaki T, Omoto R. Clinical experience with intraoperative Doppler color flow imaging in hepatectomy. J Clin Ultrasound 1987;15:9–15.

56. Hayashi N, Yamamoto K, Tamaki N, Shibata T, Itoh K, Fujisawa I, Nakano Y, Yamaoka Y, Kobayashi N, Mori K, Ozawak K, Torizuka N. Metastatic nodules of hepatocellular carcinoma: detection with angiography, CT, and US. Radiology 1987;165:61–63.

57. Tachimori Y, Makuuchi M, Asamura H, Yamazaki S, Hasegawa H, Takayasu K, Noguchi M, Hirohashi S. A case of hepatocellular carcinoma with tumor thrombi in the epiploic vein. Jpn J Clin Oncol 1988;18:269–273.

58. Makuuchi M, Hasegawa H, Yamazaki S. Ultrasonically guided subsegmentectomy. Surg Gynecol Obstec 1985; 161:346–350.

59. Shimamura Y, Gunven P, Takenaka Y, Shimizu H, Akimoto H, Shima Y, Arima K, Takahashi A, Kitaya T, Matsuyama T, Hasegawa H. Selective portal branch occlusion by balloon catheter during liver resection. Surgery 1986;100:938–941.

60. Adson MA. Resection of liver metastases—when is it worthwhile? World J Surg 1987;11:511–520.

61. Bismouth H, Castaing D, Taylor O, Villejuif. Surgery for synchronous hepatic metastases of colorectal cancers. Scan J Gastroenterology 23, supl 1988;149:144–149.

62. Brower ST, Dumitrescu O, Rubinoff S, McElhinney JA, Aufses AH Jr. Operative ultrasound establishes resectability of metastases by major hepatic resection. World J Surg 1989;13:649–657.

63. Boldrini G, de Gaetano AM, Giovannini I, Castagneto M, Colagrande C, Castiglioni G. The systematic use of operative ultrasound for detection of liver metastases during colorectal surgery. World J Surg 1987;11:622–627.

64. Machi J, Isomoto H, Yamashita Y, Kurohiji T, Shirouzu K, Kakegawa T. Intraoperative ultrasonography in screening for liver metastases from colorectal cancer: comparative accuracy with traditional procedures. Surgery 1987;101:678–684.

65. Russo A, Sparacino G, Plaja S, Cajozzo M, La Rosa C, Demma I, Bazan P. Role of intraoperative ultrasound in the screening of liver metastases from colorectal carcinoma: initial experiences. J Surg Oncol 1989;42:249–255.

66. Thomas BL, Krummel TM, Parker GA, Benator RM, Brewer WH, Cook DE, Salzberg AM. Use of intraoperative ultrasound during hepatic resection in pediatric patients. J Pediatr Surg 1989;24:690–693.

67. Onik G, Kane R, Steele G, McDermott W, Khettry U, Cady B, Jenkins R, Katz J, Clouse M, Rubinsky B, Chase B. Society of Gastrointestinal Radiologists Roscoe E. Miller Award. Monitoring hepatic cryosurgery with sonography. Am J Roentgenol 1986;147:665–669.

68. Gilbert JC, Onik GM, Hoddick WK, Rubinsky B. Real-time ultrasonic monitoring of hepatic cryosurgery. Cryobiology 1985;22:319–330.

69. Ravikumar TS, Kane R, Cady B, Jenkins RL, McDermott W, Onik G, Clouse M, Steele G Jr. Hepatic cryosurgery with intraoperative ultrasound monitoring for metastatic colon carcinoma. Arch Surg 1987;122:403–409.

70. Ferrucci JT. Liver tumor imaging: current concepts. Am J Roentgenol 1990;155:473–484.

71. Sigel B, Coelho JC, Donahue PE, Nyhus LM, Spigos DG, Baker RJ, Machi J. Ultrasonic assistance during surgery for pancreatic inflammatory disease. Arch Surg 1982;117:712–716.

72. Smith SJ, Vogelzang RL, Donovan J, Atlas SW, Gore RM, Neiman HL. Intraoperative sonography of the pancreas. Am J Roentgenol 1985;144:557–562.

73. Rindsberg S, Radecki PD, Friedman AC, Au F, Mayer DP. Intraoperative ultrasonic localization of a small pancreatic pseudocyst. Gastrointest Radiol 1986;11:339–341.

74. Plainfosse MC, Bouillot JL, Rivaton F, Vaucamps P, Hernigou A, Alexandre JH. The use of operative sonography in carcinoma of the pancreas. World J Surg 1987; 11:654–658.

75. Sigel B, Machi J, Ramos JR, Duarte B, Donahue PE.

The role of imaging ultrasound during pancreatic surgery. Ann Surg. 1984;200:486–493.

76. Sigel B, Coelho JC, Nyhus LM, Velasco JM, Donahue PE, Wood DK, Spigos DG. Detection of pancreatic tumors by ultrasound during surgery. Arch Surg 1982; 117:1058–1061.

77. Rifkin MD, Weiss SM. Intraoperative sonographic identification of nonpalpable pancreatic masses. J Ultrasound Med 1984;3:409–411.

78. Sigel B, Machi J, Kikuchi T, Yamashita Y, Anderson KW 3d, Kurohiji T, Zaren HA, Isomoto H, Kakegawa T. Intraoperative ultrasound of the liver and pancreas. Adv Surg 1988;21:213–244.

79. Lane RJ. Intraoperative B-mode scanning. J Clin Ultrasound 1980;8:427–434.

80. Lane RJ, Glazer G. Intra-operative B-mode ultrasound scanning of the extra-hepatic biliary system and pancreas. Lancet 1980;16:334–337.

81. Alexandre JH, Hernigou A, Billebaud T, Bouillot JL, Plainfosse MC. Preoperative ultrasound scanning of the pancreas. Gastroenterol Clin Biol 1985;9:572–577.

82. Lane RJ, Coupland GA. Operative ultrasonic features of insulinomas. Am J Surg 1982;144:585–587.

83. Norton JA, Sigel B, Baker AR, Ettinghausen SE, Shawker TH, Krudy AG, Doppman JL, Taylor SI, Gordon P. Localization of an occult insulinoma by intraoperative ultrasonography. Surgery 1985;97:381–384.

84. Gunther RW, Klose KJ, Ruckert K, Beyer J, Kuhn FP, Klotter HJ. Localization of small islet-cell tumors. Preoperative and intraoperative ultrasound, computed tomography, arteriography, digital subtraction angiography, and pancreatic venous sampling. Gastrointest Radiol 1985;10:145–152.

85. Doppman JL, Shawker TH, Miller DL. Localization of islet cell tumors. Gastroenterol Clin North Am 1989; 18:793–804.

86. Grant CS, van Heerden J, Charboneau JW, James EM, Reading CC. Insulinoma. The value of intraoperative ultrasonography. Arch Surg 1988;123:843–848.

87. Galiber AK, Reading CC, Charboneau JW, Sheedy PF 2d, James EM, Gorman B, Grant CS, van Heerden JA, Telander RL. Localization of pancreatic insulinoma: comparison of pre- and intraoperative US with CT and angiography. Radiology 1988;166:405–408.

88. Norton JA, Shawker TH, Doppman JL, Miller DL, Fraker DL, Cromack DT, Gorden P, Jensen RT. Localization and surgical treatment of occult insulinomas. Ann Surgery 1990;212:615–620.

89. Cromack DT, Norton JA, Sigel B, Shawker TH, Doppman JL, Maton PN, Jensen RT. The use of high-resolution intraoperative ultrasound to localize gastrinomas: an initial report of a prospective study. World J Surg 1987;11:648–653.

90. Marotel M, Hernigou A, Plainfosse MC, Alexandre JH, Chapuis Y, Dazza FE. Preoperative echography in 14 cases of pancreatic insulinoma and gastrinoma. Gastroenterol Clin Biol 1988;12:713–720.

91. Norton JA, Cromack DT, Shawker TH, Doppman JL, Comi R, Gorden P, Maton PN, Gardner JD, Jensen RT. Intraoperative ultrasonographic localization of islet cell tumors. A prospective comparison to palpation. Ann Surg 1988;207:160–168.

92. Gilbert BR, Russo P, Zirinsky K, Kazam E, Fair WR, Vaughan ED Jr. Intraoperative sonography: application in renal cell carcinoma. J Urol 1988;139:582–584.

93. Buckspan MB, Klotz PG, Goldfinger M, Stoll S, Fernandes B. Intraoperative ultrasound in the conservative resection of testicular neoplasms. J Urol 1989;141:326–327.

94. Machi J, Takeda J, Kakegawa T, Yamana H, Fujita H, Kurohiji T, Yamashita Y. The detection of gastric and esophageal tumor extension by high-resolution ultrasound during surgery. World J Surg 1987;11:664–671.

95. Machi J, Hayashida R, Kurohiji T, Nishimura Y, Edakuni S, Yamashita Y, Takeda J, Kakegawa T, Sigel B. Operative ultrasonography for lung cancer surgery. J Thorac Cardiovasc Surg 1989;98:540–545.

James E. Till

Quality of Life Measurements in Cancer Treatment

11

Within the practice of medicine there has always been dedication to enhancing the quality of life (QOL) of patients. The goals of restoration of health, relief of symptoms, and support of compromised function, all represent an intent to improve quality of life.[1] Cancer and its treatments can have detrimental impacts on QOL, so clinical oncologists are especially aware of the potential usefulness of meaningful quantitative measures of QOL.

The measurement of QOL is not confined to recent years. An example is the (hypothetical) plot of "general health" versus time presented by Roberts in 1934.[2] More recent versions of analogous plots of QOL versus time have been presented by Bush and Till.[3,4] Examples are shown in Figure 11-1. This figure illustrates two important questions. First, is it feasible (or desirable) to depict the QOL of a group at a particular point in time by a single global number? If so, health profiles of QOL versus time of the kind shown in Figure 11-1 could be constructed. Second, is it feasible (or desirable) to use such health profiles as a basis for clinical decision making? For example, would it be appropriate to conclude from Figure 11-1A (where duration of survival is equivalent) that Management I should always be preferred over Management II because the plot suggests a larger area under the health profile for the former relative

to the latter for a particular group of patients? If so, what conclusion should be drawn from Figure 11-1B, where the duration of survival was prolonged by Management III, but the QOL deteriorated inexorably such that the areas under the health profiles are equivalent?

These issues are controversial, and few statements based on any clear consensus can yet be made. Quantitative approaches to the measurement of QOL pose conceptual, methodological, and practical problems that are only beginning to be solved.

The growing interest in quantitative approaches to QOL assessment in oncology could be regarded as one component of a more general trend. Health care continues to undergo profound changes. In the past century, dramatic shifts in patterns of mortality have occurred.[5] The basis for these shifts is complex,[5,6] but, until recently, a much higher priority has been given to extension of life than to quality of life.[7,8] Currently, the goals of health care, and the roles of individual and societal values and preferences in shaping them, are being reexamined.[9,10] Increasing attention is being given to more comprehensive evaluations of the impact of diseases and interventions,[9,11] and more deliberate attempts are being made to take patients' preferences and values into account.[12–17]

The purpose of this review is to provide a re-

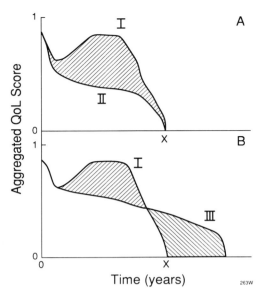

FIG. 11–1 This figure shows hypothetical plots of global (health-related) quality of life versus time, calculated for the purpose of comparing the effectiveness of different methods of management for groups of patients enrolled in a randomized clinical trial. QOL scores range from unity (equivalent to perfect health) to zero (equivalent to death). A. Health profiles are shown for two groups whose management delayed death equally. B. This figure shows health profiles for groups whose management yielded different durations of survival, but similar overall integrated QOL. (Adapted from Till JE. Uses (and some possible abuses) of quality of life measures. In: Osoba D, ed. Effect of cancer on quality of life. Boca Raton, Florida: CRC Press, 1991:137).[4]

searcher's perspective on the present status of QOL assessments with particular relevance to clinical oncology, emphasizing these three basic questions: What to measure? How to measure it? How to use the results?

Quality of Life—What to Measure? ■

When a physician asks a patient the question, "How are you?" what is being sought amounts to a simple, informal, unstructured quality of life self-assessment by the patient.[18–20] What factors ought to enter into a frank, thoughtful, thorough discussion following from this question?

The phrase "quality of life" is used in a wide variety of ways, and should be regarded as a vague, generic phrase that can encompass many different definitions, depending on the context within which it is used. Here, the phrase will not be used in a general way, but rather, in the more restricted sense of *health-related* QOL. This concept excludes such social indicators as standard of living, education, housing, and public safety.

Health-Related QOL ■

It is widely accepted that health status is a major component of the quality of life of individuals and families.[21,22] One global concept of QOL, therefore, can be based on a definition of health.[23] In 1947 the World Health Organization (WHO) defined health as "a state of complete physical, mental and social well-being and not merely the absence of disease or infirmity."[24] This definition emphasizes the multidimensional nature of health and recognizes the breadth of its determinants. A much discussed problem with such a comprehensive concept is that health defined in this way has to be affected by *all* human activity.[8] As Evans and Stoddart point out, the 1947 WHO definition has "accordingly been honored in repetition, but rarely in application."[25]

In 1984, the European region of WHO expanded on the very broad 1947 definition of health, by describing health in relation to health promotion. "The extent to which an individual or group is able, on the one hand, to realize aspirations and satisfy needs; and, on the other hand, to change or cope with the environment. Health is therefore seen as a resource for everyday life, not the objective of living; it is a positive concept emphasizing social and personal resources, as well as physical capacity."[26] This elaboration of an already very broad concept, with the inclusion of "social and personal resources, as well as physical capacity," may be contrasted with Callahan's much narrower definition (in 1973): "Health is a state of physical well-being."[27] Current approaches to the measurement of health-related QOL involve various aspects of the continuum of "health," from the extreme of well-being in the broadest sense to the other extreme of the simple absence of negative biological circumstances—disease, disability, or death.[25]

In the clinical context there is increasingly wide acceptance of the highly subjective nature of QOL, as incorporated into this definition provided by Jonsen and associates: "Quality of life may refer to the subjective satisfaction expressed or experienced by an individual in his physical, mental and social situation (even though these may be deficient in some manner)."[1]

There is also wide acceptance of the importance of taking into account the perspective of the person who is living the life being evaluated, even though that perspective may be a difficult one to assess.[1,28-30]

The final word has definitely not been heard about definitions of QOL. Different concepts of QOL, and of ways to define these various concepts, continue to be debated.[28,29,31-36] Is it a fallacy to regard QOL as a single, definable entity? Or, should one define QOL pragmatically as a kind of umbrella under which are placed those items on which the user wants to focus?[28,37]

Analogous (but much more virulent) discussions have occurred about "intelligence."[37,38] It is worthy of note that IQ measures can be used as ways to assess improvements in opportunities for learning, or as ways to justify withholding or withdrawing such opportunities. Similarly, QOL measures could be used to assess improvements in treatment, or as a justification for withholding or withdrawing treatment, as discussed later in this chapter (see Applications to Clinical Decision Making: Withholding or Withdrawing Treatment).

In the clinical context, broad agreement also exists for the following methodological themes:[39] that self-assessments of patients' health-related QOL should be obtained in ways that fulfill the measurement requirements of reliability and validity; that the use of standardized questionnaires to elicit comparable information in the same way from all patients provides clinicians with more useful information than does the use of untested *ad hoc* approaches; and that both general and disease-specific measures are important in assessing an individual's health-related QOL.

A Definition of Health-Related QOL ■

One response to the difficulties inherent in attempts to define QOL is simply to sidestep the issue of definition. Another is to focus on health status as "something useful" that is of value to users of a health care system.[36,40]

For the purposes of this review, *health-related* quality of life is defined as "the subjective experiences or preferences expressed by an individual, or members of a particular group of persons, in relation to specified aspects of health status that are meaningful, in definable ways, for that individual or group."

This concept of health-related QOL does not incorporate a definition of health status, but it does require that the aspects of health status to be measured be specified, and that they be meaningful in definable ways. For example, the phrase "meaningful in definable ways" could refer (narrowly) to "meaningful in relation to the impact of a particular disease or its treatment on physical functioning," or (much more broadly), "meaningful in the sense of realizing aspirations, or of satisfying needs, or of changing and coping with the environment" (as in the 1984 concept of health expressed by the European Region of WHO).[26]

In practice, it may be impossible to separate health-related QOL unequivocally from other aspects of QOL. For example, if a diagnosis of cancer has an impact on family relationships already under strain for other reasons, it may be quite pointless to attempt to ascertain which aspects of any changes in family relationships are health-related and which are not.

It should also be stressed that efforts to assess patients' health-related QOL in terms of subjective assessments of health status should not be confused with efforts to measure patients' satisfaction with quality of care. Subjective satisfaction with care is a separate issue.[41-44]

How to Measure QOL? ■

Issues that must be taken into account in efforts to obtain quantitative assessments of QOL have received a good deal of attention in recent years. No attempt will be made here to provide a catalogue of currently available measures and their properties, which have been discussed in several recent reviews.[20,45-49]

Discussions of the methodological issues that underlie various approaches to the development or refinement of questionnaires are of central interest to researchers in the field, but can be tedious and unrewarding for those whose primary concern is the uses of the questionnaires. However, at this early stage in the development of QOL assessment, such methodological issues, like the conceptual issues outlined in the previous section, cannot safely be ignored.

Another major point is that the measurement instruments (usually structured questionnaires) used for quantitative assessments of QOL should meet rigorous standards of quality, based on criteria analogous to those applied to all aspects of scientific measurement. In particular, the measures should be reliable (yielding reproducible results), and valid (measuring what they are supposed to measure). Criteria for assessing the reliability and validity of questionnaires are available.[50]

The assessment of validity poses some vexing problems, because it is, in essence, a process of accumulating evidence. Each application of a questionnaire involves, implicitly or explicitly, another test of its validity. Thus, anyone who uses any method for QOL assessment (including those who simply ask, "How are you?") is, wittingly or not, participating at some level in the ongoing conceptual and methodological debates about the development of instruments for QOL assessment.

Some examples of approaches to the development and characterization of questionnaires designed for QOL assessments are considered below.

Health Status Indices ∎

Attempts to describe health-related QOL have received a great deal of impetus from work on the development of indices for use in population health studies and program evaluations. For example, a multiattribute health status index provides a method for quantifying health status as a single global index.[51] Two basic steps are involved in developing a multiattribute health status index—First, the creation of a multiattribute health status classification system, and second, the use of scaling procedures to convert the health-state classification system into a single global index.[51] The second step involves asking people to make judgments about the relative desirability or "utility" of different health states. Approaches to the development of multiattribute measures of health status, and procedures for determining the weights, values, or utilities to ascribe to each attribute, are reviewed in the next two sections.

Multiattribute Health Status Classification Systems ∎

A multiattribute health status classification system provides a way of describing the health status of an individual at a point in time.[51] The development of such a classification system involves three major steps. First, a number of attributes of health status are defined. For example, the Index of Well-Being of the San Diego group[52] described a health status classification system consisting of the attributes of mobility, physical activity, social activity and symptoms/problems. Rosser and colleagues in London[53,54] used a system consisting of the attributes of disability and distress. The group at McMaster University in Canada has developed a six-attribute system applicable to children and their development.[55,56] They have applied a seven-attribute system in a study of the treatment of childhood cancer.[57] These seven attributes are sensory and communication abilities, happiness, self-care ability, pain or discomfort, learning and school abilities, physical activity, and fertility. (The last attribute was included to assess effects on fertility of therapy for some forms of childhood cancer.)

The second step in the development of a health status classification system is to define different levels of function for each attribute, ranging from the "best" to the "worst" level. An individual's health status then can be classified according to his or her function level for each of the attributes. For example, the two attributes of disability and distress in the Rosser and Watts system[54] involved eight levels and four levels for each attribute, respectively.

The third step in developing a multiattribute health status classification system is to determine the relative weights, values, or utilities to be ascribed to each attribute. The relative importance of the various attributes may be very strongly influenced by the perspective of the individual whose values are being sought, as well as by the relevant circumstances. In the clinical context, attention needs to be paid to those aspects of QOL that are of greatest importance to patients. For example, in a study of aspects of the health-related QOL of patients with metastatic breast cancer, Sutherland and colleagues[58] found that aspects of general health, such as self-care, mobility and physical activity, appetite, sleep and family relationships, were ranked more highly than items concerned directly with the common side-effects of therapy.

Measurement of Utilities ∎

Suppose that a decision maker is asked to choose which form of management would be preferred, on the basis of the results depicted in a "quality versus quality" comparison of two health profiles of the kind shown in Figure 11-1A. Suppose further that the decision maker is told the following: (1) that the duration of expected survival is exactly the same for the two profiles (X years); (2) that the area under the health profile expected for Management I is Y quality-adjusted life years (QALYs); (3) that the area under the health profile expected for Management II is Z QALYs; and (4) that Y is greater than Z. On the basis of this information, a logical decision would be to prefer the form of management that would be expected to yield the larger number of QALYs, even though the overall duration of expected survival is exactly the same. Management I might thus be preferred in this instance.

How are QALYs calculated? Weinstein and Stason[59] proposed that QALYs might be thought of as an equivalent number (less than X) of years with full health. In brief, if a health profile is plotted such that the abscissa is years of survival, and the ordinate is an aggregated QOL score, ranging from zero to one for the series of health states at each point in time, then the area under the health profile can be measured.[19,60] If an appropriate quality-adjustment factor has been applied to each point on the health profile, then the area can be expressed in QALYs. Examples of calculations of QALYs, using health state utilities as the quality-adjustment factors, are discussed by Drummond and associates.[60]

A question that immediately arises is considered equivalent by whom? When QALYs are intended for the comparison of alternatives directed at the same disorder, and not to compare the results to programs directed at other disorders, then patients are an appropriate source of preferences.[60]

Suppose that the decision maker is then asked: "How much would you prefer Management I over Management II?" The "expected utility model" provides a means to answer this question, using a procedure referred to in the jargon of the field as a "lottery," or a "standard gamble."[61,62] The basic concept of a lottery is simple—How big a risk are you willing to take to try to move from a poorer health profile to a better one? This concept thus involves attitudes toward taking risks, as well as attitudes toward the relevant health profiles.

The "lottery," illustrated diagrammatically in Figure 11-2, is formulated as follows: Suppose that you are the decision maker. You are guaranteed in advance to receive Health Profile I, with its attendant range of QOL. You are told it will last for X years of survival, and has a total area of Y

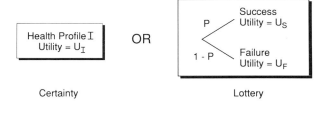

$$\text{Expected Utility } U_I = (P)\, U_S + (1 - P)\, U_F$$

FIG. 11–2 This figure shows the lottery or standard gamble approach to measuring the utility (U_I) for a health profile, relative to health profiles characteristic of perfect health (utility U_S) or unacceptable health (utility U_F).

QALYs, for an average of Y/X (less than unity) QALYs per year. You are then told, prior to the beginning of the X years of survival, that, as an alternative to remaining in Health Profile I, a (hypothetical) risky treatment is available. If accepted now, this treatment has a probability (P) of success; it could move you into a health state you perceive to be equivalent to "perfect health," lasting again for X years of survival. This state would have an area of X QALYs, or one QALY per year. However, the risky treatment also has a corresponding chance (probability Q = 1 − P) of failure; it may move you into a health state you would regard as totally unacceptable, one with an area of zero QALYs (and zero QALYs per year). You would consider it equivalent to death.

In the lottery procedure, the magnitude of the probability (P) that the hypothetical risky treatment is a success is then varied systematically, and an indifference probability is identified. That means that you are truly indifferent or unwilling to decide whether or not you wish to accept the risky treatment. The magnitude of this indifference probability then provides a quantitative measure of your preference for Health Profile I, and can be used to calculate a utility score (U_I) for that profile as shown in Figure 11-2. (The concept of utility is a general one, so that one can calculate a utility for a health profile by applying the same kind of equation that is used to calculate a utility for an individual health state. For examples of the latter calculation, see Llewellyn-Thomas, et al).[63]

A similar lottery procedure could then be used to measure your utility for Health Profile II, and the difference between the utilities for I and II would provide a quantitative measure of the extent to which you prefer Health Profile I over II (and, hence, Management I over II).

This lottery procedure is based on a theoretical concept of the way that a logical person ought to make such a risky choice. It has a strong axiomatic basis,[61] and is widely accepted by decision analysts as an idealized approach to rational decision making under conditions of uncertainty. However, as will be apparent from the above description, the details of the procedure are somewhat difficult to explain as well as cumbersome to carry out. Yet, in spite of its drawbacks, this procedure continues to be regarded as the best available way of formulating and measuring utilities.[62] It is also used as a "gold standard" against which other approaches to the assessment of preferences/values can be evaluated, including those actually based on models of decision making under conditions of certainty, rather than uncertainty.[64,65] And, because most clinical decision making is carried out under conditions of uncertainty, the lottery procedure continues to be relevant to discussions of clinical decision making.

The lottery procedure could also be applied to the "quality versus quantity" comparison illustrated diagrammatically in Figure 11-1B. This case calls for comparing two health profiles which differ in expected duration of survival. Technically, this comparison can be performed in a similar way to the lotteries outlined for the quality versus quality comparison, by obtaining utilities for the two health profiles and comparing them. In this case, however, the actual duration of expected survival differs between Health Profiles I and III. To make a comparison, some important assumptions must be made about how to combine quality and quantity of survival into a single index.[66] In particular, it must be assumed that it is justifiable to make tradeoffs between quality and quantity of survival.

Tradeoffs between quality and quantity of survival can, of course, be made only if it is assumed that prolongation of survival is not the sole objective of management. Departures from this objective raise conceptual, methodological, and ethical issues that will not be considered further here, but are discussed elsewhere.[4]

It is also beyond the scope of the present review to discuss other approaches that have been used for the assessment of preferences/values. A thorough discussion of the methodological issues is available in four review articles by Froberg and Kane,[14-17] and a more compact review has been provided by Llewellyn-Thomas and Sutherland.[67]

Multidimensional QOL Assessments ■

Attempts to describe health-related QOL, especially in the context of controlled clinical trials, are becoming increasingly dependent on the availability of structured questionnaires. Procedures for the analysis of multivariate data sets, of a kind most familiar to behavioral and social scientists, are used in the development of these questionnaires. An example of such a procedure is factor analysis.[68] This procedure provides one way to deal with the observation that if several items intended to measure different aspects of some broad concept (such as QOL) are administered to a group of people, the scores for the various items tend to be positively correlated. Can some common factors/constructs/domains/dimensions (such as physical, emotional, and social health, see Table 11-1) be identified that might be helpful in describing these associations? Do the different items emphasize different aspects of these same factors? Could the QOL of each individual, to a first approximation, be described in terms of scores for a limited number of such factors?

Questionnaire development usually involves

Table 11-1
Items Included in Factor Scales for General Health, Based on the LASA Scales Developed by Selby et al.[73]

Item*	Physical Health	Emotional Health	Social Health
Writing	0.96		
Speech	0.61		
Mobility*	0.48		0.48
Physical activity	0.47		
Depression		0.82	
Anxiety		0.75	
Concentration		0.73	
Anger		0.64	
Appetite		0.62	
Sleep		0.57	
Family relations		0.37	
Social life			0.75
Housework			0.67
Recreation and hobbies			0.46
Work			0.46

*Only items with factor loadings of greater than 0.30 are shown. "Mobility" is the only item that appears twice, as relevant to both "Physical Health" and "Social Health".

(Adapted from Ciampi A et al. Assessment of health-related quality of life: factor scales for patients with breast cancer. J Psychosoc Oncol 1988;6(1/2):1.[80])

four major phases. First, an "item pool" is assembled. The developer tries to include a broad range of items hypothesized to contribute to a description of each of the QOL factors of interest.

Second, the individual items are tested to see if they could be combined into a more limited set of multi-item scales, one for each factor of interest.[69] The techniques of factor analysis can be used for this purpose. This phase also could include an assessment of the internal consistency of the scale,[70] and tests of its reliability, such as "test-retest" reliability.[71]

In the third phase, efforts are made to examine the "construct validity" of the scales. That is, can evidence be obtained that the scales are indeed measures of the hypothesized factors of interest? In the jargon of the field, are the scales "tapping the dimensions" (or constructs or domains) of QOL that they are intended to measure? Equally important, are they *not* measuring some other factors?[69]

A fourth (and sometimes neglected) phase involves an effort to obtain information about preferences associated with each of the items or sets of items (factors). QOL questionnaires that lack information about preferences simply provide a way to gather descriptive clinical information (I. Barofsky, written communication). Incorporation of such data into a diagnosis, treatment decision, or some other clinical judgment is an additional task involving a valuation process. This task can occur either informally and implicitly, or explicitly, as a formal part of the QOL assessment. For example, the clinical data might demonstrate a decrement in the activities of daily living. If the clinical investigators made the explicit judgment that the observed decrement was unacceptable, then the patients' own preferences would not have been sought, and would not be taken into account in any use of such data in subsequent clinical decision making.

A more informal approach to this fourth phase might involve the implicit assumption that all aspects of QOL are equally important. Again, the patients' own preferences would not have been assessed. It is not possible to sidestep the valuation process. This chapter has already referred to the methods used for assessment of preferences (values or utilities).[14–17,67]

Four examples of multidimensional questionnaires specifically designed for use in oncology are outlined below, as illustrations of the approaches currently under development. For a more complete review and appraisal of the characteristics of a number of questionnaires, see Osoba, Aaronson and Till.[49]

Linear Analogue Self-Assessment ■

Linear analogue self-assessment (LASA), using visual analogue scales, is a well-established method of obtaining subjective information in an efficient way.[72] The approach is simple. Each item to be assessed is represented by a 10-cm line, "anchored" at each end by statements that define the extremes of the range of levels of function associated with that item. For example, for the item "physical activity," the range might be from "normal physical activity for me" (best) to "completely unable to move my body" (worst).[73] The patient marks the position on the line between these extremes that corresponds to his or her self-assessment for that item. A measurement of the location of the mark relative to the total length of the scale provides a quantitative score for that scale.

Priestman and Baum[74] used LASA scales to assess the QOL of patients with breast cancer, and Selby and associates[73] extended their approach. Selby's approach is based on the concept of modules of LASA scales that could, if appropriate, be combined in different ways.[75,76] General health was assessed using a core set of 16 items derived from the Sickness Impact Profile,[77] a well-known behaviorally based measure of health status. Major problems associated with breast cancer or its treatment were assessed using a 12-item module that was developed as part of the study. Each item was evaluated for reliability, feasibility, and, subsequently, relative importance.[73,58] To assess validity, the correlations between items were analyzed by factor analysis, and the observed associations seemed to fit the clinical features of breast cancer. The questionnaire was able to distinguish between clinically distinct groups of patients, and detected changes across time.[78,79]

Further work on the validation of this questionnaire using factor analysis indicated that information for 15 of the 16 items related to general health could be described in relation to three factors—physical, emotional, and social health.[80] Results of the factor analysis are shown in Table 11-1. The "factor loadings" provide an estimate of the correlation between the item and the factor. Three "factor scales" related to general health were constructed by taking the mean of all items with factor loadings greater than a chosen threshold for each factor.[80] A fourth factor scale, termed *disease-related*, incorporated 11 items related to breast cancer and its treatment. Such factor scales represent an attractive compromise between attempts to condense all the data into a single overall QOL score, and the cumbersome reporting of results for each individual item. The former approach results in a reduced ability to discriminate between groups.[80] The latter, though it permits one to seek patterns in the results for individual items, runs the risk of misinterpreting chance fluctuations as real differences in health status, because repeated tests of statistical significance must be performed. No unique, optimal statistical method for the analysis of data with multiple endpoints appears to exist at present.[81] An advantage of scores from subscales (such as factor scales) is that they can be expected to show better reliability than scores for individual items, as well as more sensitivity to differences than a single global score.[80]

The Functional Living Index—Cancer ■

The Functional Living Index—Cancer (FLIC) is a 22-item questionnaire that was designed for easy, repeated patient self-administration.[82] It was initially validated on 837 cancer patients in two cities over a three-year period. Factor analyses were interpreted in terms of items that assessed physical well-being and ability, emotional state, sociability, family situation, and nausea. The index was proposed as an adjunct to clinical trials assessment. It was intended to provide additional patient functional information on which to analyze the outcome of clinical trials, or offer specific advice to individual patients. Experience with its use illustrates the difficulties inherent in collecting QOL data in a clinical trial (see also Table 11-2, Question 5).[83,84]

The Quality of Life Questionnaire ■

The Quality of Life Questionnaire (QLQ) developed by the Study Group on Quality of Life of the European Organization for Research and Treatment of Cancer (EORTC) uses a modular approach to QOL assessment, involving both core and specific components.[76] The key elements of the 36-item core QLQ include functional status,

physical symptoms common to many malignancies and/or treatment modalities, psychological distress, social interaction, financial and economic impact, perceived health status, and overall quality of life. This questionnaire thus uses a pragmatic definition of QOL that goes somewhat beyond a focus only on health status. Reliability and validity have been assessed in an exemplary manner.

While the core QLQ is designed to be applicable across a range of tumor sites and treatment situations, tumor-specific supplements may be added to provide information on problems unique to particular groups of patients. For example, lung cancer patients were the target population for initial testing of the measurement properties of the questionnaire, so additional items were included in a supplemental QLQ module that has particular relevance to lung cancer.[76] These included two questions on coughing; a three-item scale assessing dyspnoea; four items concerned with additional side-effects of chemotherapy; and four items on pain and use of pain medications, for a total of 13 questions in the lung-cancer-specific module.

The QLQ is intended for use in cancer clinical trials. The modular system should facilitate investigations into the relationships between components of QOL and permit comparisons across trials without loss of trial-specific data.[76]

The Rotterdam Symptom Checklist (RSCL) ■

The 38-item Rotterdam Symptom Checklist (RSCL)[85] is based on analyses of data obtained from three studies done with different checklists, including a version of the Symptom Distress Scale,[86] plus eight items on functional status.

The results of factor analyses of data from three separate groups (total N = 753) revealed two main factors. The first was a psychological factor, which proved to be stable across populations. The second was a physical distress factor that appeared to be unidimensional in a heterogenous population (N = 611) of cancer patients under treatment, disease-free patients, and "normal" controls. In two smaller and more homogeneous populations of female cancer patients attending an outpatient clinic (N = 86) and patients with advanced ovarian cancer undergoing chemotherapy (N = 56), the physical distress was reflected by three factors—pain, fatigue, and gastrointestinal complaints. A scale based on the psychological distress factor was highly reliable, while the reli-

Table 11–2
Questions to Ask About QOL Assessments*

1. For what purpose will the results be used?
    —for screening or case-finding
    —to obtain health profiles
    —for the assessment of preferences
    —in clinical decision making
2. Which method of assessment is most appropriate for the purpose?
    —interview
    —questionnaire
    —self-assessment
3. What is the scope of the assessment?
    —general (includes physical, emotional, and social subscales, and a global measure of QOL)
    —specific (factor or disease-specific)
    —capable of reflecting positive aspects of QOL
4. Are adequate questionnaires available?
    —reliable (assessed for test-retest reliability)
    —valid (assessed for construct validity)
    —responsive to changes in QOL
    —used previously for a similar purpose
5. Is the intended assessment feasible?
    —acceptable to patients and health professionals
    —easily understood by patients
    —uses a clearly defined time frame
    —has a short completion time
    —easy to administer and score
    —has specially trained personnel available to administer, follow-up, monitor, and analyze the QOL assessments?
    —uses special procedures to minimize missing data and to maximize quality control
    —has policies in place to deal with sensitive issues (confidentiality of research data in relation to questions about referral or quality of care)
6. Are the results of the QOL assessments meaningful?
    —statistically
    —clinically
    —suggest actions to be taken

*Based on criteria of Osoba, Aaronson and Till.[49] See also Maguire and Selby;[46] Donovan, et al;[47] Moinpour, et al;[113] Aaronson;[28] Aaronson.[30]

ability of the physical distress scales, although not as high, was still satisfactory. Developed primarily as a tool to measure the symptoms reported by cancer patients participating in clinical research, the RSCL is also applicable for monitoring the levels of the patient's anxiety and depression.[85]

Questions to Ask About QOL Assessments ■

Because of the early stage of development of the field of QOL assessment, the challenging conceptual and methodological questions of what to measure, and how to measure it, have tended to be the main focus of attention. Some major practical issues involved in the selection and application of QOL assessments are summarized in Table 11-2, expressed as "questions to ask." The reader is referred to recent reviews for more details about the

criteria incorporated into this table (see, for example, the references in the footnote to Table 11-2). For an appraisal of a variety of QOL measures in relation to questions of the kind listed in Table 11-2, see Osoba, Aaronson and Till.[49]

How Should Results of QOL Assessments Be Used? ■

A fundamental issue in all QOL assessments is the purpose of the assessment. How will the data be used? This section provides a brief overview of the potential uses of QOL assessments (whether formal or not; see Barofsky[87]), in selected areas of particular relevance to clinical oncology. A taxonomy for specific purposes of QOL assessments has been proposed by Guyatt and associates[88] and by Osoba and colleagues.[49]

Applications to Clinical Trials: Descriptions of QOL or Evaluations of Interventions ■

At present, most QOL assessments are in a research and development phase of maturity and are not yet suitable for routine application in day-to-day clinical decision making. For this reason, applications in a research context, in randomized clinical trials (RCTs), will be considered first. Increasingly, attempts are being made to include, when appropriate, QOL assessments into the design of RCTs. For example, the Clinical Trials Group of the National Cancer Institute of Canada has formulated a policy that calls for a statement about the anticipated impact on quality of life with every proposed phase III clinical trial (and whether or not quality-of-life measures will be incorporated into the protocol).

The first type of trial includes RCTs designed primarily to evaluate the extent of changes in the QOL of individuals or groups, across time. For example, QOL data might be used as an endpoint or outcome measure in an RCT, in addition to more conventional endpoints such as duration of survival or time to relapse. The second type of trial includes RCTs designed to use QOL data to *predict* outcome or prognosis. In such trials QOL data might be used to stratify patients to be entered into an RCT.

QOL data to be used as endpoints can, in turn, be collected in two major ways. On the one hand, RCTs are usually based on clinical objectives and might be designed to obtain descriptions of the physical, emotional, and social functioning of patients before, during, and/or after application of the interventions being compared in the RCT. Measures used for data collection would usually involve patients' self-assessments of selected aspects of QOL (depending on the purposes of the study), using descriptive approaches of the kind outlined above. Well-characterized measures would already have been subjected to extensive critical appraisal to assess their reliability and validity and the feasibility of their use in the situation of interest (see Table 11-2). Detailed information about selected aspects of QOL could then be used not only as part of the quantitative assessment of the outcomes of the RCT, but *also to provide useful clues about ways to improve the interventions so that their impact on those aspects of QOL might be lessened.*

Other RCTs are increasingly being designed to evaluate the interventions from a health services perspective rather than a clinical one; they use measures more familiar to cost-effectiveness analysts and decision analysts. Measures used for data collection would be designed to assess patients' values or utilities, as discussed above.[14–17,67] The main issue in this case is an evaluation of patients' *preference* for one intervention (or its consequences) over any alternatives, rather than a description of those consequences. Again, well-characterized measures of values or utilities would have been subjected to prior critical appraisal in relation to their measurement properties. However, they would not necessarily have been designed to provide useful clues about ways in which the interventions themselves might be improved in order to reduce their impact on QOL.

Applications to Clinical Trials: Predictions of Outcome or Prognosis ■

RCTs designed to use QOL data to predict outcome or prognosis are beginning to be of interest to clinical oncologists. The potential of QOL measures as stratifying variables for patients entering RCTs is reflected in the use by the Lung Cancer Study Group (LCSG) of the Functional Living Index—Cancer (FLIC[82]) in several protocols.[89] The purpose was to test and refine the measurement of QOL in lung cancer patients. Preliminary data for 178 patients in four phase III trials indicated that the baseline QOL (FLIC) score was a strong and statistically significant prognostic indicator for survival, even after correcting for initial performance status and extent of disease.[89] Analogous findings have been reported, using a different measure of QOL, for an RCT involving 102 patients with inoperable non-small cell lung cancer, limited disease.[90] These results indicate that, at least for patients with lung cancer, a baseline QOL score might be useful as a stratifying variable.

The Spitzer Quality of Life Index,[91] which is usually based on an observer's assessment of the patient's QOL, has been shown to decrease in terminally ill cancer patients as death approaches and to be strongly associated with risk of mortality.[92] A recent report has also indicated that functional status and QOL are strong independent risk factors for subsequent mortality in patients entering treatment for end stage renal disease.[93] Thus, QOL scores might be important prognostic variables for a variety of diseases, at least for those patients for whom the prognosis is poor.

This possibility raises an ethical issue. Poor-prognosis, "high cost" patients tend to include some of the most vulnerable members of society, such as the aged, the disabled, or the poor. The use of QOL data as part of the characterization of such patients raises the possibility that such data might also be used as a basis for discrimination against vulnerable members of society.[4] This possibility becomes even more of a potential concern when QOL data are used in clinical decision making.

Applications to Clinical Decision Making: Withholding or Withdrawing Treatment ■

As QOL measures begin to be accepted by practicing clinicians as reliable and valid sources of information, it seems likely that QOL information will be used increasingly in making clinical decisions. Such information may facilitate discussion of QOL-related issues and lead to decisions about additional treatment, with an intent to improve quality of life.

However, QOL information may also be used in making decisions about withholding or withdrawing treatment. For example, as pointed out above, QOL data might provide strong support for the belief that a particular patient has a very poor prognosis. Suppose that, for medical reasons—or even for reasons based mainly on scarcity of resources—consideration is already being given to limitations on care. In such circumstances, quantitative QOL data, especially in the hands of those unfamiliar with possible pitfalls in such data, might easily tip the balance.

This type of use of QOL data is very likely to be premature because of inadequate reproducibility.[94] The currently available measures are usually unsatisfactory for application to decision making for individual patients.[95] At present, they are usually designed to be meaningful only when the results are averaged over the members of a group, such as a group of patients enrolled in a RCT. Unless new or improved measures with much higher reproducibility can be developed, application of the present generation of QOL measures to situations where decisions are being made in relation to individual patients, would, in the absence of attempts to gather further supporting data, result in far too many false conclusions. This issue will be considered further below (see Concluding Remarks).

In addition to these technical problems other considerations arise when QOL data are used in clinical decision making.[4] The possibility that QOL data might be used as a basis for discriminating among individuals raises significant ethical issues. For example, QOL assessments might be used as a justification for withholding treatment from vulnerable groups, while making the same treatment available to others judged to have a more favorable situation. This potential for discrimination needs to be borne in mind whenever QOL measures are used to label individual patients. Decisions to limit care are already being made. There are clear dangers inherent in allowing anyone, except the patient, to make decisions based on that patient's personal QOL. The limited empirical data available at present suggest that physicians, or even family members, are often not good predictors of the attitudes or preferences of individual patients.[96–99] Evidence also exists for a great deal of variation in personal values and preferences, not only from one person to another,[100,101] but perhaps, at least in some circumstances, from one time to another.[102]

Applications to Survival Analysis ■

Survival analysis is very widely used as a means of depicting and comparing the distributions of duration of survival for different groups of cancer patients. In contrast, no comparable, widely accepted way of depicting the results of QOL assessments exists. Graphs of an overall index of QOL versus time could be plotted for individual patients, in the same style as the health profiles for hypothetical groups of patients shown in Fig. 11-1. However, it is not a simple matter to depict or analyze sets of such plots for groups of patients unless a satisfactory approach to aggregation of the data is available. Issues involved in the statistical analysis of QOL data in cancer clinical trials appear in a recent paper by Olschewski and Schumacher.[103]

If detailed QOL assessments, involving data about such aspects of QOL as physical, emotional, and social functioning, are aggregated for purposes of display or analysis (Fig. 11-1), important detail could be lost. For example, a change for the worse in physical functioning might appear to be cancelled out by a change for the better in emotional functioning. Much more work needs to be done on the depiction and analysis of QOL data in ways that are intelligible to clinical oncologists. If it is necessary to rely entirely on technical experts, such as biostatisticians, for the interpretation of QOL data for groups of patients, then QOL assessments are unlikely to be widely used outside of a small coterie of researchers interested in the methodology of such assessments.

One attractive initial approach to this problem would be to incorporate QOL data into the familiar format of survival analysis.[103] Recent pioneering attempts to accomplish this aim have been reported by Goldhirsch, Gelber, and colleagues.[104] They first partitioned overall survival time (in the context of adjuvant therapy for breast cancer) into three components—time with toxicity (TOX), time without symptoms and toxicity (TWiST), and time after (systemic) relapse (REL). They then weighed TOX and REL by coefficients of utility relative to TWiST and added the results to give a period of quality-adjusted survival (Q-TWiST). Benefits measured by Q-TWiST may then be compared for different forms of therapy, taking into account a range of relative values assigned to periods with symptoms and toxicity. They recommended that quality-adjusted survival analyses of this type be used in assessing costs and benefits of toxic adjuvant therapy.[104]

The suggested equation for computing quality-adjusted survival is

$$Q\text{-TWiST} = (u_t \times \text{TOX}) + \text{TWiST} + (u_r \times \text{REL})$$

where u_t and u_r are utility coefficients to represent the value, relative to time without symptoms of disease or toxicity (TWiST), of time periods having subjective toxic effects (TOX), or time following relapse (REL), respectively. No attempt was made to measure the utility coefficients using methods such as those described earlier (see Measurement of Utilities). Instead, Q-TWiST was calculated for various arbitrarily chosen utility coefficients.

The Q-TWiST method provides a very interesting first-order approach to quality-adjusted survival analysis. However, it involves some implicit assumptions.[105]

The first assumption implicit in the equation is that the value to be given to toxicity is independent of the length of the period during which that toxicity is experienced. That is, neither u_t nor u_r are functions of time. This assumes that, for example, three months of toxicity from chemotherapy has half the value of six months of toxicity.

However, there is empirical evidence that the perceived value assigned to a health state may be related to the length of time one expects to spend in that state.[101] Indeed, Sutherland and associates[106] have reported evidence that, for some states of very poor health, there may even be a maximal endurable time that individuals not currently experiencing that health state suggest they would wish to spend in such a state. Such health states, perceived to be states "worse than death," have also been described by others.[51] (Whether or not individuals actually experiencing such states would still consider them "worse than death" needs to be examined further.) The lack of accounting for the utility for time remains one of the major criticisms of current ways of computing quality-adjusted survival.[66]

A second assumption of the Q-TWiST method is that the value of a period with toxicity is independent from the events following that period, as implied in the additive form of the equation. However, there may be an interaction between the value of a period during which toxic side-effects are experienced, and the duration of TWiST.[105] For example, six months of chemotherapy followed by ten years of TWiST might be valued quite differently from six months of chemotherapy followed by only 6 months of TWiST.

These assumptions would both be unnecessary

FIG. 11–3 This hypothetical plot of quality-adjusted survival for a group of patients is based on the individual health profiles for each of the patients in the group, plotted in order of increasing actual survival for those same patients. (Adapted from Till JE, de Haes JCJM. Quality-adjusted survival analysis (Q-TWiST). J Clin Oncol, 1991;9:525.[105])

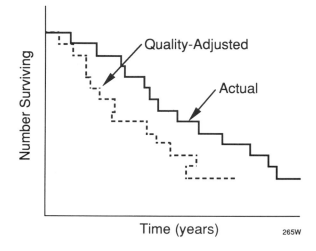

265W

if, as suggested by Mehrez and Gafni,[107] health profiles rather than individual health states are evaluated. Then, the influence of variations in relative durations of TOX and TWiST could be examined empirically, and plotted in the form of a quality-adjusted survival curve (Fig. 11-3).[105] This suggestion serves to emphasize the need for many more well-conceived studies designed to explore practical ways to obtain QOL assessments and to use them as aids in clinical decision making.

Concluding Remarks ■

An important limitation on the scope of information about subjective QOL is that, like subjective information about attitudes,[50] such information is restricted to what individuals know about their QOL and are willing to report. Numbers obtained from quantitative QOL assessments are not just like other clinical data, such as white cell counts. Although data of the latter type may be subject to measurement error, much less "fuzziness" exists about the concept of a white cell than about the concept of pain. Also, a meaningful measurement of pain requires a self-report from the patient.

Perhaps one should always take care to view QOL assessments as ways of systematically constructing answers to the basic question "How are you?" Some kind of communication must take place between the health-care professional and the patient, even if the medium of communication is a structured questionnaire. The health-care professional must provide a framework within which the patient can construct a personal report. The patient must then struggle to comprehend the framework and to take its structure into account in preparing that personal report. During the process of construction of this report, other information the patient considers relevant to QOL (but not necessarily information that might fit neatly into any preexisting framework) may be forthcoming. The professional might then incorporate the information contained in the patient's final report into some algorithm that yields a number (or numbers) intended to provide a convenient summary of some useful knowledge about the patient's QOL, abstracted from the patient's report.

It follows that it may be much more important to try to understand and learn from the process used by the patient to construct his or her report than to obtain the outcome of the process (e.g., the magnitude of the final number).[108,109] From this point of view, QOL assessments should perhaps be regarded as a process for facilitating discussion, and not merely as a process of measurement (see also Turnbull and Brunk[110]). An analogy may be made with democracy, which also should be regarded as a process for facilitating discussion and not merely as a process for counting votes.[111]

In other words, the potential of QOL assessments as means for fostering communication between patient and health-care professional may be much greater, and more rewarding, than their potential for yielding quantitative outcomes. QOL assessments provide a means to redefine and refine preferences in order to justify a course of action, and not just a way to record the preferences that already exist.

For example, a simple set of LASA scales designed to assess patients' emotional distress can permit a nurse in a busy clinical setting to look at the pattern of responses and quickly identify aspects of distress that could be explored further with the patient, as part of the assessment phase of nursing care. This kind of systematic inquiry can help patients to organize their thoughts and more clearly articulate their feelings.[112]

In conclusion, at this early stage in the development of QOL assessments, it would be premature either to dismiss them as "soft" (and therefore useless) clinical data, or to make uninformed judgments about how best to use (or not use) the data. Like any other novel approach to the acquisition of clinically relevant data, methods of QOL assessment should be developed systematically, and their uses should be evaluated critically, using the highest achievable standards of scientific rigor.

Acknowledgments. Supported by grants from the National Cancer Institute of Canada and the Medical Research Council of Canada, and by career support through the Ontario Cancer Treatment and Research Foundation.

References ■

1. Jonsen AR, Siegler M, Winslade WJ. Clinical ethics: a practical approach to ethical decisions in clinical medicine. 2nd ed. New York: MacMillan, 1986.
2. Roberts F. The radiation treatment of neoplasms—VI. Brit J Radiol. 1934;7:151.
3. Bush RS. Malignancies of the ovary, uterus and cervix. London: Edward Arnold, 1979:6.
4. Till JE. Uses (and some possible abuses) of quality of life measures. In: Osoba D, ed. Effect of cancer on

quality of life. Boca Raton, Florida: CRC Press, 1991: 137.

5. McKeown T. The role of medicine: dream, mirage or nemesis? Princeton: Princeton University Press, 1979.

6. McKinlay JB, McKinlay SM, Beaglehole R. A review of the evidence concerning the impact of medical measures on recent mortality and morbidity in the United States. Int J Health Serv 1989;19:181.

7. Fries JF. Aging, illness, and health policy: implications of the compression of morbidity. Perspect Biol Med 1988;31:407.

8. Callahan D. What kind of life: the limits of medical progress. New York: Simon and Schuster, 1990.

9. Murphy DJ, Cluff LE. Introduction: the SUPPORT study. J Clin Epidemiol 1990;43:V.

10. Schroeder SA, Zones JS, Showstack JA. Academic medicine as a public trust. JAMA 1989;262:803.

11. Cochrane AL. Effectiveness and efficiency: random reflections on health services. London: Nuffield Provincial Hospitals Trust, 1972.

12. Schwartz S, Griffin T. Medical thinking: the psychology of medical judgment and decision making. New York: Springer-Verlag, 1986.

13. Dowie J, Elstein A. Professional judgment: a reader in clinical decision making. Cambridge: Cambridge University Press, 1988.

14. Froberg D, Kane RL. Methodology for measuring health-state preferences—I: measurement strategies. J Clin Epidemiol 1989;42:345.

15. Froberg D, Kane RL. Methodology for measuring health-state preferences—II: scaling methods. J Clin Epidemiol 1989;42:459.

16. Froberg D, Kane RL. Methodology for measuring health-state preferences—III: population and context effects. J Clin Epidemiol 1989;42:585.

17. Froberg D, Kane RL. Methodology for measuring health-state preferences—IV: progress and a research agenda. J Clin Epidemiol 1989;42:675.

18. Szalai A. The meaning of comparative research on the quality of life. In: Szakai A, Andrews FM, eds. The quality of life: comparative studies. Beverly Hills, California: Sage, 1980:7.

19. Torrance GW. Utility approach to measuring health-related quality of life. J Chron Dis 1987;40:593.

20. Barofsky I, Sugarbaker PH. Cancer. In: Spilker B, ed. Quality of life assessments in clinical trials. New York: Raven Press, 1990:419.

21. Campbell A. The sense of well-being in America: recent patterns and trends. New York: McGraw-Hill, 1981:15.

22. Editorial: Independent international commission on health research for development. Lancet 1987;2:1076.

23. Till JE, McNeil BJ, Bush RS. Measurement of multiple components of quality of life. Cancer Treatment Symposia 1984;1:177.

24. World Health Organization. Constitution of the World Health Organization. WHO Chronicles 1947; 1:29.

25. Evans RG, Stoddart GL. Producing health, consuming health care. Soc Sci Med 1990;31:1347.

26. Health promotion: a discussion document on the concept and principles. Copenhagen: WHO Regional Office for Europe, 1984.

27. Callahan D. The WHO definition of health. Hastings Center Studies 1973;1:77.

28. Aaronson NK. Quality of life assessment in cancer clinical trials. In: Holland JC, Zittoun R, eds. Psychosocial aspects of oncology. New York: Springer-Verlag, 1990;97.

29. Schipper H, Clinch J, Powell V. Definitions and conceptual issues. In: Spilker B, ed. Quality of life assessments in clinical trials. New York: Raven Press, 1990:11.

30. Aaronson NK. Quality of life assessment in clinical trials: methodologic issues. Controlled Clinical Trials 1989;10:195S.

31. Van Knippenberg FCE, de Haes JCJM. Measuring the quality of life of cancer patients: psychometric properties of instruments. J Clin Epidemiol 1988;11:1043.

32. Mor V, Guadagnoli E. Quality of life measurement: a psychometric Tower of Babel. J Clin Epidemiol 1988; 41:1055.

33. De Haes JCJM, van Knippenberg FCE. Quality of life instruments for cancer patients: "Babel's Tower revisited." J Clin Epidemiol 1989;42:1239.

34. Cella DF. Quality of life in oncology: consensus views on definition and measurement [Abstract, 15th International Cancer Congress]. J Cancer Res Clin Oncol 1990 (Supplement, Part II: Lecture Abstracts); 116:947.

35. Baum M, Ebbs SR, Fallowfield LJ, Fraser SCA. Measurement of quality of life in advanced breast cancer. Acta Oncologica 1990;29:391.

36. Ware JE. Standards for validating health measures: definition and content. J Chron Dis 1987;40:473.

37. Feinstein AR. Clinimetric perspectives. J Chron Dis 1987;40:635.

38. Gould SJ. The mismeasure of man. New York: Norton, 1981.

39. Erickson P. Research roundtable. Bibliography on health indexes. 1984;2:35.

40. Evans RG. Strained mercy: the economics of Canadian health care. Toronto: Butterworths, 1984:5.

41. Ware JE, Davies-Avery A, Stewart AL. The measurement and meaning of patient satisfaction. Hlth Med Care Serv Rev 1978;1:2.

42. Cleary PD, McNeil BJ. Patient satisfaction as an indicator of quality care. Inquiry 1988;25:25.

43. Matthews DA, Feinstein AR. A new instrument for patients' ratings of physician performance in the hospital setting. J Gen Int Med 1989;4:14.

44. Wiggers JH, Donovan KO, Redman S, Sanson-Fisher RW. Cancer patient satisfaction with care. Cancer 1990; 66:610.

45. Clark A, Fallowfield LJ. Quality of life measurements in patients with malignant disease: a review. J Roy Soc Med 1986;79:165.

46. Maguire P, Selby P. Assessing quality of life in cancer patients. Br J Cancer 1989;60:437.

47. Donovan K, Sanson-Fisher RW, Redman S. Measuring quality of life in cancer patients. J Clin Oncol 1989; 7:959.

48. Cella DF, Tulsky DS. Measuring quality of life today: methodological aspects. Oncology 1990;4:29.

49. Osoba D, Aaronson NK, Till JE. A practical guide for selecting quality-of-life measures in clinical trials and practice. In: Osoba D, ed. Effect of cancer on quality of life. Boca Raton, Florida: CRC Press, 1991:89.

50. Nunnally JC. Psychometric theory. 2nd ed. New York: McGraw-Hill, 1978.

51. Boyle MH, Torrance GW. Developing multiattribute health indexes. Med Care 1984;22:1045.

52. Kaplan RM, Bush JW, Berry CC. Health status: types

of validity and the Index of Well-being. Hlth Serv Res 1976;11:478.

53. Rosser R. Issues of measurement in the design of health indicators: a review. In: Culyer AJ, ed. Health indicators. Oxford: Martin Robertson, 1983:34.

54. Rosser R, Watts V. Disability—a clinical classification. New Law J 1975;125:323.

55. Cadman D, Goldsmith C, Torrance GW. A methodology for a utility-based health status index for Ontario children. Final report to the Ontario Ministry of Health. Hamilton: McMaster University, 1986.

56. Rosenbaum P, Cadman D, Kirpalani H. Pediatrics: assessing quality of life. In: Spilker B, ed. Quality of life assessment in clinical trials. New York: Raven Press, 1990:205.

57. Feeny D, Barr RD, Furlong W, Torrance GW, Weitzman S. Quality of life of the treatment process in pediatric oncology: an approach to measurement. In: Osoba D, ed. Effect of cancer on quality of life. Boca Raton, Florida: CRC Press, 1991:73.

58. Sutherland HJ, Lockwood GA, Boyd NF. Ratings of the importance of quality of life variables: therapeutic implications for patients with metastatic breast cancer. J Clin Epidemiol 1990;43:661.

59. Weinstein MC, Stason WB. Foundations of cost-effectiveness analysis for health and medical practices. N Engl J Med 1977;296:716.

60. Drummond MF, Stoddart GL, Torrance GW. Methods for the economic evaluation of health care programmes. Oxford: Oxford University Press, 1987.

61. Von Neumann J, Morgenstern D. The theory of games and economic behavior. 3rd ed. New York: Wiley, 1953.

62. Machina MJ. Decision-making in the presence of risk. Science 1987;236:537.

63. Llewellyn-Thomas H, Sutherland HJ, Tibshirani R, Ciampi A, Till JE, Boyd NF. The measurement of patients' values in medicine. Med Decis Making 1982; 2:449.

64. Torrance GW. Social preferences for health states: an empirical evaluation of three measurement techniques. Socioecon Plann Sci 1976;10:129.

65. Mehrez A, Gafni A. Evaluating health related quality of life: an indifference curve interpretation for the time tradeoff technique. Soc Sci Med 1990;31:1281.

66. Loomes G, McKenzie L. The use of QALYs in health care decision making. Soc Sci Med 1989;28:299.

67. Llewellyn-Thomas H, Sutherland H. Procedures for value assessment. Recent Advances in Nursing 1987; 17:169.

68. Cattell RB. The scientific use of factor analysis in behavioral and life sciences. New York: Plenum Press, 1978.

69. Aaronson NK, Bakker W, Stewart AL, van Dam FS, van Zandwijk N, Yarnold JR, Kirkpatrick A. Multidimensional approach to the measurement of quality of life in lung cancer clinical trials. In: Aaronson NK, Beckmann JH, eds. The quality of life of cancer patients. New York: Raven Press, 1987:63.

70. Cronbach LJ. Coefficient alpha and the internal structure of tests. Psychometrika 1951;16:297.

71. Streiner DL, Norman GR. Health measurement scales: a practical guide to their development and use. Oxford: Oxford University Press, 1989:86.

72. Bond A, Lader MH. The use of analogue scales in rating subjective feelings. Br J Med Psychol 1974;47:211.

73. Selby PJ, Chapman JAW, Etezadi-Amoli J, Dalley D, Boyd NF. The development of a method for assessing the quality of life of cancer patients. Br J Cancer 1984;50:13.

74. Priestman TJ, Baum M. Evaluation of the quality of life in patients receiving treatment for advanced breast cancer. Lancet 1976;1:899.

75. Till JE. Quality of survival. In: Withers HR, Peters LJ, eds. Medical radiology: innovations in radiation oncology. Berlin: Springer-Verlag, 1988:25.

76. Aaronson NK, Bullinger M, Ahmedzai S. A modular approach to quality-of-life assessment in cancer clinical trials. In: Scheurlen H, Kay R, Baum M, eds. Cancer clinical trials: a critical appraisal. Berlin: Springer-Verlag, 1988:231.

77. Bergner M, Bobbitt RA, Carter WB, Gilson BS. The sickness impact profile: development and final revision of a health status measure. Med Care 1981;19:787.

78. Bell DR, Tannock IF, Boyd NF. Quality of life measurements in breast cancer patients. Br J Cancer 1985; 51:577.

79. Boyd NF, Selby PJ, Sutherland HJ, Hogg SA. Measurement of the clinical status of patients with breast cancer: evidence of the validity of self-assessment with linear analogue scales. J Clin Epidemiol 1988;41:242.

80. Ciampi A, Lockwood G, Sutherland HJ, Llewellyn-Thomas HA, Till JE. Assessment of health-related quality of life: factor scales for patients with breast cancer. J Psychosoc Oncol 1988;6(1/2):1.

81. Tandon PK. Applications of global statistics in analysing quality of life data. Stat in Med 1990;9:819.

82. Schipper H, Clinch J, McMurray A, Levitt M. Measuring the quality of life of cancer patients: the Functional Living Index—Cancer: development and validation. J Clin Oncol 1984;2:472.

83. Ganz PA, Haskell CM, Figlin RA, La Soto N, Siau J, for the UCLA Solid Tumor Study Group. Estimating the quality of life in a clinical trial of patients with metastatic lung cancer using the Karnofsky Performance Status and the Functional Living Index—Cancer. Cancer 1988;61:849.

84. Finkelstein DM, Cassileth BR, Bonomi PD, Ruckdeschel JC, Ezdinli EZ, Wolter JM. A pilot study of the Functional Living Index—Cancer (FLIC) Scale for the assessment of quality of life for metastatic lung cancer patients: an Eastern Cooperative Group study. Am J Clin Oncol 1988;11:630.

85. De Haes JCJM, van Knippenberg FCE, Neijt JP. Measuring psychological and physical distress in cancer patients: structure and application of the Rotterdam Symptom Checklist. Br J Cancer 1990;62:1034.

86. McCorkle R, Young K. Development of a symptom distress scale. Cancer Nursing 1978;1:373.

87. Barofsky I. Conceptual issues in quality of life assessment [Abstract, 15th International Cancer Congress]. J Cancer Res Clin Oncol 1990 (Supplement, Part II: Lecture Abstracts);116:948.

88. Guyatt GH, Van Zanten SJOV, Feeny DH, Patrick DL. Measuring quality of life in clinical trials: a taxonomy and review. Can Med Assoc J 1989;140:1441.

89. Ruckdeschel JC, Piantadosi S, for the Lung Cancer Study Group. Assessment of quality of life (QL) by the Functional Living Index—Cancer (FLIC) is superior to performance status for prediction of survival in patients with lung cancer [Abstract]. Proc ASCO 1989;8:311.

90. Kaasa S, Mastekaasa A, Lund E. Prognostic factors for

patients with inoperable non-small cell lung cancer, limited disease: the importance of patients' subjective experience of disease and psychosocial well-being. Radiother Oncol 1989;15:235.

91. Spitzer WO, Dobson AJ, Hall J, Chesterman E, Levi J, Shepherd R, Catchlove BR. Measuring the quality of life of cancer patients: a concise QL-index for use by physicians. J Chron Dis 1981;34:585.

92. Morris JN, Suissa S, Sherwood S, Wright SM, Greer D. Last days: a study of the quality of life of terminally ill cancer patients. J Chron Dis 1986;39:47.

93. McClellan WM, Anson C, Birkeli K, Tuttle E. Functional status and quality of life: predictors of early mortality among patients entering treatment for end stage renal disease. J Clin Epidemiol 1991;44:83.

94. Helmstadter GC. Principles of psychological measurement. New York: Appleton, 1973.

95. Addington-Hall JM, MacDonald LD. Can the Spitzer Quality of Life Index help to reduce prognostic uncertainty in terminal care? Br J Cancer 1990;62:695.

96. MacKillop WJ, Stewart WE, Ginsburg AD, Stewart SS. Cancer patients' perceptions of their disease and its treatment. Br J Cancer 1988;58:355.

97. Strull WM, Lo B, Charles G. Do patients want to participate in medical decision making? JAMA 1984; 252:2990.

98. Faden RR, Becker C, Lewis C, Freeman J, Faden AI. Disclosure of information to patients in medical care. Med Care 1981;19:718.

99. Lichtman RR, Taylor SE, Wood JV. Social support and marital adjustment after breast cancer. J Psychosoc Oncol 1987;5(3):47.

100. Boyd NF, Sutherland HJ, Heasman KZ, Tritchler DL, Cummings BJ. Whose utilities for decision analysis? Med Decis Making 1990;10:58.

101. Sackett DL, Torrance GW. The utility of different health states as perceived by the general public. J Chron Dis 1978;31:697.

102. Christensen-Szalanski JJJ. Discount functions and the measurement of patients' values: women's decisions during childbirth. Med Decis Making 1984;4:47.

103. Olschewski M, Schumacher M. Statistical analysis of quality of life data in cancer clinical trials. Stat in Med 1990;9:749.

104. Goldhirsch A, Gelber RD, Simes RJ, Glasziou P, Coates AS, for the Ludwig Breast Cancer Study Group. Costs and benefits of adjuvant therapy in breast cancer: a quality-adjusted survival analysis. J Clin Oncol 1989;7:36.

105. Till JE, de Haes JCJM. Quality-adjusted survival analysis (Q-TWiST). J Clin Oncol, 1991;9:525.

106. Sutherland HJ, Llewellyn-Thomas H, Boyd NF, Till JE. Attitudes toward quality of survival: the concept of "maximal endurable time." Med Decis Making 1982; 2:299.

107. Mehrez A, Gafni A. Quality-adjusted life years, utility theory, and healthy-years equivalents. Med Decis Making 1989;9:142.

108. Llewellyn-Thomas H, Sutherland HJ, Tibshirani R, Ciampi A, Till JE, Boyd NF. Describing health states: methodologic issues in obtaining values for health states. Med Care 1984;22:543.

109. Read JL, Quinn RJ, Berwick DM, Fineberg HV, Weinstein MC. Preferences for health outcomes: comparison of assessment methods. Med Decis Making 1984;4:315.

110. Turnbull HR, Brunk GL. Quality of life and public philosophy. In: Schalock RL, ed. Quality of life: perspectives and issues. Washington DC: American Association on Mental Retardation, 1990:193.

111. Weale A. The allocation of scarce medical resources: a democrat's dilemma. In: Byrne P, ed. Medicine, medical ethics and the value of life. Chichester: Wiley, 1990:116.

112. Sutherland HJ, Walker P, Till JE. The development of a method for determining oncology patients' emotional distress using linear analogue scales. Cancer Nursing 1988;11:303.

113. Moinpour CM, Feigl P, Metch B, Hayden KA, Meyskens FL, Crowley J. Quality of life end points in cancer clinical trials: review and recommendations. J Natl Cancer Inst 1989;81:485.

Part Three

Controversies

Nancy E. Kemeny

Is Hepatic Infusion of Chemotherapy Effective Treatment for Liver Metastases? Yes!

12

Hepatic Arterial Chemotherapy ■

Hepatic metastases are a major cause of morbidity and mortality in patients with gastrointestinal carcinomas. From 50% to 75% of patients with advanced colorectal carcinoma will develop liver metastases.[1] In an autopsy series of 1541 patients who died from colorectal carcinoma, metastatic disease in the liver was found in 672 patients (44%), of whom 46% (307/672) had metastases only in the liver.[2]

Hepatic arterial chemotherapy has been proposed for the following reasons:

1. Regional hepatic therapy has the advantage of producing high drug levels in the liver.[3] This is especially important for drugs with a steep dose-response curve such as the pyrimidine antagonists, fluorodeoxyuridine (FUDR) or fluorouracil (FU).

2. Hepatic metastases obtain most of their blood supply from the hepatic artery because metastatic lesions in the liver establish neovascular connections with the hepatic arterial circulation.[4] Normal hepatocytes derive most of their blood supply from the portal circulation. This observation was made on pathological data from both animal tumors[5] and a human study[6] using labeled FUDR. Patients with hepatic metastases were injected

with ^{3}H-FUDR (1 uCi/kg) into either the hepatic artery or the portal vein. Normal hepatocyte FUDR levels were similar whether the injections were administered into the hepatic artery or the portal vein. Tumor biopsies demonstrated that the mean tumor FUDR levels following hepatic artery or portal vein infusion were 12.4 and 0.8 nmol/g, respectively (p <0.01). Thus hepatic arterial chemotherapy increases the relative exposure of drug to tumor cells versus normal cells. In a randomized study comparing hepatic arterial infusion versus portal vein infusion in previously treated patients with liver metastases from colorectal carcinoma, there were no responses in the portal vein group while there was a 33% response rate in the hepatic arterial group.[7] Patients whose tumor failed to respond to portal vein infusion were then eligible to receive hepatic arterial infusion. Although the drug (FUDR) and the dose (0.3 mg/Kg a day for 14 days) were the same in both groups, a 33% response was seen with hepatic arterial infusion after tumor progression on portal vein infusion. This study demonstrated that regional chemotherapy for hepatic metastases from colorectal carcinoma should be administered through the hepatic artery.

3. There is a high hepatic extraction of certain drugs in the liver, allowing the use of a high che-

motherapy dose with less risk of systemic toxicity. Chemotherapeutic drugs which are most attractive for regional infusion are those extracted by the liver during the first pass, thereby producing lower systemic drug levels and consequently less systemic toxicity. Ensminger and associates[8] demonstrated that 94 to 99% of FUDR is extracted by the liver in the first pass, compared to a 19–55% hepatic extraction of FU, one of the major reasons for preferring FUDR over FU for hepatic arterial chemotherapy. Based on extraction data, the value of certain drugs for hepatic arterial infusion are listed in Table 12-1.

Collins reviewed the pharmacologic principles of regional delivery and emphasized the need for drugs with a high total body clearance.[9] The area under the concentration versus time curve (AUC) for regional therapy is a function of not only clearance of a drug, but the hepatic arterial flow. Since hepatic arterial blood flow has a high regional exchange rate (100 to 1500 mL/min), drugs with a high clearance rate are needed. Table 12-2 demonstrates the high total body clearance of such drugs as FUDR, 5-FU, and ARA-C.[10] If a drug is not cleared rapidly, it recirculates through the bloodstream numerous times, and the advantage of intra-arterial therapy over systemic therapy is mitigated.

4. Another rationale for hepatic arterial chemotherapy, especially for patients with metastatic colorectal cancer, is the concept of a step-wise pattern of metastatic progression.[11] In this concept, hematogenous spread occurs via the portal vein to the liver, then from the liver to the lungs, and then to other organs. Removal of hepatic metastases or regional hepatic infusion chemotherapy may then salvage some patients.

Table 12–2
Regional Drug Delivery Advantage for Selected Anticancer Drugs when QHA = 250 ml/min

Drug	CLTB (ml/min)	R (ml/min)
5-FUDR	25,000	101
5-FU	4,000	17
ARA-C	3,000	13
BCNU	1,000	5
Adriamycin	900	4.6
AZQ	400	2.6
cis-DDP	400	2.6
Methotrexate	200	1.8
VP-16	40	1.2

QHA: blood flow in hepatic artery

CLTB: total body clearance of drug

R: regional drug delivery advantage given CLTB and QHA and hepatic extraction of the drug

Adapted from Collins, JM. Recent Result Cancer Research 1987; 100:143.

The initial trials of hepatic artery infusion (HAI) utilized external pumps and percutaneously placed catheters which required hospitalization and patient immobilization for chemotherapy administration. Approximately 50% of patients were reported to respond to this therapeutic strategy.[12] The main problems related to this type of hepatic arterial infusion—hepatic arterial thrombosis, catheter dislodgement, and bleeding—made this method of treatment inconvenient for the oncologist and potentially harmful to the patient.[13]

The development of an implantable infusion device provided new stimulus for the further development and application of hepatic arterial delivery of chemotherapy.[14] The use of an implantable

Table 12–1
Drugs for Hepatic Arterial Infusion (HAI)

Drug	Half-Life (min)	Estimated Increased Exposure by HAI
Fluorouracil (FU)	10	5-10-fold
5-Fluoro-2-deoxyuridine (FUDR)	<10	100-400-fold
Bischlorethylnitrosourea (BCNU)	<5	6-7-fold
Mitomycin C	<10	6-8-fold
Cisplatin	20–30	4-7-fold
Adriamycin (doxorubicin hydrochloride)	60	2-fold
Dichloromethotrexate (DCMTX)	—	6-8-fold

Table 12–3
Hepatic Arterial FUDR Infusion with Internal Pump: Responses

Investigator	# Pts	% Prior Chemo	PR%	% Decrease in CEA*	Median Survival (mos.)
Niederhuber[17]	70	45	83	91	25
Balch[18]	50	40	—	83	26
Kemeny, N[19]	41	43	42	51	12
Shepard[20]	53	42	32	—	17
Cohen[21]	50	36	51	—	—
Weiss[22]	17	85	29	57	13
Schwartz[23]	23	—	15	75	18
Johnson[24]	40	—	47	—	12
Kemeny, M[25]	31	50	52	—	22

*CEA: carcinoembryonic antigen

pump offers several potential advantages over external pumps including reduction in catheter-related complications (thrombosis), precise drug administration, and greater patient acceptance.[15]

The first studies with the implantable pump and continuous FUDR therapy produced high response rates. The median response rate of ten studies involving 437 subjects (in which almost half of the patients had received prior chemotherapy) was 45%, and the median survival was 17 months (see Table 12-3).[16]

Randomized Studies of Hepatic Arterial Infusion vs Systemic Chemotherapy ∎

Seven randomized trials have been conducted to compare hepatic arterial chemotherapy to systemic therapy. The studies should have tried to address a number of questions.

Is there a higher response rate? □ In most of these studies complete response (CR) is defined as disappearance of all radiographically apparent tumor on CT scan. A partial response (PR) is defined as a reduction of at least 50% in the sum of the products of the perpendicular diameters of all lesions, and a minor response is a measurable reduction of less than 50% in tumor volume. Stable disease is described as no change in tumor volume within the first two months. Response information can be inferred from all of the studies.

Is there a difference in response duration? This question is answered in most studies.

Is there a difference in overall survival? To show a 50% increase in median survival, a study would need 100 patient deaths per study arm to provide a power of 82%.[26] None of the studies was large enough to truly answer this question.

Is there a decrease in toxicity? This question is dealt with in most of the studies.

Is there improvement in quality of life? This question has not been systematically addressed.

Memorial Sloan Kettering Cancer Center Trial ∎

One of the first trials took place at Memorial Sloan-Kettering Cancer Center (MSKCC).[27] This prospective randomized study compared hepatic arterial infusion (HAI) of FUDR with systemic FUDR, using the same drug schedule (a 14-day continuous infusion) and the same method of administration (the Infusaid pump) in both groups. The only difference was the dose of FUDR, 0.3 mg/kg/day in the HAI group and 0.125 mg/kg/day in the systemic group. FUDR was chosen for the systemic group instead of FU, so that the same drug would be used in each arm, and there would thus be fewer variables. In randomized studies comparing the two drugs, FUDR usually produced a higher response rate than 5-FU.[58]

All patients underwent exploratory *laparotomy* not only for the placement of a hepatic artery catheter and an implantable pump but also to ensure that two study groups were comparable by accurately defining the extent of liver involvement and assuring that there was no extrahepatic disease. Patients with a resectable hepatic lesion or extrahepatic disease were considered ineligible for the protocol.

Prior to randomization the patients were stratified for two important parameters—the extent of liver involvement with tumor and the baseline lactic dehydrogenase (LDH) levels.[28,29] Both of these factors have been shown to be important prognostic indicators of survival (see Fig. 12-1 and 12-2). Patients randomized to intrahepatic therapy alone had the hepatic artery catheter connected to the pump. In patients randomized to the systemic therapy, the hepatic artery catheter was connected to a subcutaneous implanted access port, and the pump was connected to an additional catheter placed in the cephalic vein. This allowed a cross-over from systemic therapy to hepatic arterial therapy in patients not responding to the systemic therapy by a minor surgical procedure (ligation of the systemic catheter followed by a pump connection to the hepatic catheter, see Fig. 12-3). One hundred seventy-eight patients were referred to the study; 162 patients were randomized since 12 refused randomization and 4 had an inadequate arterial blood supply. At laparotomy 63 patients were excluded—33 had extrahepatic disease, 25 had their tumor resected, 4 had no tumor, and 1 had an abdominal infection (Table 12-4).

Of the 99 evaluable patients, there were two complete and 23 partial responses (53%) in the group receiving HAI and 10 partial responses

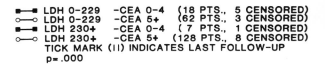

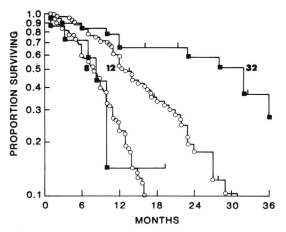

FIG. 12–2 Metastic colorectal carcinoma—survival. Survival curves based on initial LDH and CEA levels. The median survival of patients with normal LDH and CEA levels at initiation of chemotherapy was 32 months, whereas it was 8 months if both values were abnormal (p<.001). (From Kemeny N, Brown DW, Am J Med 1983;74:786–794.

FIG. 12–1 Survival distributions by percent liver involvement—medical assessment. The medial survival was 25 months for patients (pts.) with less than 20% involvement versus 6 months for greater than 60% involvement. (From Kemeny N, Niedzwicki D. Cancer 1989;63:742–747.)

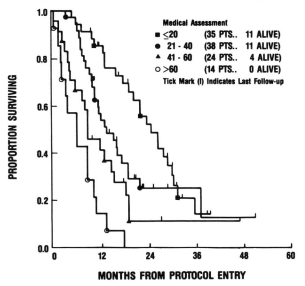

(21%) in the systemic group, p = .001 (Table 12-5). Thirty-one (60%) of the patients randomized to systemic therapy were crossed over to HAI after tumor progression. Twenty-five percent of these patients went on to a partial response after the crossover, and 60% had a decrease in carcinoembryonic antigen (CEA) levels.

Different toxicities were observed in the two groups. In the HAI group, the most frequent side-effect was hepatic enzyme elevation in 42%. In four patients (8%) changes resembling sclerosing cholangitis occurred in the bile ducts. Another frequent side-effect was ulcer disease, seen in 17%. The most frequent toxicity from systemic therapy was diarrhea, which occurred in 70% of patients, with 9% requiring admission for intravenous hydration. Twenty-three percent of patients had hepatic enzyme elevations, and 6% developed ulcers or gastritis (Table 12-5).

The median survival for the HAI and systemic groups was 17 and 12 months, respectively (p = 0.424). This is about a 40% increase in survival; however, in order to demonstrate a significant difference, more than a 100 deaths would have been necessary in each study group. The interpretation

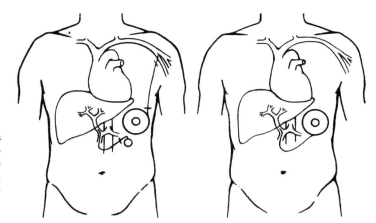

FIG. 12–3 MSKCC Study: this diagram shows conversion from systemic therapy to hepatic infusion, a crossover procedure for patients whose tumor failed to respond to systemic infusion. **Left,** minor surgical procedure required to allow crossover to intrahepatic artery. **Right,** final result. (From Kemeny N. Ann Int Med 1987;107:459.)

of survival is difficult in this study because 60% of the patients in the systemic group crossed over (that is, received hepatic arterial therapy after demonstrating tumor progression on systemic therapy). The patients who were unable to cross over (usually for mechanical reasons such as clotting of the hepatic arterial catheter) had a median survival of eight months, versus 18 months for the crossover group (p = 0.04, Fig. 12-4). Analysis of baseline characteristics in the crossover and non-crossover groups revealed no significant differences.

Commentary □ The MSKCC study clearly demonstrated a superior response rate for hepatic artery infusional chemotherapy. The two groups were comparable for all important variables including percent of liver involvement and baseline laboratory values. No patients with extrahepatic disease were included in the analysis since such patients were not randomized. A built-in flaw in the study design is that it allowed a crossover from systemic to hepatic artery infusion when the tumor progressed. Therefore, survival could not be accurately evaluated, especially since 60% of the systemic group crossed over.

Northern California Oncology Group Trial ∎

A similar randomized study conducted by the Northern California Oncology Group (NCOG) also used FUDR infusion in both the HAI and systemic groups.[30] Patients were stratified prior to

Table 12–4
MSKCC Study: Randomized HAI versus Systemic Infusion

Eligible	178
Refused Randomization	12
Inadequate Arterial Supply	4
Stratification	% liver involvement < 50% vs ≥ 50% LDH < 300 vs ≥ 300
Randomized	162
Excluded	63
Reseated	25
Extrahepatic	33
Infection	1
No Disease	4
Entered	99

Kemeny N: Ann Int Med 1987;107:459–465.

randomization by extent of liver involvement based on CT scans, baseline bilirubin values, and performance status. The doses of FUDR were 0.2 and 0.075 mg/kg/day for 14 days in the hepatic arterial and systemic groups, respectively. One hundred and forty-three patients were entered, but only 117 were eligible. They reported a 42% complete and partial response rate in the HAI group and 10% in the systemic group (p < .0001). The median time to progression was 401 days in the HAI group and 201 days in the systemic group (p = .009, see Table 12-6).

Toxicity was again different in the two groups with 16% of patients in the HAI group developing biliary tract toxicity which was reversible in all but 10% of patients. Grade 2 or greater diarrhea occurred in 40% of patients in the systemic group.

The median survival was 503 days and 484 days for the hepatic and systemic groups, respectively. Although a crossover design was not built into the

Table 12–5
MSKCC Trial: HAI vs Systemic FUDR Infusion

	HAI (n = 48)	Systemic (n = 51)	P Value
FUDR Dose Daily for 14 Days	.3 mg/kg	.125 mg/kg	
Complete Response	2	0	
	(52%)	(19.6%)	
Partial Response	23	10	0.001
≥50% Decrease in CEA	60%	25%	
Toxicity			
Ulcer	8	3	
Elevated Enzymes	20 (42%)	12	
Bilirubin >3	9	2	
Diarrhea	1	36 (70%)	
Colitis	0	4	
Biliary Sclerosis	4 (8%)	0	
Survival (Median)			
Total	17	12	0.424
Crossover		18*	
No Crossover		8	0.04

*These patients received HAI after tumor progression on systemic therapy.

Kemeny N: Ann Int Med 1987;107:459–465.

FIG. 12–4   MSKCC Study: median survivals. Triangle, entire intrahepatic group, median 17 months; diamond, systemtic non-crossover group, median 8 months; square, systemic crossover group, median 18 months. (From Kemeny N. Ann Int Med 1987;107:459.)

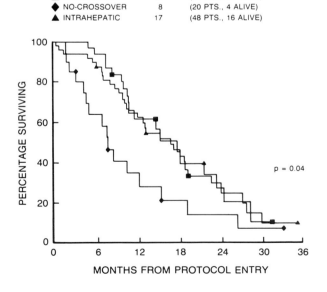

	MEDIAN (MOS.)	
■ CROSSOVER	18	(31 PTS., 12 ALIVE)
◆ NO-CROSSOVER	8	(20 PTS., 4 ALIVE)
▲ INTRAHEPATIC	17	(48 PTS., 16 ALIVE)

p = 0.04

Table 12–6
NCOG Study: Randomized HAI vs IV FUDR Infusion

	HAI n = 67	IV n = 76	P Value
FUDR dose mg/kg × 14D	0.2	0.075	
Complete response	8%	5%	
Response major	34%	5%	.0001
Biliary > grade 3	16%	0	
Irreversible jaundice	10%	0	
Diarrhea ≥ grade 3	0	18%	
Nausea, Vomiting	14%	45%	
Mucositis	0	18%	
Median time to progression (days)	401	201	.009
Median survival (days)	503	484	
No crossover		362	
Crossover		702*	

*Patients in systemic group who subsequently received hepatic arterial therapy

Hohn, D: J Clin Oncol 1989;7:1646–1654.

study, 43% of the patients in the systemic group crossed over to intrahepatic therapy after tumor progression on systemic therapy. Of the patients in the systemic group, the median survival was 23 months for those who had a crossover versus 12 months for those who did not receive hepatic therapy (Table 12-6).

Commentary □ One of the problems in this study, as in some of the other studies described below, is that patients with tumors in their hepatic lymph nodes were included in both study groups. Since the concept being tested here is whether regional therapy is effective for a certain population of patients, including patients who do not have only regional disease, interferes with interpretation of the results. Positive hepatic lymph nodes are considered a contraindication to liver resection. In a large series of patients who underwent liver resections no patients with positive hepatic lymph nodes were alive at five years.[59] These concepts should apply to patients receiving regional hepatic therapy as well. Early nonrandomized pump studies showed that patients with positive hepatic lymph nodes had a worse survival rate. The number of patients in the NCOG trial with extrahepatic disease in the two groups was not reported. Another problem with the study is that a crossover was permitted, although it was not built into the study design. Therefore, as in the MSKCC study, any true improvement in survival associated with HAI might have been overlooked.

National Cancer Institute Trial ■

A National Cancer Institute (NCI) study compared hepatic arterial to systemic infusion using FUDR in both treatment groups.[31] Sixty-four patients were entered into the study and analyzed for survival. However, 26% of the patients entered never received chemotherapy — 11 (34%) of the HAI group and 3 (9%) of the systemic group. Of the 21 patients treated in the HAI group 8 (38%) had positive hepatic lymph nodes. The study reported a significantly higher response rate for HAI—62% versus 17% for systemic therapy (Table 12-5). The toxicity for the arterial group was considerable—chemical hepatitis (79%), biliary sclerosis (21%), peptic ulcers (16%), and gastritis (21%). In the systemic group severe diarrhea occurred in 59% (Table 12-7). The survival data are based on all randomized patients. The median sur-

Table 12–7
NCI Study: Randomized HAI vs Systemic Chemotherapy

	HAI n = 32	IV n = 32	P Value
Dose FUDR mg/kg	.3	.125	
Treated	21	29	
+ Hepatic Nodes	8*	7	
Complete Response	1	1	
Partial Response	12 (62%)	4 (17%)	.003
>50% Reduction in CEA	12/20	3/26	
Toxicity			
Chemical Hepatitis	79%	7%	
Bilirubin >3	33%	0	
Biliary sclerosis	21%	0	
Ulcer	16%	0	
Diarrhea		59%	
Hospitalization for diarrhea		21%	
Survival (Median)	22m	12m	
Actuarial 2 year	34%	17%	.06
Actuarial 2 year without + Nodes	47%	13%	.03

*For patients without + hepatic lymph nodes

Chang A: Ann Surg 1987;206:685–693.

vival was 22 months for the HAI group, despite the fact that 53% of patients had extrahepatic disease and 34% of patients never received intrahepatic therapy (Fig. 12-5). In the systemic group 10% were not treated and the median survival was 12 months. In the subset of patients without extrahepatic disease, the two-year survival was 47% in the HAI group versus 13% in the systemic group (p = 0.03, see Fig. 12-6).

Commentary □ One of the main problems with this study is the small sample size; only 13 patients were in the HAI group if patients who were not treated or who had positive hepatic lymph nodes are excluded. The authors of the NCI study concluded that patients with positive hepatic lymph nodes should be excluded from regional therapy.

Mayo Clinic Trial ■

Another small study (69 patients) was conducted by the Mayo Clinic and compared hepatic arterial FUDR 0.3 mg/kg × 14 days to systemic bolus FU 500 mg/m² IV × 5 days.[32] Patients were stratified by baseline PS, extent of hepatic metastases, and the presence of measurable disease. The trial permitted entry only of symptomatic patients and did not allow a crossover to an alternative treatment. The response rate was 48% in the HAI group and 21% in the systemic group (p = 0.02). The time to hepatic progression was 15.7 and 6 months, respectively (p = 0.0001, see Fig. 12-7). The median survival was 12.6 and 10.5 months for the hepatic arterial and the systemic groups, respectively (p = 0.53).

Twenty percent of patients in the HAI group developed severe clinical hepatitis and 13% developed gastritis. The systemic group toxicity consisted of severe stomatitis in 30%, diarrhea in 18%, and leukopenia in 45%. The investigators reported an improvement in symptoms in 61% of patients treated with HAI and in 45% of the patients in the systemic group (Table 12-8).

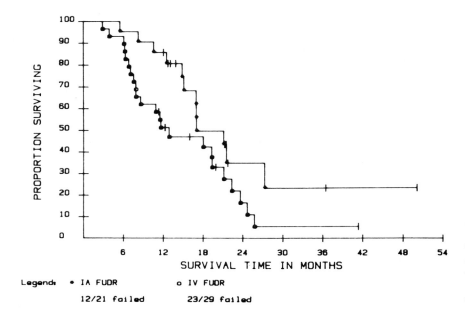

FIG. 12–5 NCI Study: survival of all randomized patients who received the assigned treatment. The two-year survival rates for IA (top line) and IV (bottom line) treatment groups were 34% and 17%, respectively (p = 0.06). (From Chang A. Ann Surg 1987;206:695.)

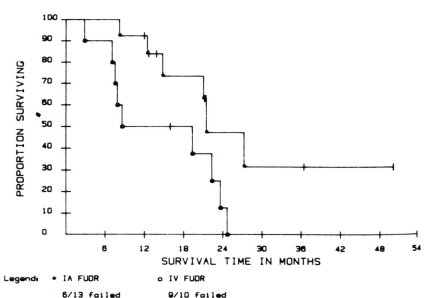

FIG. 12–6 NCI Study: survival of patients with documented negative hepatic lymph nodes who were randomized for IA (top line) and IV (bottom line) treatment. The two-year actuarial survival rates for IA and IV reatment groups were 47% and 13%, respectively (p = 0.03). (From Chang A. Ann Surg 1987;206:695.)

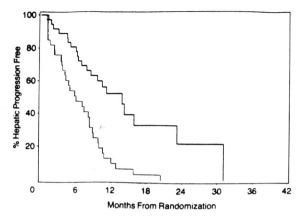

FIG. 12–7 Mayo Clinic Study: time to tumor progression in the liver is shown for patients receiving floxuridine (thick line) and fluorouracil (thin line). There is a significant difference for the floxuridine arm (two-sided p<.0001). (From Martin J. Arch Surg 1990;125:1022.)

Commentary □ Although this trial may permit a comparison of the response rates, it cannot adequately address survival. Only 36 patients were included in the HAI group, of whom five (14%) had never received treatment, seven (20%) had extrahepatic disease, three (9%) had hepatic artery thrombosis, and two (6%) had pump malfunction. All of these patients were included in the survival analysis, although 47% either were not adequately treated or had extrahepatic disease. The investigators report that the survival of patients with extrahepatic disease is significantly shorter than of those without extrahepatic disease (p = 0.04); therefore inclusion of these patients in the HAI

group will have a negative impact on survival. No comment appears in the report about the survival in the adequately treated patients.

Multicenter French Trial ■

In a trial by a multicenter group in France, 163 patients were randomized to hepatic arterial FUDR for 14 days versus systemic bolus FU daily × 5 every four weeks.[33] The groups of patients had comparable clinical and laboratory characteristics, including percent of liver involvement and baseline LDH levels. The response rate in patients with measurable disease was 49% in the HAI group and 14% in the systemic group (Table 12-9). Extensive hepatic toxicity occurred in the HAI group, with 35% of the patients experiencing sclerosing cholangitis by one year and 50% by two years. Crossovers were not allowed in this trial. Median time to hepatic progression was 15 months for the HAI group and 6 months for the systemic group (Fig. 12-8). Median survival was 14 months for the HAI group and 10 months for the systemic group. The two-year survival was 22% for the hepatic group and 10% for the systemic group (p<0.02, see Fig. 12-9).

Commentary □ The size of this trial and the lack of crossover in the design, make it possible to compare survivals. A significant increase occurred in two-year survival for the HAI group. Unfortunately, the toxicity was excessive, with a higher incidence of biliary sclerosis than reported

Table 12–8
Mayo Clinic Trial: Randomized HAI vs Systemic Chemotherapy

	HAI n = 36*	Sys n = 33	P Value
Chemotherapy dose	FUDR 0.3 mg/kg	FU 500 mg/m² × 5	
Tumor response	48%	21%	.02
Toxicity			
Chemical Hepatitis	26%	0	
Gastritis	13%	0	
Stomatitis	0	30%	
Diarrhea	0	18%	
Leukopenia	0	45%	
Hepatic progression (months)	15.7	6	.0001
Survival (months)	12.6	10.5	.31
Improved symptoms	61%	45%	.3

*53% of patients were not adequately treated or had extrahepatic disease.
Martin, J: Arch Surg 1990;125:1022–1027.

Table 12–9
French Trial: Randomized HAI vs Systemic Chemotherapy

	HAI n = 81	S n = 82	P Value
Chemotherapy Dose	FUDR 0.3/kg	FU 500 mg/^{m} × 5	
CR	13%	2%	
PR	36%	12%	
Median time to progression (mos)	15	6	
Extrahepatic Metastases	44%	39%	
Sclerosing Cholangitis	35%*	0	
Median Survival (mos)	14	10	
1-year survival	61%	44%	
2-year survival	22%	10%	<.02

*at 1 year

Rougier P: ASCO 1990;9:104.

by any other group. Insufficient information was provided to determine if dose adjustment for enzyme elevations was appropriately made. Despite the toxicity in the HAI arm, there remained an increase in survival compared to systemic FU. Another possible criticism is that systemic treatment did not always start immediately, since some physicians waited until patients were symptomatic.

Other Studies ∎

A study comparing HAI FUDR therapy with systemic FU treatment in symptomatic patients is being conducted in England.[34] It is designed to recruit 100 patients. Because of careful dose reduction for hepatic enzyme elevation, no liver toxicity has been observed in the 52 patients entered to

date. We do not yet have data on the number of responses but we have information about the percentage of tumor replacement in the liver. There has been a substantial decrease in the HAI group and an increase in the systemic group (Fig. 12-10). No crossover has been allowed, and the study will address both survival and quality of life issues.

In an intergroup study,[35] participants compared three types of treatment: HAI, combined intrahepatic and systemic therapy, and systemic. However, they were able to accrue only 43 patients. The response rates were 58%, 56%, and 38%, respectively, for the three treatments. The small sample size makes it difficult to discuss response and survival.

Another randomized study, conducted at the City of Hope,[36] asked a different question—Does HAI added to hepatic tumor resection increase the time to progression and improve overall survival? Ninety-one patients were entered in three different groups (Table 12-10). In group A, after solitary metastasis resection, patients were randomized to re-

FIG. 12–8 French Study: time to hepatic progression for the intrahepatic therapy group (solid line) and the systemic group (broken line). (From Rougier P. ASCO: 1990;9:104.)

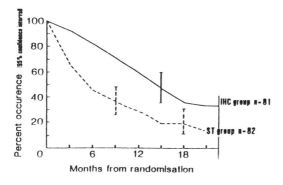

FIG. 12–9 French Study: survival curves for the intrahepatic (solid line) and the systemic groups (broken line). (From Rougier P. ASCO: 1990;9:104.)

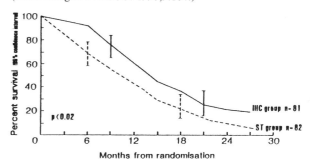

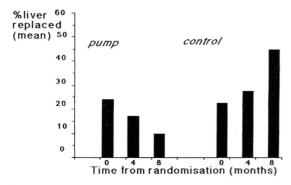

FIG. 12–10 English Study: percent of tumor replacement in the HAI (pump) group and the systemic chemotherapy group (control) over an eight-month period. At eight months tumor replacement is substantially down to 15% in the pump group and up to 50% in the control group. (Allen-Mersch: personal communication.)

ceive either no further treatment (A1) or HAI (A2). In group B, after resection of multiple metastases, the patients were randomized to receive no further treatment (B2) or HAI (B1). In group C there was no resection; patients were randomized to HAI (C1) or systemic FU followed by HAI (C2). If one looks at the group with solitary liver metastasis (Table 12-10), time to failure was 9 months in Group A1 (resection alone) and 31 months in Group A2 (resection plus HAI), p < 0.03. In the B group, 30% of patients who had resection plus HAI were alive at five years versus 7% of those receiving resection alone.

Commentary □ The English study will be one of the few studies that will look at quality of life issues, measuring anxiety and depression scores as well as using the Rotterdam physical score symptom checklist. This study, like the French trial, will hopefully address the survival issue since no crossover is permitted and the larger sample sizes may provide interpretable results. The City of Hope trial suggested a possible benefit from HAI treatment after resection since disease-free intervals increased. The numbers of patients in each group, however, are too small to generate significant information about survival. The Eastern Cooperative Oncology Group (ECOG) has embarked on a similar trial to see if HAI after resection of hepatic metastases improves survival.

Summary of Randomized Studies ■

Seven randomized trials demonstrate a significantly higher response rate with intrahepatic infusion versus systemic infusion in the treatment of hepatic metastases from colorectal carcinoma (Table 12-11). In every study the complete and partial response rates were higher for the HAI groups. Most of the investigators checked technetium 99 macroaggregated albumin perfusion (MAA) scans to be sure that there was perfusion of the liver. Figure 12-11 demonstrates a normal perfusion scan. A response from hepatic arterial chemotherapy depends on good hepatic perfusion. There may be perfusion of the stomach or other organs and not the liver (as depicted in Fig. 12-12), which increases toxicity and decreases response.

Because of the early successes with intrahepatic infusion, some of these studies allowed patients in the systemic arm to receive intrahepatic therapy

Table 12–10
Randomized Study of Resection ± HAI

Groups	# Pts	Time to Failure (Months)	P Value	Survival (Months)
Solitary met resection				
A1 resection only	6	9	≥.03	28
A2 resection + HAI	5	31		37
Multiple resection				
B1 resection + HAI	10	15	.18	19
B2 resection only	14	9		22
Unresectable				
C1 HAI	31	9		14
C2 Systemic than HAI	10	8	.94	12
C3 + Portal nodes, HAI	15	6		9

Wagner L, Kemeny M. J Clin Oncol 1990;8:1885.

Table 12–11
Randomized Studies of Intrahepatic vs Systemic Chemotherapy for Hepatic Metastases

| Group | # Pts | HAI | | Systemic | | P |
		Drug	% Response	Drug	% Response	
MSKCC[27]	162	FUDR	52	FUDR		0.001
NCOG[22]	143	FUDR	42	FUDR	10	0.0001
NCI[31]	64	FUDR	62	FUDR	17	.003
Consortium[35]	43	FUDR	58	5-FU	38	–
City of Hope[36]	41	FUDR	56	5-FU	0	–
Mayo Clinic[32]	69	FUDR	48	5-FU	21	0.02
French[33]	163	FUDR	49	5-FU	14	–

–: not available

after tumor failure on systemic therapy; therefore, the impact of intrahepatic treatment on survival is difficult to infer (Table 12-12). The studies demonstrate a survival advantage for the patients who received subsequent hepatic arterial treatment, with a mean one-year survival of 69% for the patients who had crossed over from systemic therapy to HAI versus 35% for the group who did not cross over (Table 12-12). The major flaw in these trials is the relatively small numbers of patients. The studies may have been large enough to dem-

onstrate a difference in response rate, but were too small to address survival. An analogous situation is the issue of adjuvant chemotherapy in colorectal carcinoma. For many years, patients with Dukes C colon cancer did not receive chemotherapy because the many small studies available failed to show a significant increase in survival. When a large study was finally completed, a significant increase in survival suggested a benefit of adjuvant therapy.[37] Since we not yet have a large enough randomized study of intrahepatic infusion versus systemic therapy, we should try to maximize response rates (especially complete responses) in an

FIG. 12–11 MSKCC Trial: survival curves of intrahepatic FUDR and LV treated patients compared retrospectively to patients treated with intrahepatic FUDR alone. (All patients had non-resectable disease.)

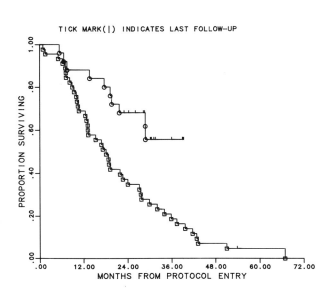

FIG. 12–12 Normal macroaggregated albumin perfusion scan.

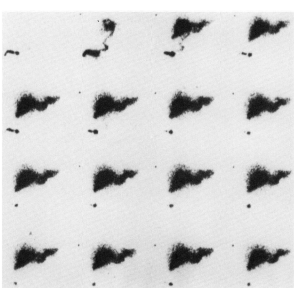

Table 12–12
Randomized Study of Hepatic (HA) vs Systemic (SYS) Chemotherapy

	Survival % Alive				Survival % Alive			
	1 year		*2 year*		*1 year*		*2 year*	
	HA	*SYS*	*HA*	*SYS*	*Crossover*	*No Crossover*	*Crossover*	*No Crossover*
MSKCC	60	50	25	20	60	28	25	14
NCOG	60	42	30	20	78	42	40	17
NCI*	85	60	44	13				
FRANCE	61	44	22	10				
MEAN	66	49	30	18	69	35	37	15

*Excluding patients with + hepatic lymph nodes

attempt to have an even more definitive impact on survival.

Toxicity of Intrahepatic Therapy ∎

A summary of the gastrointestinal toxicities noted by investigators using the implantable pump appears in Table 12-13. The side-effects of systemic chemotherapy are almost never observed with hepatic arterial infusion. Myelosuppression does not occur with intrahepatic FUDR.[16,19,27] Although intrahepatic mitomycin-C or BCNU may depress platelet counts, the absolute depression and frequency of depression occur to a lesser degree than with systemic administration. Nausea, vomiting, and diarrhea do not occur with HAI of FUDR. If diarrhea does occur, shunting to the bowel should be suspected.[38] The most common problems with HAI are ulcer disease and hepatic toxicity.[16,19] The most likely mechanism for gastric toxicity from hepatic arterial infusion is inadvertent perfusion with drug of the stomach and duodenum via small branches from the hepatic artery. Hohn and colleagues[39] did not observe ulcer disease in their patients, and they attribute this state to their surgical technique, which involved careful denuding of the vessels arising from the hepatic artery (distal to the cannulation) that supply the stomach and duodenum.[39] Other attempts to modify this toxicity include careful reduction of the dose with any gastrointestinal symptoms.

Hepatic toxicity in the different studies is outlined in Table 12-13. Approximately one-fourth of patients developed an elevated bilirubin. Investigators disagree about the nature of hepatic toxicity. Some feel it is similar to hepatitis because of documented hepatocyte necrosis and cholestasis on liver biopsy.[40] Others believe the hepatic toxicity is due to pericholangitis and fibrosis of biliary radicals. In early stages of toxicity, hepatic enzyme elevations will return to normal when the

Table 12–13
Hepatic Arterial FUDR Infusion with Internal Pump: Toxicity

Investigator	# Pts	Gastritis (%)	Ulcer (%)	Increased SGOT (%)	Increased Bilirubin (%)	Diarrhea (%)	Biliary Sclerosis (%)
Niederhuber[17]	70	56	8	32	24	—	—
Balch[18]	50	—	6	23	23	0	—
Kemeny N[19]	41	29	29	71	22	0	5
Shepard[20]	53	—	20	49	24	—	—
Cohen[21]	50	—	40	10	25	—	—
Weiss[22]	17	50	11	80	23	23	—
Schwartz[23]	23	53	—	77	20	10	—
Johnson[24]	40	—	8	50	13	0	5
Kemeny, M[25]	31	17	6	47	—	8	19
Hohn[30]	61	35	2	0	78	11	29

drug is withdrawn and the patient is given a rest period. In some patients, however, jaundice does not improve. These patients may develop biliary strictures, most commonly at the site of hepatic bile duct bifurcation, but also in the common bile duct or intrahepatic radicals. Necrosis of the main bile ducts in patients treated with hepatic arterial FUDR has been documented. In an autopsy series from Lausanne, Switzerland,[41] involving patients who had received HAI, the most remarkable feature was gross bile duct damage associated with histological blood vessel changes. Inflammatory and atrophic changes occurred as well as necrosis of the walls of small arteries. These changes may lead to ischemic injury of the bile ducts.

The exact mechanism of the biliary sclerosis is not clear. The bile ducts, like hepatic tumors, derive most of their blood supply from the hepatic artery and not the portal vein.[42] Therefore the bile ducts, like the tumor, are being exposed to a higher concentration of drug when it is perfused via the hepatic artery. Evidence suggests ischemia alone as a cause of bile duct strictures.[43] Ischemia may enhance the cytotoxic effect of the hepatic arterial drug on the bile duct.

Radiographically, these lesions resemble idiopathic sclerosing cholangitis. Since the ducts are sclerotic, sonograms are usually normal and the diagnosis must be made by endoscopic retrograde cholangiopancreatography (ERCP) to exclude metastatic lesions as a cause of strictures. In some patients the strictures are more centralized, and drainage procedures either by ERCP or by transhepatic cholangiogram may be helpful. Computerized tomography (CT) of the liver should be done to exclude metastatic lesions as a cause of strictures.

Close monitoring is necessary to avoid biliary sclerosis. If the serum bilirubin becomes elevated, no further treatment should be given until it returns to normal, and then only with a small test dose (0.05 mg/kg/day). In some patients who cannot tolerate even a low dose for two weeks, it may be possible to continue treatment by giving the FUDR infusion for one week rather than the usual two weeks. The rate of biliary sclerosis in the various trials is listed in Table 12-13.

At MSKCC it was found that serum SGOT was a useful laboratory test to monitor hepatic toxicity.[12] A review of the liver function tests obtained every two weeks revealed a certain pattern of SGOT elevation in 23 of the original 45 patients; the SGOT increased at the end of FUDR infusion (two weeks after treatment began) and then re-

Table 12–14
Dose Modification for Hepatic Toxicity

SGOT	BILI	ALKPHOS	FUDR Dose
2× baseline	—	—	80%
3× baseline	or 2×	2×	50%
>3× baseline	or 3×	3×	Hold

turned to normal or near-normal levels prior to the next dose (four weeks after treatment began). This pattern occurred in all of the patients who later developed severe hepatic toxicity (bilirubin >3 mg/ml). Alkaline phosphatase values should also be followed carefully. The NCOG investigators now never retreat patients in whom alkaline phosphatase levels double after therapy. At MSKCC we reduce dose or hold dose as outlined in Table 12-14.

A major problem in comparing toxicity among the randomized studies is differences in toxicity criteria. Biliary toxicity in some studies is interpreted as an increase in hepatic enzymes, whereas in other studies it requires the presence of biliary sclerosis. There are also degrees of biliary sclerosis; a patient who has an elevated bilirubin that returns to normal is certainly different from a patient whose bilirubin never returns to normal and may or may not improve with stent placement.

Another side-effect of HAI chemotherapy is the development of cholecystitis, which has been reported to occur in as many as 33% of patients.[57] In more recent series, the gallbladder has been removed at the time of catheter placement to prevent this complication and to avoid the confusion of these symptoms with other hepatic side-effects from pump treatment.

Commentary ∎

A major advantage of HAI is the lack of systemic toxicity. The lack of nausea and vomiting, hair loss, diarrhea, and dermatologic toxicity is gratifying to the patient. The gastrointestinal complications (ulcer and gastritis) of HAI can virtually be eliminated with very careful monitoring of arteriograms and careful surgical denuding of appropriate blood vessels.

Biliary toxicity is the limiting side-effect of HAI. Careful monitoring of enzymes, especially SGOT, alkaline phosphatase, and bilirubin with appropriate dose modification decrease the toxicity.

New Approaches to Decrease the Hepatic Toxicity ■

New approaches are being taken in order to decrease the hepatic toxicity induced by hepatic arterial FUDR. Since inflammation of the portal triads may lead to ischemia of the bile ducts, the hepatic arterial administration of dexamethasone was evaluated and found to decrease elevated liver function tests in patients who developed hepatic toxicity from HAI.[44] A prospective double-blind randomized study of intrahepatic FUDR with dexamethasone (D) versus FUDR was conducted at MSKCC in order to confirm these earlier findings and to determine whether the simultaneous administration of dexamethasone with FUDR would allow for the administration of higher doses of chemotherapy. The patients were stratified before randomization by the percentage of liver involvement and the perfusion pattern on MAA perfusion scan. Although no significant increase in tolerable dose was documented, the response rate in 49 evaluable patients was 71% for the FUDR + D and 40% for FUDR alone (p = 0.03).[45] There was a trend towards decreased bilirubin elevation in patients receiving FUDR + D compared to the group receiving FUDR alone (9% vs 30% p = 0.07).[37] There was also a trend toward increased survival in the FUDR + D, 23 months versus 15 months for FUDR alone (Table 12-15).

Circadian modification of hepatic intra-arterial (IA) FUDR infusion has been reported to produce less hepatic toxicity than a constant infusion rate. In a retrospective, non-randomized study at the University of Minnesota,[46] a comparison of constant (flat) infusion versus circadian modified (CM) hepatic arterial FUDR infusion was conducted in 50 patients with metastatic colorectal carcinoma. The initial dose was 0.25–0.3 mg/kg/day for a 14-day infusion. The group with circadian modification received 68% of each daily dose between 3 pm and 9 pm, 2% between 3 am and 9 am, and 15% in each of the adjacent six-hour periods. Over nine courses of treatment the patients with CM infusion tolerated almost twice the daily dose of FUDR (0.79 mg/kg/day vs 0.46 mg/kg/day). CM infusion resulted in 46% of patients having no hepatic toxicity versus 16% of patients after flat FUDR infusion. Unfortunately, the authors do not present information on response rates achieved in both groups.

Another approach to decrease toxicity from HAI has been to alternate IA FUDR with IA FU. Weekly IA bolus of FU has similar activity to IA FUDR and does not cause hepatobiliary toxicity; however, it frequently produces treatment limiting systemic toxicity or arteritis. Stagg and associates[47] conducted a phase II study, alternating hepatic infusion of FUDR and hepatic infusion of FU. The following regimen was administered: HIA FUDR 0.1 mg/kg/d × 7 days followed by hepatic artery bolus FU 15 mg/kg via the pump side port on days 14, 21, 28, repeating this cycle every 35 days. The response rate was 51%, and only 14/69 patients (8 due to liver toxicity and 6 due to systemic toxicity) required modification of their treatment.

Commentary ■

Although the results obtained with the addition of dexamethasone should be confirmed, it is interesting that a small dose of dexamethasone will increase response, decrease toxicity, and perhaps increase survival without any added harm to the patient. The use of FU into the sideport of the pump allows the use of less FUDR and therefore, possibly less biliary toxicity. Patients treated with this approach, however, will experience more systemic side-effects, and a new toxicity, arteritis. The use of circadian rhythm seems to decrease toxicity but this study needs to be confirmed at other institutions and with a prospective randomized trial design. Since this University of Minnesota study was retrospective, the decrease in toxicity may be due to the physician's improvements

Table 12–15
Randomized Trial of HAI FUDR in FUDR plus Dexamethasone

	FUDR n = 25	FUDR + D n = 24	P Value
CR + PR	40%	71%	.03
>50% reduction in CEA	64%	84%	
Bil >3	30%	9%	.07
Sclerosing Cholangitis	8%	8%	
Time to Prog (mos)	12	19	
Survival (mos)	15	23	.06

Kemeny N: Cancer 1990;65:2446.

in recognizing and managing toxicity, rather than a real decrease in toxicity. One cannot recommend circadian infusion yet without confirmation, since it requires a much more expensive pump and more sophisticated machinery.

Methods to Increase Response Rate ■

As with systemic chemotherapy, combinations of drugs given either simultaneously or sequentially may increase response rate. In an early study using Mitomycin C, BCNU, and FUDR, Cohen and associates[48] produced a 70% partial response rate. In a randomized study of the three drugs versus FUDR alone, presently being conducted at MSKCC, a slight increase occurs in response rate and survival with the three drugs. The 67 patients in this trial had all received previous systemic chemotherapy. The median survival from the initiation of HAI is presently 18.9 months with the three-drug regimen and 14.9 for FUDR alone. The response rates are presently 45% and 32%, respectively for the two treatment groups (Table 12-16).[49] The data are too preliminary at present to draw conclusions.

In another attempt to improve survival and response rate, a combination of hepatic arterial FUDR and leucovorin (LV) was evaluated.[50] The rationale for this trial was that laboratory studies have shown enhanced cytotoxicity of FUDR when used with high doses of LV, related to enhanced binding of the FUDR to thymidylate synthetase.[53] Also, clinical trials in patients receiving systemic chemotherapy demonstrated increased response rates with FU and LV compared to FU alone.[16] Twenty-four patients were treated at three dose levels. The first eight patients were treated with LV 30 mg/m2/d and FUDR 0.3 mg/kg/d, both for a 14-day infusion via the pump, alternating with two weeks of saline. All eight patients had a partial response (PR), but two developed sclerosing cholangitis within four months. The next group of patients were treated with a lower dose of FUDR (0.2 mg/kg/d) and the same dose of LV, both for 14 days. Four of seven patients had a PR, and no biliary sclerosis was seen. A third dose schedule employed FUDR 0.3 mg/kg and LV 30 mg/m², both for only seven days, alternating with one week of saline. Six of nine patients had a PR and three developed cholangitis.

The overall response rate was 72%, with 75% of patients alive after one year, 66% alive after two years, and 33% at three years (Fig. 12-13). FUDR plus LV appears to have a high response rate in the treatment of hepatic metastases from colorectal carcinoma, but hepatic toxicity appears greater than previously reported with FUDR alone.[50] Presently the four-year survival is 23%.

Commentary ■

In patients whose tumor fails to respond to one form of systemic chemotherapy, another form of systemic therapy rarely produces a response. Hepatic arterial therapy, however, produces at least a 33% response rate after tumor growth on systemic therapy.

One might infer from this data that intrahepatic treatment is needed only after failure of systemic treatment. Arguments against this viewpoint include (1) the lack of systemic side-effects, (2) the ease of administration of continuous infusion via

Table 12–16
A Randomized Trial of Hepatic Arterial FUDR (F) + Mitomycin + BCNU (FMB) vs FUDR Alone in Previously Treated Patients with Liver Metastases from Colorectal Cancer

Response	FMB (N = 29)	F (N = 34)	P Value
PR	45%	32%	.31
Median Duration of Response (months)	15.0	9.1	.04
Median Survival (months)	18.8	14.9	.05
Toxicity:			
Bilirubin >3 mg/dl	38%	21%	.52
Biliary Sclerosis	10%	3%	.23
WBC < 3,000/mm³	14%	9%	.41
Platelet < 100,000/mm³	28%	6%	.02

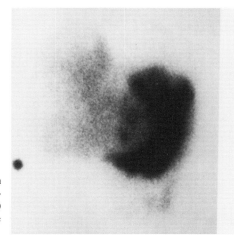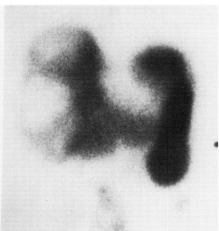

FIG. 12–13   Abnormal flow scan demonstrating uptake in stomach (on the right of each figure) and very poor uptake in the liver, on the left of each figure.

an implantable pump; and (3) the likelihood that delaying HAI until a patient fails on systemic treatment will reduce the number who can tolerate surgery for hepatic artery cannulation. One might also argue that a percutaneous catheterization of the hepatic artery could be performed prior to pump placement because this would allow one to see if there is a tumor response prior to laparotomy. This step, however, could lead to artery thrombosis and eliminate further opportunities for hepatic infusion.

The addition of LV to FUDR for HAI seems to increase response rate and survival, but it is also associated with greater biliary toxicity. Even with the increase in toxicity, 66% of these patients are alive at two years and 33% at three years, and 23% at four years, which is an impressive number. As with systemic chemotherapy, it seems that combinations of drugs or biochemical modulation of drugs may improve the response rate and perhaps survival.

Comparative Survival of Intrahepatic vs Systemic Chemotherapy ■

The use of systemic FU and LV has been suggested as standard treatment for metastatic colorectal carcinoma because of improved response rates compared to systemic FU alone, as demonstrated in Table 12-17. The mean response rate for the FU and LV groups versus the FU treated groups is 38% and 12%, respectively. At one year, 52% of the FU and LV treated patients were alive versus 43% of the FU treated patients. At two years, 19% of the combined treatment patients and 16% of the FU treated patients were alive (Table 12-18). If we compare the percentage of patients alive from the randomized studies using intrahepatic FUDR to studies using systemic FU and LV, the percent alive at one year and at two years is greater for those receiving HAI. At two years, 30% of the HAI patients were alive versus 19% of

Table 12–17
Randomized Studies of Systemic FU + LV vs FU Alone

Investigator	# Pts	% Response		% Diarrhea		% Leukopenia	
		LV + FU	FU	LV + FU	FU	LV + FU	FU
Valone[51]	162	18	17	24	12	12	4
Erlichman[52]	130	43	7	25	5	22	17
GITSG[53]	343	30	12	48	34	39	58
NCCTG[54]	208	43	10	61	43	19	48
Doroshow[55]	79	44	13	22	18	26	18
Petrilli[56]	44	48	11	23	12	10	37
Mean		38	12	34	20	21	30

Table 12–18
Survival Comparison of Systemic FU + LV Trials to Trials of Hepatic Arterial Infusion of FUDR

	Systemic FU + LV Survival %		Systemic FU Survival %			HAI FUDR Survival %	
	1 year	2 year	1 year	2 year		1 year	2 year
Valone[51]	46	18	48	18	MSKCC	60	25
Erlichman[52]	55	18	32	16	NCOG	60	30
GITSG[53]	58	18	50	16	NCI	85	44
NCCTG[54]	51	20	36	15	France	61	20
Doroshow[55]	61	25	58	12			
Petrilli[56]	42	18	35	18			
Mean	52	19	43	16		66	30

the patients treated with systemic FU and LV (Table 12-18). One might argue that these studies do not contain comparable patient groups, and therefore the HAI treated patients have a better survival rate. In fact, the patients treated in the systemic therapy trials should have a better survival rate because they included patients with lung metastases. Patients with lung metastases have a median survival of 12 months, while those with only liver metastases have a median survival of eight months, and those with lung plus liver metastases have a median survival of 10.7 months.[29] The two-year survivals for these three groups of patients (liver alone, lung and liver, and lung alone) were 0, 10%, and 30%, respectively. Some of the patients selected for HAI have very advanced disease, which often make them poor candidates for systemic therapy (Fig. 12–14).

Cost and Quality of Life ■

Does this treatment improve quality of life? For investigators who see a large number of these patients, it is clear that the patients treated with HAI feel better than the systemically treated patients. They experience none of the irritating side-effects of systemic therapy. The HAI patients do experience side-effects, but the severe symptomatic hepatic toxicity is seen in only 8% of them.

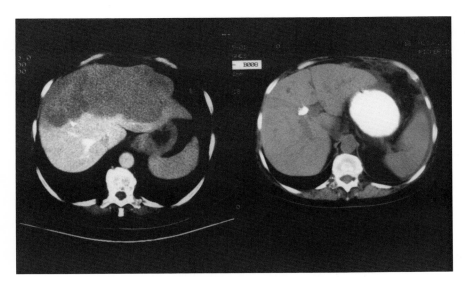

FIG. 12–14 Patient's CT before treatment (left), demonstrating massive liver involvement; patient's CT after intrahepatic therpy (right), showing an excellent partial response.

The opponents of HAI therapy argue that the patient must undergo an additional laparotomy. This statement is correct, but 15% of patients (roughly 20,000 patients per year) with colorectal carcinoma have hepatic metastases at presentation. In many of these patients pump placement at the time of initial surgery would decrease cost and avoid another laparotomy.

A theoretical disadvantage of HAI chemotherapy would be the potential development of extrahepatic metastases. Actually, randomized studies of HAI versus systemic chemotherapy have not demonstrated a significant increase in extrahepatic metastases in the intrahepatic therapy groups. A cogent argument has been made for early intensive treatment of hepatic metastases by resection and/or intra-arterial infusion to prevent the step-wise spread of colorectal carcinoma to other organs.

Another objection to pump therapy is the high initial cost of the surgery and the pump. The initial cost to a patient is approximately $14,000 (if laparotomy, surgeon's professional fees, hospitalization, and the pump are included). After a year of treatment the total cost is $21,000. For systemic FU and LV the cost is $1,948 a month (if chemotherapy administration, physician's fees, and drug costs are included) or approximately $23,400 a year. After one year, therefore, the costs are quite similar.

Conclusion ■

This chapter has tried to delineate the advantages of HAI. From a pharmacologic standpoint, HAI has several theoretical advantages, and prospective randomized studies clearly demonstrate an improvement in response rate over systemic therapy.

From a pharmacologic standpoint, intrahepatic infusional therapy is likely to be more effective than systemic therapy since higher drug levels are achieved at the sites of metastatic disease. Utilizing agents with high hepatic extraction virtually eliminates the systemic toxicity observed with "standard" therapy (intravenous FU or FU and LV).

In clinical trials involving over 600 patients, the 50% response rate produced with intrahepatic FUDR therapy has, to date, not been matched by systemic therapy. Some of the randomized studies do not clearly evaluate the issue of whether there is a survival advantage because a crossover design was allowed in some of the studies, and patients with positive nodes were included in the HAI treated groups. Patients who received HAI treatment either originally or after crossover had a longer survival.

Severe toxicity may occur with either intrahepatic or systemic therapy. Intrahepatic therapy produces severe gastrointestinal or hepatic toxicity in roughly 10% of patients, whereas FU and LV produced a mortality of 6% in one study and severe gastrointestinal toxicity (diarrhea, mucositis, nausea, and vomiting) and myelosuppression in roughly 20% of patients. The toxicity of intrahepatic therapy may be minimalized with better surgical technique, close monitoring of liver function tests, and perhaps circadian dose adjustment, and intrahepatic dexamethasone.

Because the liver is often the initial site of metastatic disease in patients with colorectal carcinoma, early intensive therapy with surgical resection and/or intrahepatic infusion at a time when the tumor burden is small may prevent the progression of metastases to other sites. While intrahepatic therapy is only applicable to a minority of patients with metastatic colorectal carcinoma (those with only hepatic metastases), it may be the best available therapy for these patients, often the ones with the worst prognosis.

The preliminary study of HAI FUDR and LV, with a response rate of over 70%, is promising, although more work will have to be done to limit its toxicity. The use of HAI dexamethasone in combination with FUDR or circadian modification of hepatic arterial FUDR infusion may help decrease hepatic toxicity. To improve response and decrease toxicity, trials in the future may use one or more of these modalities, with or without systemic therapy.

References ■

1. Coller FA. Cancer of the colon and rectum. New York: Am Cancer Soc, 1956.
2. Weiss L, Grundmann E, Torhorst J, et al. Haematogenous metastatic patterns in colonic carcinoma: An analysis of 1541 necropsies. J Pathol 1986;150:195–203.
3. Chen HSG, Gross JF. Intra-arterial infusion of anti-cancer drugs: theoretic aspects of drug delivery and review of responses. Cancer Treat Rep 1980;64:31–40.
4. Breedis C, Young C. The blood supply of neoplasms in the liver. Am J Pathol 1954;30:969.
5. Cohen A, Schaeffer N, Higgins J. Treatment of metastatic colorectal cancer with hepatic artery combination chemotherapy. Cancer 1986;57:1115–1117.

6. Sigurdson ER, Ridge JA, Kemeny N, Daly JM. Tumor and liver drug uptake following hepatic artery and portal vein infusion. J Clin Oncol 1987;5:1936–1940.

7. Daly J, Kemeny N, Sigurdson E, Oderman P, Thom A. Regional infusion for colorectal hepatic metastases: A randomized trial comparing the hepatic artery versus the portal vein. Arch Surg 1987;122:1273–1277.

8. Ensminger WD, Rosowsky A, Raso V. A clinical-pharmacological evaluation of hepatic arterial infusions of 5-fluoro-2'-deoxyuridine and 5-fluorouracil. Cancer Res 1978;38:3784–3792.

9. Collins JM. Pharmacologic rationale for regional drug delivery. J Clin Oncol 1984;2:498–504.

10. Collins JM. Pharmacologic rationale for hepatic arterial therapy. Recent Results Cancer Res 1986;100:140–148.

11. Weiss L. Metastatic inefficiency and regional therapy for liver metastases from colorectal carcinoma. Reg Cancer Treat 1989;2:77–81.

12. Sugarbaker P, Kemeny N. Treatment of metastatic cancer to liver. In: DeVita V, Hellman S, Rosenberg S, eds. Cancer: Principles and Practice of Oncology, 3rd Edition. Philadelphia: Lippincott, 1989:2275–2293.

13. Tandon RN, Bunnell IL, Copper RG. The treatment of metastatic carcinoma of the liver by percutaneous selective hepatic artery infusion of 5-fluorouracil. Surgery 1973;73:118.

14. Buchwald H, Grage TB, Vassilopoulos PP, et al. Intra-arterial infusion chemotherapy for hepatic carcinoma using a totally implantable infusion pump. Cancer 1980; 45:866–869.

15. Ensminger W, Niederhuber J, Dakhil S, et al. Totally implanted drug delivery system for hepatic arterial chemotherapy. Cancer Treat Rep 1981;65:393.

16. Kemeny N. Role of chemotherapy in the treatment of colorectal carcinoma. Sem in Surg Oncol 1987;3:190–214.

17. Niederhuber JE, Ensminger W, Gyves J, et al. Regional chemotherapy of colorectal cancer metastatic to the liver. Cancer 1984;53:1336.

18. Balch CM, Urist MM. Intra-arterial chemotherapy for colorectal liver metastases and hepatomas using a totally implantable drug infusion pump. Recent Results Cancer Res 1986;100:123–147.

19. Kemeny N, Daly J, Oderman P, et al. Hepatic artery pump infusion: Toxicity and results in patients with metastatic colorectal carcinoma. J Clin Oncol 1984;2:595–600.

20. Shepard KV, Levin B, Karl RC, et al. Therapy for metastatic colorectal cancer with hepatic artery infusion chemotherapy using a subcutaneous implanted pump. J Clin Oncol 1985;3:161.

21. Cohen AM, Kaufman SD, Wood WC, et al. Regional hepatic chemotherapy using an implantable drug infusion pump. Am J Surg 1983;145:529–533.

22. Weiss GR, Garnick MB, Osteen RT, et al. Long-term hepatic arterial infusion of 5-fluorodeoxyuridine for liver metastases using an implantable infusion pump. J Clin Oncol 1983;1:337–344.

23. Schwartz SI, Jones LS, McCune CS. Assessment of treatment of intrahepatic malignancies using chemotherapy via an implantable pump. Ann Surg 1985;201:560–567.

24. Johnson LP, Wasserman PB, Rivkin SE. FUDR hepatic arterial infusion via an implantable pump for treatment of hepatic tumors. Proceedings Am Soc Clin Oncol 1983;2:119.

25. Kemeny MM, Goldberg D, Beatty JD, et al. Results of a prospective randomized trials of continuous regional chemotherapy and hepatic resection as treatment of hepatic metastases from colorectal primaries. Cancer 1986;57:492.

26. Lesser ML, Cento SJ. Chron Dis 1981;34:533–544.

27. Kemeny N, Daly J, Reichman B, Geller N, Botet J, Oderman P. Intrahepatic or systemic infusion of fluorodeoxyuridine in patients with liver metastases from colorectal carcinoma. Ann Intern Med 1987;107:459–465.

28. Kemeny N, Daly J, Oderman P, Niedzwiecki D, Shurgot B. Prognostic variables in patients with hepatic metastases from colorectal cancer: Importance of medical assessment of liver involvement. Cancer 1989;63:742–747.

29. Kemeny N, Braun DW. Prognostic factors in advanced colorectal carcinoma: The importance of lactic dehydrogenase, performance status, and white blood cell count. Am J Med 1983;74:786–794.

30. Hohn D, Stagg R, Friedman M, et al. A randomized trial of continuous intravenous versus hepatic intraarterial floxuridine in patients with colorectal cancer metastatic to the liver: the northern California oncology group trial. J Clin Oncol 1989;7:1646–1654.

31. Chang AE, Schneider PD, Sugarbaker PH. A prospective randomized trial of regional versus systemic continuous 5-fluorodeoxyuridine chemotherapy in the treatment of colorectal liver metastases. Ann Surg 1987; 206:685–693.

32. Martin JK Jr, O'Connell MJ, Wieand HS, Fitzgibbons RJ Jr, Mailliard JA, et al. Intra-arterial floxuridine versus systemic fluorouracil for hepatic metastases from colorectal cancer: A randomized trial. Arch Surg 1990; 125:1022.

33. Rougier PH, Hay JM, Olivier JM, Escat J, Laplanche A, et al. A controlled multicentric trial of intra-hepatic chemotherapy (IHC) vs standard palliative treatment for colorectal liver mestastases. Proceedings ASCO 1990; 9:104.

34. Mersh A. Personal Communication. London, England.

35. Niederhuber JE. Arterial chemotherapy for metastatic colorectal cancer in the liver. Conference Advances in Regional Cancer Therapy. Giessen, West Germany, 1985.

36. Wagman LD, Kemeny MM, Leong L, Terz JJ, et al. A prospective randomized evaluation of the treatment of colorectal cancer metastatic to the liver. J Clin Oncol 1990;8(11):1885–1893.

37. Moertel CG, Fleming TR, MacDonald JS, Haller DG, Laurie JA, Goodman PJ, Glick JH, Veeder MH, Mailliard JA. Levamisole and fluorouracil for adjuvant therapy of resected colon carcinoma. N Engl J Med 1990;322:352–358.

38. Gluck WI, Akwari OE, Kelvin FM, et al. A reversible enteropathy complicating continuous hepatic artery infusion chemotherapy with 5-fluoro-2-deoxyuridine. Cancer 1985;56:2424.

39. Hohn DC, Stagg RJ, Price DC, et al. Avoidance of gastroduodenal toxicity in patients receiving hepatic arterial 5-fluoro-2'-deoxyuridine. J Clin Oncol 1985;3:1257–1260.

40. Doria MI Jr, Shepard KV, Levin B, et al. Liver pathology following hepatic arterial infusion chemotherapy. Cancer 1986;58:855–861.

41. Pettavel J, Gardiol D, Bergier N, et al. Necrosis of main bile ducts caused by hepatic artery infusion of 5-fluoro-2-deoxyuridine. Reg Cancer Treat 1988;1:83–92.

42. Northover JM, Terblanche J. A new look at the arterial supply of the bile duct in man and its surgical implications. Br J Surg 1979;66:379–384.

43. Doppman JL, Girton ME. Bile duct scarring following ethanol embolization of the hepatic artery. An experimental study in monkeys. Radiology 1984;152:621–626.

44. Paquette P, Campos LT, Flax I, et al. Prevention and treatment of sclerosing cholangitis related to chemotherapy delivered by Infusaid pump. Proceedings Amer Soc Clin Oncol 1987;6:89.

45. Seiter K, Kemeny N, Berger M, Niedzwiecki D, et al. A randomized trial of intrahepatic (IH) infusion of FUDR with dexamethasone (D) vs FUDR alone in the treatment of metastatic colorectal cancer. Proceedings ASCO 1990;9:108.

46. Wesen C, Olson G, Roemeling R, Grage T, Hrushesky WJM. Circadian modified intra-arterial treatment of colo-rectal carcinoma metastatic to the liver allows higher dose intensity to be safely given. ASCO 1989; 8:105.

47. Stagg RJ, Venook AP, Chase JL, Lewis BJ, Warren RS, Roh M, Mulvihill SJ, Grobman BJ, Rayner AA, Hohn DC. Alternating hepatic intra-arterial floxuridine and fluorouracil: A less toxic regimen for treatment of liver metastases from colorectal cancer. J Clin Oncol J National Cancer Inst 1991;83:423–428.

48. Cohen AM, Schaeffer N, Higgins J. Treatment of metastatic colorectal cancer with hepatic artery combination chemotherapy. Cancer 1986;57:1115–1117.

49. Seiter K, Kemeny N, Cohen A, Sigurdson E, Niedzwiecki D. A randomized trial of hepatic arterial FUDR + mitomycin + BCNU (FMB) versus FUDR alone in previously treated liver metastases from colorectal cancer. Proceedings ASCO, 1991;140.

50. Kemeny N, Cohen A, Bertino JR, Sigurdson ER, Botet J, Oderman P. Continuous intrahepatic infusion of floxuridine and leucovorin through an implantable pump for the treatment of hepatic metastases from colorectal carcinoma. Cancer 1990;65:2446–2450.

51. Valone FH, Friedman MA, Wittinger PS, et al. Treatment of patients with advanced colorectal carcinoma with fluorouracil alone, high-dose leucovorin plus fluorouracil, or sequential methotrexate, fluorouracil, and leucovorin: A randomized trial of the North California Oncology Group. J Clin Oncol 1989;7:1427–1436.

52. Ehrlichman C, Fine S, Wong A, Elhakim T. Randomized trial of fluorouracil and folinic acid in patients with metastatic colorectal carcinoma. J Clin Oncol 1988;6:469–475.

53. Petrelli N, Douglass HO, Herrera L, Russell D, Stablein DM, et al. The modulation of fluorouracil with leucovorin in metastatic colorectal carcinoma: A prospective randomized Phase III trial. J Clin Oncol 1989;7:1419–1426.

54. O'Connell MJ. A phase III trial of 5-fluorouracil and leucovorin in the treatment of advanced colorectal cancer. Cancer 1989;63:1026–1030.

55. Doroshow JH, Multhauf P, Leong L, et al. Prospective randomized comparison of fluorouracil versus fluorouracil plus high-dose continuous infusion leucovorin calcium for the treatment of advanced measurable colorectal cancer in patients previously unexposed to chemotherapy. J Clin Oncol 1990;8:491–501.

56. Petrelli N, Herrera L, Rustum Y, et al. A prospective randomized trial of 5-fluorouracil versus 5-fluorouracil and high-dose leucovorin versus 5-fluorouracil and methotrexate in previously untreated patients with advanced colorectal carcinoma. J Clin Oncol 1987;5:1559–1565.

57. Kemeny M, Battifora H, Blayney D, et al. Sclerosing cholangitis after continuous hepatic artery infusion of FUDR. Ann Surg 1985;202:176.

58. Ansfield FJ, Curreri AR. Further comparison between 5-fluorouracil (5-FU) and 5-fluoro-2'-deoxyuridine 95-FUDR). Cancer Chemother Rep 1963;32:101–105.

59. Hughes KS. Hepatic Metastases Registry. Resection of the liver for colorectal metastases: a multi-institutional study of patterns of recurrence. Surgery 1986;100:278–284.

Michael J. O'Connell

Is Hepatic Infusion of Chemotherapy Effective Treatment for Liver Metastases? No! 13

In spite of an appealing pharmacologic rationale, improvements in drug delivery systems that facilitate prolonged intra-arterial therapy, and enthusiastic reports from early clinical trials, hepatic infusion chemotherapy has not been established to be the preferred method of treatment for patients with liver metastases. Since the only controlled clinical trials directly comparing hepatic infusion chemotherapy with systemic chemotherapy have been conducted in patients with colorectal cancer metastatic to the liver, the following discussion will focus specifically on this category of patients.

Early Clinical Experience and Uncontrolled Clinical Trials ■

Historically, the investigation of hepatic arterial chemotherapy for the treatment of colorectal liver metastases was entirely appropriate, given the lack of effective systemic chemotherapy for this condition. A scientifically valid pharmacologic rationale existed that would support a greater therapeutic effect on colorectal liver metastases with direct regional chemotherapy administration.[1,2] The fluorinated pyrimidines 5-fluorouracil (5FU)

and 5-fluorodeoxyuridine (FUDR) were the most active cytotoxic agents against metastatic colorectal carcinoma. FUDR, in particular, has a very high hepatic extraction ratio—roughly 95 percent of this drug is cleared by the liver on the first pass following administration into the hepatic artery. Total body clearance is very rapid, with a serum half-life of only a few minutes following systemic drug administration. These pharmacologic features allow delivery of much higher concentrations of FUDR to the liver when given directly by the arterial route compared to the amount delivered to the liver when maximally tolerated doses are given intravenously.

Technical problems greatly limited the early use of arterial infusion chemotherapy. Inadequate perfusion of the liver and inadvertent perfusion of other upper abdominal organs due to dislodgement of the catheter tip, sepsis, bleeding, damage to peripheral arteries at the site of puncture, and need for prolonged hospitalizations were major problems associated with use of percutaneous catheters.

The development of surgically implanted arterial catheters and infusion pumps was a major technical advance that made possible administration of intra-arterial chemotherapy for prolonged periods of time on an outpatient basis with a substantial reduction in infectious and vascular complications.[3,4] Based on sound pharmacologic principles and armed with an innovative new technology, Ensminger and associates reported a striking tumor response rate of 83 percent and an impressive median survival of approximately two years in a selected group of patients treated with prolonged intra-arterial infusions of FUDR for colorectal liver metastases at the University of Michigan.[5,6] The favorable survival experience in these patients was difficult to assess, of course, since this population of patients was highly selected. Only patients who were fit to undergo a major surgical procedure for implantation of the arterial infusion system, and who were free of extrahepatic metastases or jaundice, were candidates for therapy. Thus, comparison of survival in this select group of patients with historical series of patients with colorectal liver metastases treated with systemic chemotherapy would not be correct.

As might be expected, subsequent reports[7-10] of tumor response rates associated with intra-arterial FUDR for colorectal liver metastases varied widely from the 80% range to as low as 20% (Table 13-1). This disparity may be accounted for by one or more of the following factors: adequacy of establishing complete perfusion of the liver; differences in dose intensity of chemotherapy administered, criteria used to document tumor response, and prognostic features in the patients selected for study; prior chemotherapy exposure; and small numbers of patients treated. Clearly controlled clinical trials were indicated to evaluate this new treatment method adequately.

Table 13-1
Summary of Uncontrolled Clinical Trials of Hepatic Arterial Infusion Chemotherapy with FUDR for Colorectal Liver Metastases

Institution	No. of Patients	Tumor Response Rate	Reference
University of Michigan	93	78%	6
University of Alabama	81	88%	7
Memorial Sloan Kettering	41	37%	8
Sidney Farber	21	29%	9
University of Chicago*	40	20%	10

*Mitomycin C 15 mg/m² given through pump side port on day 15 of every other course of FUDR

Randomized Clinical Trials ■

Four randomized clinical trials have been reported which compare arterial infusion therapy with FUDR versus systemic therapy with single agent FUDR or 5FU.[11-14] All four studies were designed to test the intra-arterial FUDR regimen originally described by Ensminger (0.3 mg/kg/d × 14 days alternating with two-week rest periods), although the dose of FUDR was reduced due to severe hepatobiliary toxicity during the course of two of the trials.[12,13] In three of the trials FUDR given by the same schedule (14 days of continuous infusion alternating with two-week rest periods) but a different route of administration (intravenous) was used as the control.[11-13] The fourth trial used systemic 5FU given by rapid IV push for five consecutive days repeated every five weeks as the control.[14] All patients in the Memorial study underwent surgical staging.[11] Sixty-three of the 162 patients randomized (39%) were excluded from the study based on operative findings (tumor was resectable; extrahepatic metastases were identified; or tumor was not present at all). In the other three trials, clinical staging, including CT scanning of the abdomen, was used and only patients randomized to receive intra-arterial FUDR were required to undergo laparotomy. In the Northern California Oncology Group (NCOG) study, 14 of 64 eligible patients (22%) randomized to intra-arterial FUDR were excluded from analysis based on operative findings or other technical factors.[12] In the National Cancer Institute (NCI) study[13] and Mayo/North Central Cancer Treatment Group (NCCTG) study,[14] all eligible patients randomized to intra-arterial FUDR were included in survival analyses although 11 of 32 patients (34%) in the NCI study and 5 of 36 patients (14%) in the NCCTG study did not in fact receive intra-arterial therapy. Eight patients (38%) in the NCI study and seven patients (26%) in the NCCTG study who received intra-arterial FUDR had evidence of extrahepatic tumor discovered at laparotomy. Two of the trials (Memorial and NCOG) allowed "crossover" of patients who failed systemic chemotherapy to receive intra-arterial FUDR at the time of tumor progression.

The therapeutic results of these four randomized trials are summarized in Table 13-2. In spite of the differences in methodology among the four trials, a remarkable consistency appears in the major results. All studies indicated a highly significant improvement in tumor response rates for patients receiving intra-arterial FUDR; time-to-

Table 13–2
Summary of Randomized Clinical Trials of Hepatic Arterial Infusion Chemotherapy with FUDR for Colorectal Liver Metastases

Institution or Cooperative Group	No. of Evaluable Patients	Tumor Response Rate (%)			Patient Survival Median (mo.)		
		IA	IV		IA	IV	
Memorial Sloan Kettering[11]	99	50	20	p = 0.001	17	12	p = 0.42
NCOG[12]	115	42	10	p = 0.0001	16.8	16.1	p = NS
NCI[13]	64	62	17	p < 0.003	17	12	p = 0.27
Mayo/NCCTG[14]	69	48	21	p = 0.02	12.6	10.5	p = 0.53

hepatic-tumor-progression was significantly prolonged with intra-arterial FUDR in the two studies that reported this endpoint (NCOG, Mayo/NCCTG); none of the studies documented a significant difference in patient survival when all evaluable patients randomized were analyzed. Two of the trials (Memorial, NCOG) allowed crossover of patients from systemic to intra-arterial chemotherapy at the time of tumor progression, which may have had a confounding effect on survival analyses in those trials. Neither of the trials without a crossover (NCI, Mayo/NCCTG) demonstrated a significant improvement in survival for intra-arterial FUDR. Although neither of these studies had sufficient numbers of patients to rule out a small survival advantage for FUDR, the Mayo/NCCTG trial could exclude a doubling in median survival (from 10.5 to 21 months) with a p value < 0.05.

Subset analyses within the NCI trial suggested a survival advantage for patients treated with intra-arterial FUDR who did not have metastases to perihepatic lymph nodes. These subset analyses should clearly be regarded as exploratory in nature and would require confirmation in a separate controlled trial to determine whether these observations were anything more than the well-known statistical variability associated with subset analyses within randomized trials.[15] In both the Memorial and NCOG trials, patients crossed over to intra-arterial FUDR at the time of tumor progression lived longer than patients initially treated with intravenous FUDR who did not subsequently receive intra-arterial FUDR. However, as pointed out by the authors of the NCOG trial, these differences in survival could be attributed to more favorable selection factors in patients undergoing crossover. The authors of the Memorial study also indicated that their study was primarily designed to look at tumor response rate, and that statistical comparison of survival in patients who did not cross over with those who did would not be appropriate.

Toxicity associated with intra-arterial FUDR in these trials was substantial. The dose of FUDR was decreased to 0.2 mg/kg/d in both the NCI and NCOG trials because of unacceptable hepatobiliary toxicity. In the NCI study, 79% of patients developed chemical hepatitis, 21% had biliary sclerosis, and 17% developed peptic ulcers. In the NCOG study, 10 of 25 patients (40%) treated at the 0.3 mg/kg/d FUDR dose developed biliary strictures, and 3 of these patients developed permanent jaundice. Toxicity was decreased by reducing the FUDR dose, but 26 of the 50 patients receiving intra-arterial FUDR had treatment terminated because of drug toxicity. In the Mayo/NCCTG trial jaundice attributed to intra-arterial FUDR was seen in 26 percent of patients, and one patient developed multiple biliary strictures. The Memorial experience documented ulcer disease in 17% of patients, biliary sclerosis in 8%, and jaundice in 19%.

Formal assessment of quality of life among patients treated with intra-arterial FUDR or systemic chemotherapy has not been reported. We were not able to document more frequent improvement in performance status, relief of tumor-related symptoms, or weight gain in patients treated with intra-arterial FUDR compared to systemic 5FU.[14] Morbidity from laparotomy, gastrointestinal ulcers, and hepatobiliary toxicity also must be considered when evaluating the impact of intra-arterial FUDR on quality of life.

Treatment of Colorectal Liver Metastases with Systemic 5FU Plus Leucovorin ∎

Results of the controlled trials of intra-arterial FUDR summarized above are no longer clinically relevant because they used a single agent—5FU or FUDR—as the systemic therapy for comparison. The objective tumor response rates were very low (10%–21%), consistent with previous experience with single-agent systemic chemotherapy in this disease. A number of recent controlled clinical trials, however, have indicated significantly improved response rates and prolongation of patient survival with systemic 5FU plus leucovorin combination chemotherapy compared to single agent 5FU or combination chemotherapy with high-dose methotrexate plus 5FU.[16–21]

Summarized in Table 13-3 is our experience with the 5FU plus low dose leucovorin regimen in patients with advanced measurable colorectal cancer who had hepatic metastases as their primary indicator lesion of metastatic disease.[20,21] Also indicated in Table 13-3 is our experience with intra-arterial FUDR from our randomized trial using the same criteria for assessing objective tumor response.[14] We have included only patients with good performance status (ECOG performance status 0 or 1) in this table. Although these data are not from a prospectively randomized comparison of the two treatment methods, the results are quite similar. Any slight improvement in median survival for patients treated with intra-arterial FUDR could be related to exclusion of patients with any clinical evidence of extrahepatic metastases from receiving intra-arterial therapy, whereas patients treated with systemic 5FU plus leucovorin may have had multiple sites of extrahepatic tumor in addition to liver metastases.

Summary of Limitations of Intrahepatic Infusion Chemotherapy for Colorectal Liver Metastases ∎

Based upon all available clinical trials data, we do not believe that intrahepatic infusion chemotherapy has been established to be the preferred method of treatment for colorectal cancer metastatic to the liver for the following reasons:

1. Intrahepatic infusion chemotherapy with FUDR is not effective in controlling occult extrahepatic metastatic disease. In the original University of Michigan series[16] 73% of patients whose metastatic tumor was clinically confined to the liver at the time of presentation died of uncontrolled extrahepatic malignant disease. Indeed, this should not be surprising when one realizes that intra-arterial FUDR is a regional treatment being given for a systemic disease process.

2. It is currently not possible to select prospectively the subset of patients with colorectal liver metastases who will remain free of disseminated extrahepatic tumor for a prolonged period of time. Only these patients would benefit to a significant extent from an effective regional therapy. Many additional patients would be needlessly subjected to a major surgical procedure and the toxicities of intra-arterial therapy which, with currently available drugs, is ineffective in treating extrahepatic malignant disease.

3. Improvement in patient survival with intra-arterial FUDR has not been documented. Retrospective subset analysis within the completed controlled trials is inadequate to prove survival benefit with intra-arterial FUDR. The available data do not rule out a possible small gain in median survival for intra-arterial therapy. However, the clinical value of any putative survival gain

Table 13–3
Mayo/NCCTG Experience with Hepatic Arterial Infusion Chemotherapy with FUDR or Systemic Chemotherapy with 5FU plus Low-Dose Leucovorin in Patients with Colorectal Liver Metastases and Good Performance Status*

Treatment Method	No. of Patients	Tumor Response (%)	Time-to-Progression Median (mo.)	Survival Median (mo.)
Hepatic Arterial FUDR	31	48	6.0	12.6
Systemic 5FU + Low-Dose Leucovorin	40	50	5.4	10.5

*ECOG Performance Status 0 or 1

must be weighed against the complexity, expense, and toxicity of prolonged therapy with intra-arterial FUDR.

4. Intra-arterial FUDR is associated with substantial risk for severe hepatobiliary toxicity and gastrointestinal ulcer formation. Although the risk of hepatobiliary toxicity can be decreased by reducing the dose of FUDR,[22] such dosage modification may also diminish the effectiveness of hepatic tumor control. Meticulous devascularization of the stomach and duodenum from tributaries of the gastroduodenal artery at the time of catheter placement may greatly reduce the incidence of chemotherapy-induced ulcer formation.[23] The requirement for considerable surgical expertise and experience to establish arterial access safely greatly limits the widespread use of this technique in general clinical practice.

5. A major surgical procedure with its attendant morbidity and risk is required to establish arterial access for infusion chemotherapy.

6. Substantial financial cost (conservatively estimated at $15,000–$20,000) is associated with hepatic arteriography and hospitalization for laparotomy, purchase of implantable infusion systems, and arterial flow studies required to carry out prolonged intrahepatic infusion chemotherapy.

7. Randomized studies have not been conducted to compare intra-arterial FUDR and systemic 5FU plus leucovorin. We have not observed substantial differences in efficacy between these two treatment methods in patients participating in Mayo/NCCTG clinical trials. Systemic 5FU plus leucovorin is a vastly less complex and less expensive treatment (approximately $375.00 per month for drugs and administration) and would be preferred in clinical practice unless a substantial benefit for intra-arterial therapy could be documented.

Prospects for the Future ∎

In spite of the limitations of hepatic infusion chemotherapy with FUDR summarized above, we must keep in mind the potential pharmacologic advantages of intrahepatic chemotherapy to improve local tumor control. Perhaps in the future new chemotherapeutic agents will be discovered that have substantially more regional activity against colorectal liver metastases, less toxicity, and unlike FUDR can provide control of extrahepatic metastases when given by the intra-arterial route of administration.

An alternative strategy, which we are presently pursuing on a research basis, is the use of systemic chemotherapy with 5FU plus low-dose leucovorin sequenced between cycles of intra-arterial FUDR with the intent of controlling or eradicating occult extrahepatic metastases, as well as improving the tumor response rates within the liver. We also hope to avoid the cumulative hepatobiliary toxicity characteristic of prolonged intra-arterial FUDR by limiting the number of cycles given in conjunction with systemic 5FU plus leucovorin. If this treatment strategy is documented to be safe and yields promising therapeutic results, controlled trials against the most effective contemporary systemic chemotherapy will be required to establish any advantage for the intrahepatic infusion chemotherapy regimen.

References ∎

1. Ensminger WD, Rosowsky A, Raso V, et al. A clinical-pharmacological evaluation of hepatic arterial infusions of 5-fluoro-2'-deoxyuridine and 5-flourouracil. Cancer Res 1978;38:3784–3792.
2. Collins JM. Pharmacologic rationale for regional drug delivery. J Clin Oncol 1984;2:498.
3. Buchwald H, Grage T, Vassilopoulos PP, et al. Intra-arterial infusion chemotherapy for hepatic carcinoma using a totally implantable infusion pump. Cancer 1980;45:866.
4. Ensminger W, Niederhuber J, Dakhil S, et al. Totally implanted drug delivery system for hepatic arterial chemotherapy. Cancer Treat Rep 1981;65:393.
5. Ensminger W, Niederhuber J, Gyves J, et al. Effective control of liver metastases from colon cancer with an implanted system for hepatic arterial chemotherapy. Proceedings ASCO 1982;1:94.
6. Niederhuber J, Ensminger W, Gyves J, et al. Regional chemotherapy of colorectal cancer metastatic to the liver. Cancer 1984;53:1336.
7. Balch CM, Urist MM, Soong SJ, et al. A prospective phase II clinical trial of continuous FUDR regional chemotherapy for colorectal metastases to the liver using a totally implantable drug infusion pump. Ann Surg 1983;198:567.
8. Kemeny N, Daly J, Oderman P, et al. Hepatic artery pump infusion: Toxicity and results in patients with metastatic colorectal carcinoma. J Clin Oncol 1984;2:595.
9. Weiss GR, Garnick MB, Osteen RT, et al. Long-term hepatic arterial infusion of 5-fluorodeoxyuridine for liver metastases using an implantable infusion pump. J Clin Oncol 1983;1:337.
10. Shepard KV, Levin B, Karl RC, et al. Therapy for metastatic colorectal cancer with hepatic artery infusion chemotherapy using a subcutaneous implanted pump. J Clin Oncol 1985;3:161.

11. Kemeny N, Daly J, Reichman B, et al. Intrahepatic or systemic infusion of fluorodeoxyuridine in patients with liver metastases from colorectal carcinoma. Ann Intern Med 1987;107:459–465.

12. Hohn DC, Stagg RJ, Friedman MA, et al. A randomized trial of continuous intravenous versus hepatic intra-arterial floxuridine in patients with colorectal cancer metastatic to the liver: The Northern California Oncology Group Trial. J Clin Oncol 1989;7:1646–1654.

13. Chang AE, Schneider PD, Sugarbaker PH, et al. A prospective randomized trial of regional versus systemic continuous 5-fluorodeoxyuridine chemotherapy in the treatment of colorectal liver metastases. Ann Surg 1987;207:685–693.

14. Martin JK, O'Connell MJ, Wieand HS, et al. Intra-arterial floxuridine versus systemic fluorouracil for hepatic metastases from colorectal cancer. Arch Surg 1990; 125:1022–1027.

15. Fleming TR, Green SJ, Harrington DP. Considerations for monitoring and evaluating treatment effects in clinical trials. Controlled Clin Trials 1984;5:55–66.

16. Erlichman C, Fine S, Wong A, et al. A randomized trial of fluorouracil and folinic acid in patients with metastatic colorectal carcinoma. J Clin Oncol 1988;6:469–475.

17. Petrelli N, Herrera L, Rustum Y, et al. A prospective randomized trial of 5-fluorouracil versus 5-fluorouracil and high-dose leucovorin versus 5-fluorouracil and methotrexate in previously untreated patients with advanced colorectal carcinoma. J Clin Oncol 1987;5:1559–1565.

18. Petrelli N, Douglass HO, Herrera L, et al. The modulation of fluorouracil with leucovorin in metastatic colorectal carcinoma: A prospective randomized phase III trial. J Clin Oncol 1989;7:1419–1426.

19. Doroshow JH, Bertrand M, Multhauf P, et al. Prospective randomized trial comparing 5FU versus 5FU and high dose folinic acid for treatment of advanced colorectal cancer. Proceedings ASCO 1987;6:96.

20. Poon MA, O'Connell MJ, Moertel CG, et al. Biochemical modulation of fluorouracil: Evidence of significant improvement of survival and quality of life in patients with advanced colorectal carcinoma. J Clin Oncol 1989;7:1407–1417.

21. O'Connell M, Poon M, Wieand H, et al. Biochemical modulation of 5-fluorouracil (5FU) with leucovorin (LV): Confirmatory evidence of improved therapeutic efficacy in the treatment of advanced colorectal cancer. Proceedings ASCO 1990;9:106.

22. Hohn D, Melnick J, Stagg R, et al. Biliary sclerosis in patients receiving hepatic arterial infusions of floxuridine. J Clin Oncol 1985;3:98.

23. Hohn DC, Stagg RJ, Price DC, et al. Avoidance of gastroduodenal toxicity in patients receiving hepatic arterial 5-fluoro-2'-deoxyuridine. J Clin Oncol 1985;3:1257.

Thomas C. Chalmers

Joseph Lau

Meta-Analysis
of Randomized Control
Trials Applied
to Cancer Therapy

14

The utility of meta-analysis of randomized control trials for the saving of lives has been established in most fields of medicine, especially cardiovascular disease[1-4] and cancer.[5] The latter is the subject of this review of the published data.

Background ■

The randomized control trial remains the most reliable method of determining efficacy of different methods of treatment of patients with cancer. This is especially true in areas such as adjuvant therapy where the selection of patients to receive a new therapy may be a more important determinant of outcome than the actual therapy, especially when the adjuvant treatment may be harmful. In these cases the differences in terms of long-term survival may be quite minor, and exquisite care in making certain that experimental and control groups are similar at the time of intake into the study is necessary. Only by randomization can one be assured of that similarity.

The facts of life, however, seem to be that the great majority of randomized control trials in the field of adjuvant therapy of cancer do not include enough patients to ensure that a clinically effective treatment is not being missed. Although highly effective treatments can be established with relatively small numbers, these are still very rare in the field of cancer. Small differences must therefore be defined, which requires large numbers of patients.

A primary justification of meta-analysis of randomized control trials, that is, the pooling of data from multiple trials, is that, in this manner, adequate numbers of patients may be achieved. The process is reliable because the control and treated groups in each randomized control trial are carried into the analysis as individual studies, and the differences of interest are not likely to be obscured by comparing the treatment with an improper control.

A legitimate criticism of meta-analysis is that the errors and biases of original research may be perpetuated and the results "fixed in stone" by meta-analysis. That situation is certainly something to be wary of, but it is a problem well in hand. The most important method of control available is to confine the meta-analyses to randomized control trials so that the patients being compared are most likely to be similar before the start of treatment. Opportunities for bias, however, remain in the conduct of individual randomized control trials. Some groups ignore these and include all patients that are randomized; others attempt to measure the impact by applying various methods of assessing quality. Unfortunately, the absence of a fixed standard and random variations due to chance do not allow the development of a precise method of detecting errors due to bias, but a quantitative assessment of quality is still useful.[6,7] It allows the ranking of trials included in a meta-analysis according to their quality so that the authors or the reader may do sensitivity analyses, that is, measure the impact of leaving out the poorer quality studies.

In the individual trial one of the most important sources of errors due to bias is an improper randomization procedure that gives the clinician admitting patients to the trial an opportunity to suspect which treatment will be up next, so that the benefit of randomization is obviated by the rejection of some patients and acceptance of others with knowledge of what treatment they will be receiving.[8] This defect is easily overcome by making sure that the randomization process is blinded; that is probably a more important quality-control procedure than blinding of the therapies, especially since the latter is so hard to achieve in patients receiving cancer therapy.

Choice of endpoint is relevant to the opportunity for misinformation. For instance, the duration of adjuvant therapy and the long follow-up necessary leads to a temptation to measure disease-free survival rather than total survival because the former will provide an answer much more quickly. The former is also much more subject to bias in situations in which the physicians caring for the patients may suspect whether the patient has received the active or inactive, favored or unfavored therapy. Opportunity for bias also exists in the agreement that patients can drop out of studies if they know which therapy they have received, and this may likewise destroy the efficacy of a randomization procedure.

Many of these defects have been highlighted because of their importance in interpreting meta-analyses. One should not "shoot the messenger" when dealing with the problem. A better meta-analysis will be done when better primary trials are carried out.

A source of misleading conclusions of meta-analyses resulting from bias is the selection and rejection of papers for inclusion. This problem became apparent when we were trying to explain differences in the apparent relationship between peptic ulcer and corticosteroid therapy in meta-analyses done by two different groups.[9–12] We believe that this problem is minimized by blinding the source and the results of individual trials before determining acceptance or rejection by two different people.[13]

Heterogeneity of results, a source of concern to the critics of meta-analysis, is handled in several ways. The tests for heterogeneity are routinely done but are insensitive. One can deal with the problem by carrying out all meta-analyses both according to a fixed affects model (Mantel-Haenzel)[14,15] or a random effects model (DerSimonian and Laird).[16] It has been shown that the random affects model has larger variances when heterogeneity exists and is thus more conservative.[17] However, conservatism may not be advantageous, as is illustrated by the fact that the adoption of some highly effective therapies studied in heterogeneous trials may be delayed if one is conservative by using only the random affects model. Thrombolytic drugs in the treatment of acute myocardial infarction are a good example of that phenomenon. The reduction of 20–30% in hospital mortality was shown by 1973 in the fixed effects model combination of the published randomized control trials, but did not become apparent until 1979 in the random affects model.

Probably the most serious objection to meta-analysis—serious because there is no adequate method of handling the problem—is the possible power of publication bias to increase the likelihood of type one errors. An inclination to publish positive trials and leave the negative ones in file drawers has been established by many different means.[18–20] Short of requiring registration of all trials at the time they are started, no adequate method exists of reducing this danger to interpretation of meta-analyses that have borderline positive outcomes. It is clear that when efficacy is well established in a meta-analysis, it would require too many negative trials in peoples' file drawers to obviate the conclusion.

Examples of Meta-Analysis of Cancer Therapy ■

The following examples of application of the method to the cancer field include only data from published meta-analyses; it should be emphasized that not all of them were done by our bias minimizing method. The extensive studies carried out by the Oxford group, however, include careful documentation of individual patient responses, something which our group does not believe in because of the possibilities that personal communications are more apt to include inaccurate data. Instead of contacting individual investigators, we have put our extra efforts into determining quality of the published trials.

Both the Oxford and Boston groups have worked on this problem. Figures 14-1 and 14-2 reveal the data on multi-drug chemotherapy as of 1987. The impressive difference suggested by the disease-free survival data in our study has been totally borne out by overall survival data reported more recently by the Oxford group.[5] Since most of the individual trials were not large enough to detect the lengthening of life by chemotherapy, meta-analysis was crucial in demonstrating the effect. This situation is especially true in distinguishing between the sizes of the effect of chemotherapy in the premenopausal and postmenopausal women. Only with meta-analysis could it have been demonstrated that the reverse situation applies to tamoxifen, more effective in postmenopausal than premenopausal patients.

Figure 14-2 requires some explanation. It is a technique called cumulative meta-analysis which we have developed to determine when a treatment

has been demonstrated by successive randomized control trials to be either effective or ineffective. The difference between this and the usual meta-analysis is that we perform a separate meta-analysis every time a new trial is published. With this method we can demonstrate fluctuations around statistical significance in therapies that eventually are proven to be effective. Retrospectively, we can determine when a new treatment was effective by the usual standards of statistical significance, and prospectively, with some concern about false positives, we can determine when to stop further trials.

An example of what can be shown by meta-analysis of too-small trials is presented in Figures 14-3, 14-4, and 14-5, from data presented by Stell and Rawson.[22] There is no evidence of efficacy of adjuvant chemotherapy for head and neck cancer. In Figure 14-3 the data are presented by drug group, and the overall effect is nil, with an apparent random scatter of the control death rate and the differences between the experimental and the control treatments. There are two statistically significant trials, one favoring drug and one the con-

(text continues on page 240)

FIG. 14–1 Meta-analysis of randomized control trials of adjuvant chemotherapy for patients (Pts) with breast cancer, disease-free survival at two to three years as the endpoint. Each study and the overall pool of the studies are presented as the odds ratios with their 95% confidence intervals, using the Mantel-Haenszel method (fixed effects model).

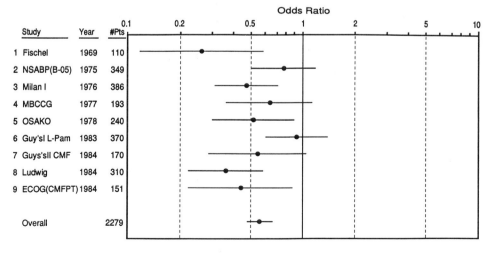

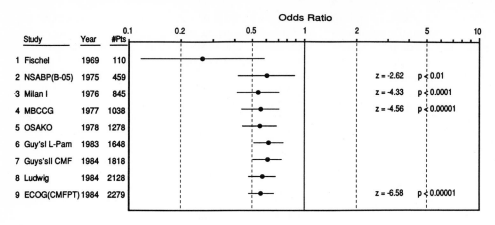

FIG. 14–2   The same data as in Figure 14-1 presented as a cumulative meta-analysis. With the publication of each new trial a new meta-analysis is performed. The average effect stays about the same, around a 40% reduction, as the confidence intervals narrow and the statistical significance increases.

FIG. 14–3   Meta-analysis of 23 trials of adjuvant chemotherapy for head and neck cancer; data expressed as rate difference and 95% confidence intervals, by the DerSimonian and Laird method (random effects model); trials are grouped by therapy as presented by the authors of the original meta-analysis.[22]

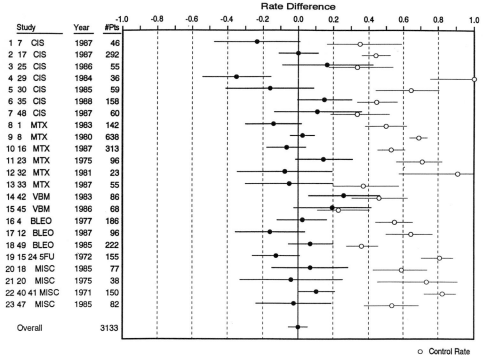

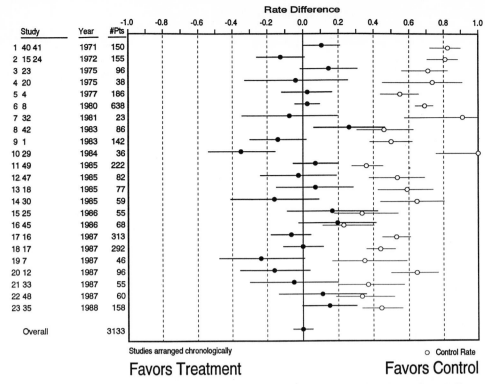

FIG. 14–4 Same trials as in Figure 14-3, here ordered by year of publication and revealing an interesting drop in the control death rate over time with no apparent change in the treatment effect.

FIG. 14–5 Cumulative meta-analysis of the data in Figure 14-4. The scale has been enlarged to show the steady progression towards null, with narrowing confidence intervals.

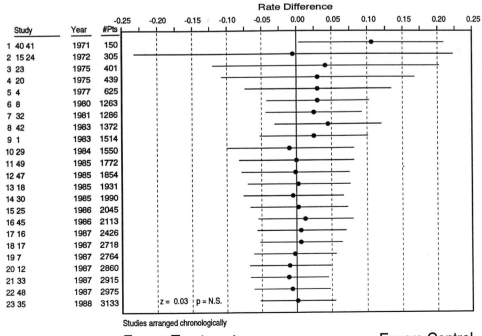

239

trol treatment, and none of the "negative" trials is large enough to rule out an effect of clinical interest.[23] Figure 14-4 presents the same data in the order of publication, and the following important information is supplied: although the mean difference between treatments is nil, a striking decrease occurs in the control death rate over the years. In Figure 14-5 the same data are presented as a cumulative meta-analysis revealing wide confidence intervals in the beginning, no false positives, and steadily falling confidence intervals around the null hypothesis.

The results of meta-analyses of the randomized control trials of adjuvant radiotherapy are in sharp contrast to the results of the chemotherapy trials. As long ago as 1974 the technique was applied by Stjernsward and the conclusion reached that although radiotherapy had an effect on local metastases, it resulted in a shortening of life.[24] Although this information was received with derision, there has been little adverse reaction to the more detailed meta-analysis—including individual patient data—carried out by the Peto group.[25] This study clearly demonstrates that ten years of follow-up radiotherapy has resulted in a statistically significant shortening of life. The information could only have been obtained by careful follow-up of all of the patients in the pooled randomized control trials.

The adjuvant radiotherapy experiences clearly illustrate one of the bases for rejection of meta-analyses of randomized control trials—bias of the evaluator. Such bias is illustrated by a study of review articles of controversial therapeutic topics in which there was a clear answer from the meta-analyses of clinical trials.[26] In the case of adjuvant radiotherapy in the days when radical mastectomy was routine, 21 of 29 radiotherapists favored the therapy in spite of the trials, and 29 of 34 other cancer specialists did not ($p < .001$). This background could explain the recent "Sounding Board" article in the *New England Journal of Medicine*,[27] which clearly goes against the tide favoring randomization when it is not known whether one treatment is better than another; the first author used to be a radiotherapist.

In conclusion, there are over 15 meta-analyses of randomized control trials of cancer therapy in the English language and over 20 of epidemiologic topics related to cancer. No doubt these have fulfilled a useful function. When properly conducted, meta-analysis is a new scientific discipline of the greatest importance.

Acknowledgments. Supported by grant # ROIHS-05936 from the Agency for Health Care Policy and Research; United States Public Health Service.

References ∎

1. Chalmers TC, Levin H, Sacks HS, Reitman D, Berrier J, Nagalingam R. Meta-analysis of clinical trials as a scientific discipline. I: Control of bias and comparison with large cooperative studies. Stat Med 1987;6:315–325.
2. Chalmers TC, Berrier J, Sacks HS, Levin H, Reitman D, Nagalingam R. Meta-analysis of clinical trials as a scientific discipline. II: Replicate variability and comparison of studies that agree and disagree. Stat Med 1987;6:733–744.
3. Yusuf S, Wittes J, Friedman L. Overview of results of randomized clinical trials in heart disease. I. Treatments following myocardial infarction. JAMA 1988;260:2088–2093.
4. Yusuf S, Wittes J, Friedman L. Overview of results of randomized clinical trials in heart disease. II. Unstable angina, heart failure, primary prevention with aspirin, and risk factor modification. JAMA 1988;260:2259–2263.
5. Early Breast Cancer Trialists' Collaborative Group (EBCTCG). Treatment of early breast cancer. Worldwide evidence 1985–90, vol. 1. Oxford: Oxford University Press, 1990.
6. Emerson JD, Burdick E, Hoaglin DC, Mosteller F, Chalmers TC. An empirical study of the possible relation of treatment differences to quality scores in controlled randomized clinical trials. Controlled Clin Trials 1990; 11(5):339–352.
7. Chalmers TC, Smith H, Blackburn B, Silverman B, Schroeder B, Reitman D, Ambroz A. A method for assessing the quality of a randomized control trial. Controlled Clin Trials 1981;2(1):31–49.
8. Chalmers TC, Celano P, Sacks HS, Smith H Jr. Bias in treatment assignment in controlled clinical trials. N Engl J Med 1983;309(22):1358–1361.
9. Conn HO, Blitzer BL. Nonassociation of adrenocorticosteroid therapy and peptic ulcer. N Engl J Med 1976; 294:473.
10. Messer J, Reitman D, Sacks HS, et al. Association of adrenocorticosteroid therapy and peptic ulcer disease. N Engl J Med 1983;309:21.
11. Conn HO, Poynard T. Adrenocorticosteroid administration and peptic ulcer: A critical analysis. J Chronic Dis 1985;38:457.
12. Chalmers TC. Meta-analysis in clinical medicine. Trans Am Clin Climatol Assoc 1987;99:144–150.
13. Chalmers TC. Problems induced by meta-analyses. Stat Med 1990;10:971–980.
14. Mantel N, Haenszel W. Statistical aspects of the analysis of data from retrospective studies of disease. J Natl Cancer Inst 1959;22:719.
15. Yusuf S, Peto R, Lewis J, et al. Beta blockade during and after myocardial infarction: An overview of the randomized trials. Prog Cardiovasc Dis 1986;27:335.

16. DerSimonian R, Laird N. Meta-analysis in clinical trials. Controlled Clin Trials 1986;7:177.
17. Berlin JA, Laird N, Sacks HS, Chalmers TC. A comparison of statistical methods for combining event rates from clinical trials. Stat Med 1981;8:141–152.
18. Rosenthal R. The file drawer problem and tolerance for null results. Psycholog Bull 1979;86:638–641.
19. Dickersin K, Chan S, Chalmers TC, Sacks HS, Smith J Jr. Publication bias and clinical trials. Controlled Clin Trials 1987;8:343–353.
20. Begg CB, Berlin JA. Publication bias: a problem in interpreting medical data. J Royal Stat Soc, Series A 1988; 151:419–453.
21. Himel HN, Liberati A, Gelber R, Chalmers TC. Adjuvant chemotherapy for breast cancer. A pooled estimate based on published randomized control trials. JAMA 1986;256(9):1148–1159.
22. Stell PM, Rawson NSB. Adjuvant chemotherapy in head and neck cancer. Br J Cancer 1990;61:779–787.
23. Freiman JA, Chalmers TC, Smith H, Kuebler RR. The importance of beta, the type II error and sample size in the design and interpretation of the randomized control trial. Survey of 71 "negative" trials. N Engl J Med 1978; 299:690–694.
24. Stjernsward J. Decreased survival related to irradiation postoperatively in early operable breast cancer. Lance 1974;ii:1285–1286.
25. Cuzick J, Stewart H, Peto R, Baum M, Fisher B, Host H, Lythgoe JP, Ribeiro G, Scheurien H, Wallgren A. Overview of randomized trials of postoperative adjuvant radiotherapy in breast cancer. Cancer Treat Rep 1987; 71:1;15–29.
26. Chalmers TC, Frank CS, Reitman D. Minimizing the three stages of publication bias. JAMA 1990;263(10): 1392–1395.
27. Hellman S, Hellman DS. Of mice but not men. N Engl J Med 1991;324:22:1585–1589.

Karin B. Michels

Quo Vadis Meta-Analysis? A Potentially Dangerous Tool if Used Without Adequate Rules

15

In recent years, a boom in the use of a new research tool, called meta-analysis, has been observed. Critically perceived after its introduction in 1976 in the psychometric field[1] and only hesitantly applied in clinical medicine in the years thereafter, meta-analysis has lately become popular, especially in the areas of cancer and cardiology.

But first, what is meta-analysis? Here the controversy begins. No clear definition exists of meta-analysis, nor do many rules. The players can set many of their own standards—which makes meta-analysis a sometimes doubtful enterprise.

Meta-analysis has been unusually controversial. Its potential for misuse is high. A carelessly done meta-analysis can have disastrous consequences if treatment recommendations are based on it. Reliability and validity of a meta-analysis, however, are hard to determine. Bias and error might find easier access to a combination of several studies than to one large study. The statistical methods used to achieve an overall estimate of association are far from being uniform and accepted.

In psychology, meta-analysis has been called "mega-silliness"[2] and "an abuse in research integration."[3] It is surrounded by enough uncertainty to have its status questioned as "science or religion."[4] While many clinicians and epidemiologists have begun to favor the seemingly easy-to-apply technique of pooling results of different studies, critics have not yet accepted meta-analysis as a form of serious science.

An Effortless Way to Combine Data? ■

Meta-analysis—also referred to as overview[5]—is the combination of results from several studies (not the combination of raw data!). But where lies the justification for throwing together results of individual randomized clinical trials or epidemiological studies in order to come up with an overall estimate of effect? The single studies, in fact, might have important differences in design and may be carried out under different conditions and with different populations, which makes it questionable to compare, and even more questionable, to combine results. Furthermore, different treatment doses might have been applied for different lengths of time or even different endpoints pursued.

Goldman and Feinstein maintain that the pooling of data from different sources can be valid only if the component studies contain patients who are sufficiently similar in diagnosis, clinical severity,

243

principal treatment, and outcome events.[6] Yet, no rules exist as to what can be combined in a meta-analysis, and it is up to the meta-analyst to decide which studies he or she perceives as "combinable."

A test, generally applied when conducting a meta-analysis, examines heterogeneity of outcome. Heterogeneity of outcome, of course, can be—at least in part—explained by differences in study design.[7] Interpretation of heterogeneity is again up to the meta-analyst.

What to do if the test for heterogeneity comes out positive? Data are usually combined anyway. According to Peto, standard statistical tests for heterogeneity among many different trials are of limited value, partly because they are statistically insensitive, and partly because some heterogeneity of the real effects of treatment in the different trials is likely to exist, no matter what a formal test for heterogeneity may indicate.[8] Consequently, whether or not there is some real heterogeneity is not considered to invalidate the statistical techniques for a meta-analysis. Other analysts are reluctant to pool data if there is heterogeneity of treatment effects and question the meaning of the overall results of a meta-analysis when there is heterogeneity across studies.[9]

As Fleiss and Gross[10] point out, the Food and Drug Administration (FDA)—skeptical in its approach to meta-analysis in general—is critical of combining clinical trials that have considerable differences in their estimated treatment effects, especially if the measure of association shows a difference in direction.[11,12] Fleiss and Gross, in contrast, see a justification for meta-analysis, especially when studies differ in respect to the magnitude of treatment effects.[10]

It remains unsolved what is sensible to combine and call meta-analysis. This disturbing problem goes well beyond the homogeneity–heterogeneity issue. Should all available studies be included in an overview, or should only the "good" ones be combined? And how does one decide which are "good"? Peer review gives no quality assurance, for studies that have passed peer review can be flawed.[13] Restricting attention to studies that have appeared in peer reviewed journals, as some meta-analysts recommend, therefore does not seem to add to the validity of the process.

Stick to the published literature? Here we run into the problems of "file drawer bias" and "publication bias." Some researchers will not even submit their findings for publication if the results are negative or if they found no association or effect.[14] The manuscript remains in the file drawer and no public record exists indicating that the study has ever been conducted. Also, reviewers and editors tend to favor studies that show an effect; studies with positive results are more likely to be published than studies with negative results.[15–18] The resulting bias might have a serious impact on meta-analyses, particularly leading to an overestimate of the effect size.[19,20]

Some meta-analysts, lead by the Clinical Trial Service Unit at the University of Oxford, have made great efforts in trying to identify unpublished randomized clinical trials and include them in their overviews.[8,21,22] While some have applauded the strategy of including all studies that can be found, even if they are flawed,[23] others have criticized this procedure.[24] Alternatively, statistical adjustments have been proposed to account for bias if only published studies are combined.[18,25] The accuracy of an adjustment for a bias of unknown magnitude, however, is difficult to evaluate.

Similar to the choice of including unpublished studies in a meta-analysis, although less controversial, is the decision to combine only randomized clinical trials or to allow inclusion of nonrandomized trials as well. Although most meta-analysts favor restricting overviews to randomized studies,[26,27] one review of meta-analyses found that nearly 30% combined results from randomized and nonrandomized studies.[28]

The decision about which studies go into a meta-analysis determines the outcome of the overview. Depending on sample size and variance, a single study can change the overall measure of association dramatically. A good example for this phenomenon is given by Fleiss and Gross in their insightful review of meta-analysis.[10] They describe an overview of randomized trials of the effect of aspirin in preventing death after myocardial infarction. The first five trials published between 1974 and 1980 resulted in a statistically significant overall odds ratio indicating the effectiveness of aspirin. When a sixth trial was included in 1980 the picture changed, eliminating any significance. It was not until a seventh trial was conducted and added eight years later that significance in favor of aspirin was reestablished.

Thus, meta-analysis must not be seen as simple aggregation of data. Many choices have to be made by the investigator beforehand, and many sources of measurement error threaten reliability and validity of such an enterprise.

Accuracy of the Combined Results Approach ■

Some might think of meta-analysis as similar to a multicenter study. A study that is carried out at various centers simultaneously, however, at least has a common protocol for all participating institutions. Yet even when this is true there may be huge center-to-center variation. Outliers may be observed even with a single study protocol.

This situation suggests that subtle differences in protocol execution may affect results. If this is true, how much more variation must there be when diverse studies with different protocols are combined. Outliers are even more difficult to distinguish from large sampling errors, especially if sample sizes are small. Yet outliers have a dramatic inflationary effect on the variance. What should be done with them in a meta-analysis?

Combining the results of individual studies must raise the question of accuracy. How "good" is the overall estimate that results from such pooling across studies? What inferences can be drawn? Random error and bias are clearly more threatening to the validity in a combined approach than in one large study.

Two statistical methods to combine results of various studies have dominated the meta-analytic field. The "fixed effects model," as suggested by Peto, concentrates on the studies at hand and bases its estimates exclusively on the studies included in the overview.[8,22] The association studied holds only for the trials selected for the meta-analysis, therefore questions arise on the degree of generalizability of the results to other studies.

Alternatively, the method proposed by Der-Simonian and Laird tries to account statistically for interstudy variation and is referred to as the "random effects model."[29] Although it may allow predictions whether a treatment will have an effect in general, it requires one to assume that the different trial designs adopted would have to be randomly selected from some underlying universe of trials or set of possibilities that include the populations about which predictions are to be made.

Considerable debate has taken place as to which method of analysis is preferable.[10] It must be emphasized that both methods, however, are only approximations for the overall effect size.

The meta-analyst still has the chance to reduce measurement error of the individual studies when conducting an overview and, thus, increase reliability and validity.[30] This requires considerable effort since raw data might have to be reanalyzed within the individual studies. It might be sensible to do so in some instances, for example, when the intention-to-treat principle has not been followed. Few meta-analyses have gone this far.[31]

What Is the Role of Meta-Analysis? ■

With the growing popularity of a new research tool such as meta-analysis the following questions have to be asked: "What impact does it have? What are its immediate consequences? Does meta-analysis influence related research methods? Does meta-analysis change clinical practice? What role is it supposed to play?

Concerns have been raised that meta-analysis might deemphasize the need for large multicenter studies and encourage small single-investigator trials which are then included in a meta-analysis to reach sufficient statistical power.[4] It has been stated that "pooling exercises" or combining after the fact must never be viewed as substitute for simple, well-designed prospective clinical trials.[9]

Despite the fact that meta-analysis is beginning to gain acceptance in medicine, it has yet to leave its mark on clinical practice. Meta-analyses have been published and reported in the media, but meta-analysis has not changed clinical practice. It seems that findings from meta-analysis have been less successful in being incorporated into clinical care than those from large multicenter trials. When, for example, a meta-analysis indicated ten years ago that Streptokinase reduced mortality from myocardial infarction,[32] thrombolysis was still hesitantly used until European multicenter trials gave evidence that was obviously considered more reliable. The only meta-analysis that is considered to have influenced treatment recommendations is probably the overview of treatment of early breast cancer.[8] This meta-analysis was presented immediately before a Consensus Development Conference of the National Cancer Institute took place in 1985. The treatment recommendations given by the panel resembled the results of the overview and are likely to have been led by them.[33]

But then again: is it the goal of meta-analysis to affect care? Fleiss and Gross describe the purposes of meta-analysis as to increase statistical power, resolve controversy when studies disagree, improve estimates of effect size, and answer new questions that were not previously posed in individual studies.[10] Peto argues that the idea of an overview is not to govern the treatment of individual patients but rather to provide a context in which to view the patient and in which to view individual trials.[34] Meanwhile, the Federal Agency for Health Care Policy and Research funds efforts to evaluate the effectiveness of treatments on the basis of meta-analysis. The quality assessment group is developing guidelines for patient care that will be influenced largely by the results of meta-analyses.

Conclusions ■

Meta-analysis has become fashionable lately. It is "in" just to have done a "little meta-analysis." This is where its dangers lie. Meta-analysis is still a "free art," and few rules are attached to it. There seems no easy or obvious recipe for conducting a sensible meta-analysis; researchers tend to favor their own set of rules. This preference results in a diversity of data combinations that appear under the global name of meta-analysis.

Yet it is not some simple data pooling that results in interpretable analyses. General standards are needed to guide the clinician as much as the epidemiologist in conducting a meta-analysis while leaving sufficient room for professional judgment. Certainly, before meta-analysis is used to set guidelines for health care and affect national payment policy, standards must be developed.

A satisfactory environment for the conduct of meta-analysis must be established before this new research tool can achieve enough credibility to affect patient care. Among necessary steps to be taken is the establishment of a registry for clinical trials as well as epidemiological studies.[4,35] It has been suggested that internal review boards and ethics review committees responsible for reviewing human research proposals could serve as a basis for a national system of study registration.[4]

A second "environmental" need is to improve access to data. Once appropriate studies are identified, the meta-analyst should not restrict attention to published or publicly available data but must have access to and work with the principal investigators of the individual studies to collect missing information, improve accuracy of data included in the overview, include corrected results in the meta-analysis, and ensure follow-up of the study population. The collaboration between meta-analyst and study investigators is extremely important; at the same time immense tensions are to be expected and have been observed in the past. Investigators may well be concerned that their results will be buried in an anonymous meta-analysis for which the meta-analyst will receive all the credit. Meta-analysts can easily acquire the reputation of "parasites" in the world of studies and trials. It is the responsibility of the meta-analyst to ensure that proper credit is given to the trial investigators.

It has to be kept in mind that meta-analyses can only give rather global answers and crude estimates pointing out directions of treatment effects. *Post-hoc* analysis must be avoided and a specified design should be established beforehand. Meta-analyses may confirm an existing treatment principle or generate new hypotheses which thereafter have to be confirmed in specifically designed research. Too many unknown variables are involved in a meta-analysis to make it reliable enough for treatment decisions for the individual patient to be based solely on it. The meta-analysis, again, like every single trial, represents only a fraction of the population for which inferences are sought. How generalizable are the results obtained on this fraction remains unclear, since the fraction cannot necessarily be assumed to be random. Interstudy variations which have to be considered in an overview, effect measures which might point into opposite directions but are nevertheless combined, adding some element of uncertainty. Finally, the statistical analysis can only approximate the effect size.

Meta-analysis can be a useful tool in oncology as well as other areas of medicine to obtain an overall impression of the effect of treatment or the association between exposure and outcome. A meta-analysis, however, can answer only global questions; subgroup analyses are considered invalid. Meta-analysis seems most appropriate for very clearly defined endpoints such as mortality, which has little room for interpretation. But meta-analysis can not replace the carefully designed clinical trial, much less the epidemiological study. Many decisions in medicine involve specific questions that cannot be addressed by an overview and require a more sophisticated study design tailored for a limited patient population.

Since study-to-study variation is even more significant in epidemiological research than in clinical trials, meta-analysis might not be very applicable to this type of research. As Fleiss and Gross point out, meta-analysis is much more carefully applied to the results of clinical trials, whereas the quality of epidemiological studies does often not hold to lead to scientifically valid results when combined.[10] In addition, issues of misclassification and confounding come into play.

Indeed, often a statistical synopsis of results is not even necessary. If results of individual studies are convincing and mutually confirmatory evidence is provided, several individual studies can be forceful enough to be the basis for treatment recommendations. This was seen with three studies on adjuvant systemic treatment in breast cancer patients which resulted in the first clinical alert sent out by the National Cancer Institute in 1988.[36]

As Jenicek puts it, meta-analysis in medicine is still in its "embryonic stage." It might be too early at this stage to base general treatment recommendations on meta-analysis, which is certainly not mature enough to be the basis for textbook chapters, as recently suggested by Chalmers.[37] Much remains to be developed and discovered about this young research technique.

Acknowledgments. The author is indebted to Joseph L. Fleiss, PhD, and Gerald A. Faich, MD, MPH, for helpful comments on the manuscript.

References ∎

1. Glass GV. Primary, secondary, and meta-analysis of research. Educational Researcher 1976;5:3–8.
2. Eysenck HJ. An exercise in mega-silliness. Am Psychol 1978;33:517.
3. Eysenck HJ. Meta-analysis: An abuse of research integration. J Spec Educ 1984;18:41–59.
4. Meinert CL. Meta-analysis: Science or religion? Contr Clin Trials 1989;10:257S–263S.
5. Peto R. Discussion of Light RJ. Accumulating evidence from independent studies: What we can win and what we can lose. Stat Med 1987;6:229.
6. Goldman L, Feinstein A. Anticoagulants and myocardial infarction: The problem of pooling, drowning, and floating. Ann Intern Med 1979;90:92–94.
7. Bailey KR. Inter-study differences: How should they influence the interpretation and analysis of results? Stat Med 1987;6:351–358.
8. Early Breast Cancer Trialists' Collaborative Group (EBCTCG). Treatment of Early Breast Cancer. Worldwide evidence 1985–1990. Oxford, Oxford University Press, 1990:17.
9. DeMets DL. Methods for combining randomized clinical trials: strength and limitations. Stat Med 1987;6:341–348.
10. Fleiss JL, Gross AJ. Meta-analysis in epidemiology, with special reference to studies of the association between exposure to environmental tobacco smoke and lung cancer: a critique. J Clin Epidemiol 1991;44:127–139.
11. Dubey S. Regulatory considerations on meta-analysis, dentifrice studies and multicenter trials. Proceedings Biopharmaceutical Section of the Am Stat Assoc, 1988;18–27.
12. Stein RA. Meta-analysis from one FDA reviewer's perspective. Proceedings Biopharmaceutical Section of the Am Stat Assoc, 1988;34–38.
13. Selected proceedings from the First International Congress on Peer Review in Biomedical Publication. JAMA 1990;263:1317–1441.
14. Rosenthal R. The "file drawer problem" and tolerance for null results. Psychol Bull 1979;86:638–641.
15. Coursol A, Wagner EE. Effect of positive findings on submission and acceptance rates: A note on meta-analysis bias. Professional Psychology, 1986;17:136–137.
16. Dickersin K, Chan SS, Chalmers TC, Sacks HS, Smith H. Publication bias in randomized controlled trials. Contr Clin Trials 1987;8:343–353.
17. Begg CB, Berlin JA. Publication bias and dissemination of clinical research. J Natl Cancer Inst 1989;81:107–115.
18. Berlin JA, Begg CB, and Louis TA. An assessment of publication bias using a sample of published clinical trials. J Am Stat Assoc 1989;84:381–392.
19. McNemar Q. At random: Sense and nonsense. Am Psychol 1960;15:295–300.
20. Rosenthal R. Meta-Analysis Procedures for Social Research. Beverly Hills: Sage, 1984:41–45.
21. Yusuf S. Obtaining medically meaningful answers from an overview of randomized clinical trials. Stat Med 1987; 6:281–286.
22. Yusuf S, Peto R, Lewis J, Collins R, Sleight P. Beta blockade during and after myocardial infarction. An overview of the randomized trials. Prog Cardiovasc Dis 1985;27:335–371.
23. Fleiss JL. Discussion of Light RJ, Accumulating evidence from independent studies: What we can win and what we can lose. Stat Med 1987;6:230.
24. Light RJ. Accumulating evidence from independent studies: What we can win and what we can lose. Stat Med 1987;6:221–228.
25. Iyengar S, Greenhouse JB. Selection models and the file drawer problem. Stat Sci 1988;3:109–117.
26. Peto R. Why do we need systematic overviews of randomized trials? Stat Med 1987;6:233–240.
27. O'Rourke K, Detsky AS. Meta-analysis in medical research: Strong encouragement for higher quality individual research efforts. J Clin Epidemiol 1989;42:1021–1029.
28. Sacks HS, Berrier J, Reitman D, Ancona-Berk VA, Chalmers TC. Meta-analysis of randomized controlled trials. N Engl J Med 1987;316:450–455.
29. DerSimonian R, Laird N. Meta-analysis in clinical trials. Contr Clin Trials 1986;7:177–188.
30. Michels KB. Unpublished observation.
31. Early Breast Cancer Trialists' Collaborative Group (EBCTCG). Treatment of Early Breast Cancer. Worldwide Evidence 1990 (in preparation).
32. Stampfer MJ, Goldhaber SZ, Yusuf S, Peto R, Henne-

kens CH. Effect of intravenous streptokinase on acute myocardial infarction. Pooled results from randomized trials. N Engl J Med 1982;307:1180–1182.

33. DeVita VT. Personal Communication.

34. Peto R. Discussion of Wittes RE, Problems in the medical interpretation of overviews. Stat Med 1987;6:279.

35. Boissel JP, Sacks HS, Leizorovicz A, Blanchard J, Panak E, and Peyrieux JC. Meta-analysis of clinical trials: Summary of an international conference. Eur J Clin Pharmacol 1988;34:535–538.

36. Clinical Alert from the National Cancer Institute. May 18, 1988.

37. Chalmers TC. Oral Presentation. Annual Meeting of the Association of American Physicians, Seattle, May 5, 1991.

Index

Index

Numbers followed by an f *indicate a figure;*
t *following a page number indicates tabular material.*

ISBN 0-397-51157-4

90000